CHILDHOOD CANCER AND THE FAMILY
Meeting the Challenge
of Stress and Support

CHILDHOOD CANCER AND THE FAMILY

Meeting the Challenge of Stress and Support

By

Mark A. Chesler, Ph.D.

and

Oscar A. Barbarin, Ph.D.

BRUNNER/MAZEL Publishers • New York

We acknowledge permission received from the following two sources to reprint excerpts that appear throughout this volume:

Roach, N. *The Last Day of April.* American Cancer Society, Inc., 1974.
Pendleton, E. *Too Old to Cry . . . Too Young to Die.* Nashville, Tenn: Thomas Nelson, 1980.

Library of Congress Cataloging-in-Publication Data

Chesler, Mark A.
    Childhood cancer and the family.

    Bibliography: p. 311
    Includes index.
    1. Tumors in children – Social aspects. 2. Cancer –
Patients – Family relationships. 3. Tumors in children –
Psychological aspects. I. Barbarin, Oscar A.
II. Title. [DNLM: 1. Neoplasms – in infancy & childhood.
2. Neoplasms – psychology. 3. Social Environment.
4. Stress, Psychological.   QZ 200 C524c]
RC281.C4C44 1987   155.9′16   86-21627
ISBN 0-87630-441-2

Published by
BRUNNER/MAZEL, INC.
19 Union Square
New York, New York 10003

Acknowledgments

We appreciate the assistance of several groups of people in the conduct of this work. First, our families, our wives and children, have been constant sources of support and inspiration. Joan and Millie have been professional colleagues as well as emotional partners. Deborah and Naomi Chesler, and Andrea and Oscar David Barbarin, have helped us keep this research grounded in the real experience of children and families. We have learned much about coping and social support in these intimate settings. Our close friends also provided us with critical emotional and practical assistance as we wrestled with, became submerged in, or were delighted with this work.

Several medical and social scientific colleagues have been extraordinary sources of help and support. Through work with medical colleagues we have learned many details about the care of children with cancer. As the study neared completion, we shared preliminary results with Raymond Hutchinson (MD) and Mary Waskerwitz (CPNP), and with other professionals and scientists in meetings across the country. We have been rewarded by them with new data, new insights, and richer interpretations of the complex phenomena of childhood cancer. Only the constraints of protecting the anonymity of patient populations and medical sites prevent us from naming more of these cherished colleagues individually.

Minna Nathanson is an especially valued colleague. She took the time to apply her considerable conceptual and editorial skills, as well as her personal and professional experience, to make this manuscript more meaningful and more readable. Friends in the national office of the Candlelighters Childhood Cancer Foundation, Grace Ann Powers Monaco and Julie Sullivan, as well as members of the Board of Directors of Candlelighters, encouraged us regarding the importance of this work.

The efforts of the local self-help group of parents of children with cancer were essential in helping to identify the population pool, publicize the study, and provide feedback on instruments and procedures.

Several students have been valued assistants from design to data collection to analysis to writeup. A group of 12 undergraduates did a marvelous job of interviewing parents and children. Their response to the people and the issues in this study, as well as their work with the interview data, was a thrilling experience for ourselves as instructors. Eve Reider, Sheryl Lozowski, Adam Plotnick, Carol Lindsay, and Jan Paris constantly provided proof of the commitment and excitement that bright and mature undergraduates can bring to work that touches their hearts and minds . . . and that they touch in return. Graduate students and professionals who also contributed skillfully to data analysis include Diane Hughes, Judy Lebo-Stein, Karin Elliot, Marcene Root, and Elaine Selo.

Able and dedicated secretarial help was rendered by Danielle Hogston, Carol Crawford, and Shiela Wilder. Donna Beuerle also made it possible for other members of the Sociology Department's secretarial staff to assist us during a long hot summer of interview reconstruction.

The University of Michigan, through a grant from the Committee on the International Year of the Child, and the Spencer Foundation financially supported various portions of this work. The Center for Research on Social Organization housed us, our data, and our many assistants.

Finally we thank the parents and children, as well as friends and educators, who participated in this study as informants. Their willingness to share portions of their lives with us has been both exciting and humbling. We hope we serve them well. And we hope this work also serves others who are now struggling to improve the quality of life of children and families of children with cancer – children, parents, professionals, friends, and family members.

We dedicate this work to the families of children with cancer – past, present, and future.

Ann Arbor   Mark A. Chesler
Michigan   Department of Sociology
1986   University of Michigan

and

Oscar A. Barbarin
School of Social Work
University of Michigan

Contents

Introduction

This book is about childhood cancer. It is about families' efforts to meet the challenge posed by this illness and to make the best of an undesirable and disruptive situation. To understand their responses, we must look at the problems and opportunities, the joys and sorrows, and the continuing struggles experienced by families of children with cancer. It is not a medical book. Although it deals with a medical condition, it is primarily about the psychosocial issues faced by children with cancer and their families and friends. It is not a sad book. Although it describes stress, sadness, and pain, it also discusses joy and courage. It is a book about families – about parents and their children. It is about how ordinary people manage to respond to an extraordinary challenge.

WHAT HAVE WE LEARNED ABOUT
PSYCHOSOCIAL ISSUES IN CHILDHOOD CANCER?

Research into the lives of children with cancer and their families is relevant and important for many families with this experience. We hope that not only parents but also medical and social service professionals will read this book. In addition, many of the experiences of families with childhood cancer are similar to those of families with other chronic and serious childhood illnesses, such as cystic fibrosis, muscular dystrophy, diabetes, lupus, and multiple handicapping conditions. Much of this volume is relevant to people concerned with chronic and serious illnesses affecting adults as well.

In the pages of this book you will see people in great emotional pain and sadness. Parents faced with a threat to their child's life, the potential or actual death of their child, and the suffering of a child undergoing vigorous treatment often come to a new understanding of the meaning of a cruel and often tragic illness. Nothing fundamentally erases parental pain or the raw sense of futility, waste, and unfairness that often accompanies childhood cancer. But you will also see examples of people courageously and lovingly going on with their lives and teaching themselves and their children new and important lessons about the meaning and quality of life. In meeting this challenge, parents constantly search for ways to live with the pain or sadness of this illness, to make sense of this experience, and to find ways to enrich and improve their own and their children's lives.

Survivors of childhood cancer (children who survive their illness and parents and siblings of these children) often grow in ways neither we nor they can predict. For instance, many youngsters report, and their parents often agree, that they are more mature and have clearer goals than their peers. Many husbands and wives, and siblings of children with cancer, report they have drawn together, relied on each other in new ways, and love and care for each other more strongly and overtly. Of course, no set of positive outcomes compensates for the tragedy of serious childhood illness. No parents would "choose" to have their child be seriously ill or die. But the message from these parents is quite clear: If this is what life brings, "You go on," "You deal with it as best you can," "You survive and maybe you grow."

Our studies and other recent research reveal the importance of hope and optimism in creating positive forms of coping with the illness and its side effects or aftereffects. We also observe the importance of open communication among family members, between parents and children and the medical staff, and between the family and classmates, educators, and friends. The importance of a vigorous struggle, tempered by the acceptance of things that cannot be altered, emerges as a key to positive personal coping and a successful family life.

Many parents of children with cancer tell us that they try to normalize their own and their children's lives. This quest for normalcy takes many different paths, and it is represented in a variety of struggles or dilemmas. One struggle is with the expectation of psychological normalcy. Despite earlier research studies, there is now increasing evidence that children with cancer are not psychologically abnormal; neither they nor their families consistently or inevitably develop severe psychological problems. Although children and parents are likely to experience mood swings, anxiety, and depression, these are normal reactions to an abnormal situation. Whereas alertness and hard work are required, these families are not predestined for extreme conflict and dissolution.

A second struggle is with the confusion between "being normal" and "being like everyone else." Although children with cancer and their families are generally psychologically healthy and normal, they are not "just like" everyone else. They are experiencing a difficult situation, a series of stressful circumstances, and are facing unique challenges. It would be a mistake to deny or overlook this reality. We must understand these different experiences and their impact if we are to appreciate how families of children with cancer reconstruct their lives.

A third struggle with normalcy involves rethinking continuity with the past and adapting to future possibilities. Most families initially try to establish normalcy by keeping their own and their child's life as much as possible as it was before the illness. Since this is an impossible task, it is important to create new ways of living that are more concerned with growth than with preservation and that look to the future instead of to the past.

Because childhood cancer affects more than the young patient, it has become fashionable to discuss it as a "family disease." But cancer affects more than the immediate family; it truly is a "community disease," affecting relatives, friends, and even casual acquaintances. Everyone who touches the lives of young patients with cancer, everyone who cares about these children, is likely to be affected deeply by the illness and illness-related issues. As parents reach out to other family members and friends for support and help, they encounter people who also care and feel deeply, and who are moved by their own experience with the illness. Even medical staff and school personnel are not immune from these strong feelings. Thus, not only do family members need help and support from other people, but other people also need support and education from the family. Many parents also educate professionals while they are educated and served by them. Together they engage in a mutual struggle with a common set of concerns about the ill child, about their own reactions, and about the integrity of family and community relationships.

In a number of communities, parents have formed organizations to help other families of children with cancer deal with the illness and its impact. "Giving to others is a way of getting" and family self-help groups reflect both the needs and the new-found strengths of families. Many other programs, both formally established and voluntary, staffed by professionals or parents, located in the medical system or the community, are needed to help everyone deal most positively with the challenges of childhood cancer.

PLAN OF THE BOOK

The chapters of this book focus sequentially on stress, coping, and social support/services. Chapters 2, 3, and 4 examine the *stresses* or challenges of childhood cancer. Chapter 1 discusses the nature of childhood cancer and its treatment and briefly describes the research procedures utilized in preparing this volume. Chapter 2 focuses upon medical stresses accompanying the disease, through discussion of a series of events or stages in the illness. Chapter 3 focuses upon the psychosocial stresses of childhood cancer, examining several different kinds of stress experienced by family members, and ways in which social relationships may make life more difficult for the parents of children with cancer. Chapter 4 focuses upon the family's relations with the medical staff, exploring positive and negative dimensions of these relationships.

Chapters 5, 6, 7, and 8 discuss the *coping strategies* people use to meet these challenges. Chapter 5 examines the coping strategies individual parents utilize, exploring the differences between internally directed strategies that seek to establish some psychological comfort and externally directed strategies that seek to alter the nature of the stress or the stressful situation itself. Chapter 6 examines family coping strategies, exploring the ways in which the family as a unit coordinates its responses to the stresses of childhood cancer. Chapter 7 focuses explicitly upon raising or parenting the child with cancer; it pinpoints some of the problems and opportunities involved in trying to normalize the child's life, in avoiding spoiling the ill child or wreaking havoc among siblings and spouses. Chapter 8 discusses coping strategies from the point of view of youngsters with cancer; it utilizes children's reports of how they deal with this illness, their parents, siblings, friends, and futures.

Chapters 9, 10, and 11 discuss various *social supports and services* available to and utilized by many families of children with cancer. Chapter 9 focuses upon parents' relations with their close friends, the special dilemmas the illness creates for such relationships, and the many ways in which friends are and can be helpful. Chapter 10 focuses upon the ways in which some families with childhood cancer reach out to other such families, and how participation in self-help or mutual support groups proves helpful. Chapter 11 discusses families' relations with school systems, ways in which parents and educators may orchestrate the child's return to school, and problems many youngsters encounter as they reenter the normal school environment.

Finally, Chapter 12 summarizes the findings of the study by suggesting some important ways in which parents can play an active role in the health care of their children, and answers a series of practical questions raised by parents. These suggestions reflect the determination of many families who respond to the demands and stresses of the illness as a series of challenges rather than as overwhelming threats. The ideas are drawn partly from parents' own reports of their experiences and actions and partly from our interpretations of the research data.

CHILDHOOD CANCER AND THE FAMILY
Meeting the Challenge of Stress and Support

CHAPTER 1

Childhood Cancer and Its Treatment

Cancer refers to a process in the body in which a cell, or group of cells, has developed the ability to grow in an abnormal and uncontrolled fashion. Although the single term "cancer" is used, it actually refers to a variety of different diseases, each affecting different tissues and organs. These diseases are dangerous because the abnormal cells, or tumors, grow in dangerous sites in or near vital organs, or because they may spread to other parts of the body, disrupting normal organ function.

Cancer in children is a relatively rare disease. However, it strikes over 6,000 American children a year and is the largest nonaccidental cause of death in people between 2 and 16 years. It occurs in newborn babies, toddlers, preschool children, and school-age children well into their teens. For our purposes, "children" includes young people from 2 minutes to 20 years old. Young people over 20 years are more likely to be considered adults, often are separated from their parents, and usually are treated in adult oncology centers.

Because the presenting symptoms of cancer may be quite varied and nondramatic, such as joint pain or swelling, low-grade fever of long duration, or fatigue and loss of skin tone and pallor, cancer may develop in a child for some time before it is recognized or diagnosed with certainty. The diagnosis of a suspected cancer is confirmed by a series of procedures that establish the existence of a malignancy and assess its type and extent. In addition to routine physical examinations, physicians may conduct blood tests, bone marrow aspirations, spinal taps, tissue biopsies, and various X-ray examinations.

We can distinguish various kinds of childhood cancer by the part of the body or organ system they attack; the most common forms of childhood cancer are listed in Table 1.1.[1] The age of the child is often associated with the type of cancer (Potter, 1974; Sutow, 1984). For instance, retinoblastoma, neuroblastoma, and Wilms' tumor are most likely to occur in very young children – at a median age of less than three years. Brain tumors and cancers of the central nervous system are found with greatest frequency in the five- to nine-year age group. Bone cancers (sarcomas) and lymphatic cancers are more likely to occur in prepubescent and adolescent youngsters. Although the link between age and leukemia, the most common form of childhood cancer, is not as clear-cut, most children diagnosed with leukemia are between the ages of 2 and 12 years.

There is no general scientific agreement on the causes of childhood cancer and no certain knowledge of the cause operating in any particular individual's situation. There is some evidence for the operation of genetic or hereditary factors, especially in some forms of retinoblastoma. There also is some evidence for the influence of environmental factors, such as diet, air and water pollutants, or heavy metal toxicity. And there is some evidence for the operation of a virus, one that compromises the immune system of vulnerable individuals.

Once a diagnosis of childhood cancer has been made, the child usually spends a few days in the hospital, sometimes as much as several weeks,

Table 1.1
Common Forms of Childhood Cancer

Type of Childhood Cancer	Cell System of Origin	Percent of All Childhood Cancers
Leukemias	Bone marrow and blood system	33%
Brain and spinal cord	Central nervous system	20
Lymphomas (e.g., Hodgkin's disease)	Lymph system	11
Soft tissue (e.g., rhabdomyosarcoma)	Skeletal muscles and connective tissue	6
Neuroblastoma	Sympathetic nervous system	8
Wilms' tumor	Kidney	6
Osteogenic and Ewing's sarcomas	Bone	5
Retinoblastoma	Eye	3
Miscellaneous or other		8

while treatment is initiated. During this period the child may undergo surgery and almost certainly is treated with radiation and/or chemotherapy (drugs). These treatments have toxic effects on the body, and most children experience considerable physical discomfort as well as fear and anxiety. After this early period, some patients may return to the hospital for several days at a time, but many children receive treatment as outpatients. The majority spend most of their lives at home, in the neighborhood, and, it is hoped, in school. While the disease is in remission (arrested), most children are able to participate regularly in family and school activities.

Active outpatient treatment often continues for one to three years. If the child relapses, intensive treatments are reinitiated and treatment is extended over a longer period of time. The response to subsequent relapses is more intensive and experimental treatment, perhaps leading to extended hospitalization and death. For many children, however, the years bring less intensive treatment, fewer side effects, and greater likelihood of passage into normal adulthood. Recent progress in understanding these diseases and determining how best to treat them has been advanced greatly by cooperative efforts among many children's cancer centers and by the standardization and evaluation of treatment for many children at once. While standard protocols exist for treatment of the common types of childhood cancer, actual treatments vary considerably, taking into account the stage and severity of each child's illness, and the uniqueness of each patient.[2]

Table 1.1 indicates that the most common form of childhood cancer is leukemia. There are several different types of childhood leukemia; the most common is acute lymphoblastic (or lymphocytic) leukemia (ALL), but there is also a variety of non-lymphocytic forms (ANLL). Leukemia is a cancer of the blood system, originating in the bone marrow where blood cells are formed. The overgrowth of leukemic cells in the marrow crowds out healthy blood cells and infiltrates the bloodstream and other organs.

The standard initial treatment (induction) for ALL consists of a multidrug regimen, often including vincristine, prednisone, and L-asparaginase, to reduce the number of leukemic cells and gain a remission of the disease. When the disease is brought under control (for 95% of the patients within a few weeks), a new chemotherapeutic regimen (maintenance), usually adding methotrexate and 6-mercaptopurine, is begun. In addition to these chemotherapeutic agents, preventive cranial radiation therapy is given to prevent the spread of the disease to the brain and spinal cord. Children with poorer initial prognoses will be given more intensive chemotherapy, perhaps including cytoxan and anthracycline agents (daunorubicin or adriamycin). The mode, extent, and duration of treatment for this disease vary, as research continues to modify and improve medical care, but most children who do well are in treatment for at least two years. If they have a relapse, treatment will extend over several more years, possibly with a bone marrow transplant (if a suitable donor can be found) and more experimental drugs.

A second major form of childhood cancer is osteogenic sarcoma, a cancer of the bone that typically affects teenagers. This disease usually is discovered in the long bones of the leg. Treatment generally involves surgical removal of the tumor, often including amputation of the limb, although in some cases limb-salvage procedures can be employed. Subsequent chemotherapy involves agents such as high-dose methotrexate, cisplatin, and adriamycin. Within a short time after amputation most patients are outfitted with a prosthesis. Some children wear a prosthesis all the time, whereas others substitute crutches or leave off their prosthesis. Children with osteogenic sarcoma are hospitalized for surgery, and most of their remaining treatment, stretching out over a year, also involves brief hospitalizations. Another form of bone cancer, Ewing's sarcoma, generally occurs in young adolescents. Usually it is treated with surgery, intensive radiation therapy, and subsequent multidrug chemotherapy.

A third form of childhood cancer, also one that usually affects teenagers, is Hodgkin's disease. This is a cancer of the lymph system, the network of glands which creates and circulates lymphatic material to fight infections throughout the body. The standard treatment for minimal stage Hodgkin's disease involves radiation, with chemotherapeutic combinations such as MOPP (nitrogen mustard, oncovin-vincristine, procarbazine, and prednisone), or ABVD (adriamycin, bleomycin, vinblastine, and DTIC) used with patients with more advanced stages of the disease. Diagnosis of Hodgkin's disease patients often involves surgical removal of the spleen and abdominal lymph nodes. They are hospitalized for short periods during the initial phases of their treatment, and then continue treatment as outpatients.

Two other forms of childhood cancer occur most often in much younger children. Wilms' tumor, a cancer of the kidney, is most common in two- to three-year olds. Recent advances in treatment for these patients have been so successful that many children recover completely and have no noticeable effects by the time they enter school. Wilms' tumor is treated surgically by the removal of the diseased kidney and by follow-up chemotherapy (actinomycin-D and vincristine). In higher stages of the disease, radiation therapy and other chemotherapeutic agents are added. Since humans have two kidneys, and one can function for both, general kidney function usually remains intact with a single, healthy kidney.

Neuroblastoma also affects very young children. It occurs in sympathetic nerve cells, usually located in the abdomen, neck, or chest. Tumors are removed surgically, if possible, often with radiation therapy as well. Chemotherapy, including cyclophosphamide, vincristine, and DTIC, is utilized with higher stages of the disease. Bone marrow transplantation is also possible in a number of cases.

Rhabdomyosarcoma develops from muscle tissue and is the most common soft tissue tumor of childhood. It is most likely to occur among young adolescents. Surgical removal of the tumor is the typical initial treatment, followed by one to two years of chemotherapy (with drugs such as adriamycin, vincristine, cyclophosphamide, and actinomycin). Radiation therapy sometimes is also utilized.

Brain tumors, the second most common form of childhood cancer, are generally diagnosed in 5- to 10-year-olds. Their treatment involves surgery, if the tumor is operable, and then radiation therapy. If the tumor is inoperable, radiation therapy is used (perhaps chemotherapy as well). Hospitalization for both diagnosis and surgery is necessary. The recuperative period may be lengthy, but continuing treatment can be received as an outpatient. Depending on the site and size of the tumor, there are likely to be lasting neurological and motor system effects.

The aim of all treatment for childhood cancer is to do maximum damage to cancerous cells while not overly compromising the general health of the patient. However, the treatments do damage healthy cells and have a variety of toxic side effects. These effects are temporarily physically disabling or uncomfortable, and a number present lasting impediments to normal functioning. Although the specific side effects experienced by each child vary with the specific disease and its treatments, most radiologic and chemotherapeutic agents produce some side effects. For instance, children who are receiving initial or intensive dosages of chemotherapy often have nausea, vomiting, and loss of appetite, usually lasting only a few days beyond the administration of the drug. With some types of radiation therapy, a longer loss of appetite may be more common. Children undergoing intensive and aggressive therapy often report loss of energy and fatigue, which makes it difficult for them to sustain concentration on schooling, household chores, and friendships. Although these side effects may be severe enough for the child to remain at home for several days, they generally do not require extensive absence from school.

Drugs effective against cancer are especially targeted for fast-growing tumor cells; they often have potent effects on other fast-growing cells in the body, such as mucous membranes and hair. Cranial radiation also causes hair loss. This is of greater concern to some patients than to others and to adolescents most of all. Cranial radiation also may cause hearing loss or intellectual impairments. Prednisone, which is most often used with leukemic patients, causes weight gain and facial puffiness.

All children treated for cancer are likely to experience suppression of their immune system and blood counts, rendering them more vulnerable to infection and hemorrhage. Three different kinds of blood cells are involved: white cells, which fight infection; red cells, which carry oxygen through the bloodstream to tissues and organs; and platelets, which form the body's basic clotting mechanisms and fight injury or wounds. If the absolute white blood count is too low, patients may be kept at home or isolated until they are more resistant to infection. Similarly, if the platelet count is too low, children may be kept home or temporarily restricted from participating in gym and in other forms of physical contact. If the red blood cell, or hemoglobin, count is too low, children will be fatigued and listless. Although most of these side effects are temporary, they have a variety of important cosmetic, emotional, behavioral, and health impacts.

Those children who have surgery as part of their treatment may have more permanent side effects, depending upon the site of the surgery. Brain surgery may leave children with various cognitive or motor deficits. Children who have lost a limb to treatment have visible side effects and often face motor skill problems, despite the assistance of prostheses.

The results of childhood cancer treatment have improved so notably over the past 10 to 20 years that the long-term side effects of treatment can now begin to be assessed. In the next few years we may have more definitive data, but recent studies suggest some neurologic deficits for young children treated with cranial radiation and subsequent cancers or organ damage for those treated with extensive radiation or chemotherapy.[3] These long-term side effects are, ironically, now a cause of concern because more children are surviving long enough to reveal them. Finding a balance between lifesaving treatment and treatment-induced problems is one of the next research frontiers in pediatric oncology.

RECENT ADVANCES IN TREATMENT

New drugs, novel combinations of existing drugs, and the use of drugs in combination with radiation therapy have led to more effective arrest of cancerous growth. Developments in radiation therapy have enabled radiologists to focus with more control on the cancerous site(s). Improvements in surgical technique have been combined with drug and radiation therapies. The use of bone marrow transplants also offers new hope to young cancer patients.

These treatment innovations are available in most major cancer centers, but are less likely to have been disseminated to smaller community hospitals. Therefore, the experiences of children in large childhood cancer research centers are likely to be different from those of children in hospitals that are not a part of this network. Miller and Miller (1984) report that a series of studies demonstrates that children with various forms of childhood cancer do better when treated at university cancer centers or specialized hospitals than at community hospitals.[4] This is especially true when the form of cancer is one in which new methods have made gains. For childhood cancers that have a good prognosis with standard therapy, or for which little effective therapy exists, the place of treatment makes little difference in the outcome. Specialty centers have the latest research results on treatment modalities and protocols available; they are the centers of systematic inquiry, and they generally have a pediatric intensive care unit, a blood bank with the capability of doing pheresis, facilities for parenteral nutrition and protective isolation, radiation oncologists familiar with pediatric patients, advanced laboratories for diagnosis of critical disease markers, and so on (Miller & Miller, 1984).

As treatment for childhood cancer has become more standardized and effective, competent care often can be provided and monitored on an outpatient basis at local community hospitals or in pediatricians' offices. This is especially likely for children with less complicated forms of the illness or who are doing well. Such localized options are far more convenient for families who might have to travel long distances to major children's cancer centers and are consistent with efforts to control hospital costs and decentralize medical care. They also permit the best combination of specialized care at major cancer centers and general care by a familiar physician in the local community. Research to monitor and evaluate how this pattern of medical care affects mortality, disease control, and quality of life is essential.

When the most advanced treatment modalities are available and used, they have resulted in dramatic increases in rates of survival. Figure 1.1, prepared by the National Cancer Institute, shows the improvement from 1960 to 1980 in the two-year survival rates, differentiated by each type of children's cancer. Similarly, five-year survival rates for children with cancer are greater for children diagnosed between 1970 and 1973 than for children diagnosed between 1960 and 1963. From the early part of the 1960s to the 1970s, the five-year survival rates for children diag-

nosed with the most common form of childhood cancer, acute lymphocytic leukemia, improved from 4% to 34%. For the second most common, brain tumors, five-year survival rates improved from 48% to 59%;
and for neuroblastoma, comparable rates improved from 25% to 40%.
Despite such progress, the data presented in Table 1.2 show clear differences in the five-year survival prospects of children with bone cancer
(30%) or leukemia (34%), compared with retinoblastoma (85%) or Hodgkin's disease (90%). We still have a long way to go, since no survival
rate can be described as acceptable until it is 100%. However, the long-
term and short-term outlooks for children with most forms of cancer
have become considerably brighter.[5]

These data indicate that what was once an almost universally fatal
childhood disease is now not only not universally fatal, but that treatment and survival extend well beyond childhood. As recently as 1973,
child psychiatrist C. M. Binger could write that:

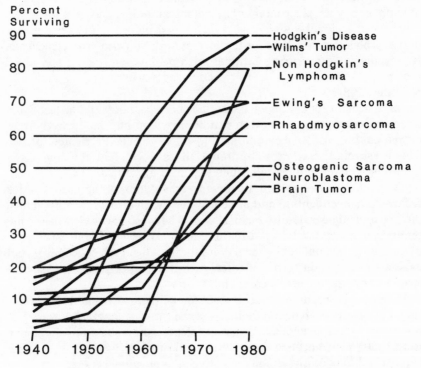

Figure 1.1. Proportion of children with solid tumors
surviving two years from diagnosis*

Decade of Discovery, 1981.

Table 1.2
Percentage of Children with Cancer who
Survive Five Years After Diagnosis*

Cancer Group	% Survival at Five Years
Bone cancer	30
Acute lymphocytic leukemia	34
Neuroblastoma	40
Glioma cancer (brain)	59
Wilms' tumor (kidney)	70
Retinoblastoma (eye)	85
Hodgkin's disease (lymph glands)	90

Cancer Facts and Figures, 1984.

Diagnostic tests revealed that Jimmy had a fatal disease — acute leukemia . . . As the hematologist proceeded to answer their questions concerning the diagnosis, anticipated course of illness, treatment, and its fatal prognosis . . . .(p. 172)

By 1975, however, Wilbur noted that:

Many people . . . treat children with cancer as though they will all have a fatal outcome. Out of this has evolved a particular emphasis on helping families and children prepare for their expected death. The expectation of a frequently successful outcome with eradication of disease, and a recognition of the importance of rehabilitation, has just begun to emerge. (p. 809)

As parents and families celebrate medical advances in treatment, they also encounter new issues in the care and management of the child, and in the maintenance of family and other social relationships. With a greater chance of "life," many families are now more concerned with enhancing the "quality of life" of those affected by childhood cancer. The medical community is also giving more attention to this issue. Wilbur argued, as early as 1975, that, "Without successful emotional rehabilitation, neither the successful treatment of the tumor nor the successful correction of physical problems will have great meaning" (p. 811). And Van Eys (1977b) has pressed his concern for "a truly cured child," a child free of cancer and of the secondary physical, psychological, and social side effects of the disease and treatment. In the past few years increased attention has been given to these issues, with the appearance of more scholarly articles and books on the psychosocial aspects of childhood cancer.[6]

THE RESEARCH REPORTED IN THIS BOOK

The extended life span and potential cure of a greater number of children with cancer has led to increased concerns about the quality of their lives. As the focus has shifted from an emphasis on families' preparations for or reactions to death, it has begun to deal with the problems of *living* with childhood cancer. This requires an emphasis upon the whole child – the child as an emotional and social being, not merely as a physical object with a dread disease. It requires an emphasis on the mental as well as the physical health of the whole family, not merely on the ill child and his/her immediate caretakers. It also requires attention to the whole community of people involved in the life and care of the child with cancer – family, friends, medical staff, school staff.

In our research on psychosocial aspects of childhood cancer, we applied recent developments in sociology and psychology to those issues. A *stress-coping-support* paradigm (illustrated in Figure 1.2) was utilized. We sought to discover the *stresses* that parents (and children) face as they experience childhood cancer. Some of these stresses are direct outgrowths of the illness and its required treatments and side effects. Other stresses are rooted in the social environment, in the reactions of others, or, perhaps, in the emotional and psychological characteristics of each person. We also were interested in understanding people's *coping strategies*, the ways in which they deal with these stresses. Parents and children utilize a variety of strategies to alter the impact that stress has upon them to control their emotional reactions to the roller-coaster rides of fear and joy, anxiety and relief. Some even find ways to alter stressful family or medical environments or situations. One major coping pattern is an attempt to gain *social support* from a variety of informal sources and *special services* from a range of professional agencies.

To investigate these issues we needed to talk at length with families of children with cancer. We selected our informants from the total population of childhood cancer families treated over a 10-year period at a major Midwestern hospital. We stratified this population by age and life status (living or deceased) of the child with cancer. Using this information, we drew a representative sample of families. To maximize other important comparisons, we made substitutions to ensure adequate representation within each category of: (1) male and female patients and (2) children with different kinds of cancer. In each family we planned to talk with both parents, with children with cancer over six years of age, and with some siblings.

The study was announced in a quarterly newsletter sent to several hundred families of former and current patients treated at the hospital.

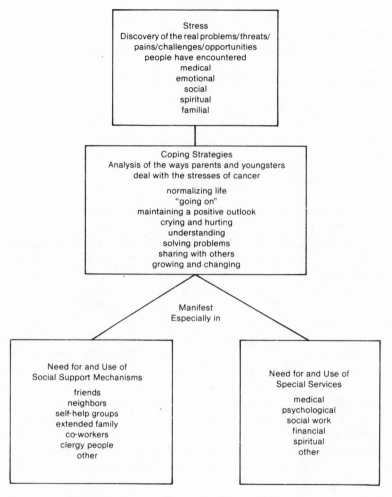

Figure 1.2. What this research is about

Then, each of the 85 families in the projected sample was sent a letter describing the study. The mailing included child and adult consent forms. Of the 85 families in the original pool, 15 families could not be located, and another 15 families declined to be interviewed. The final sample, described further in the Appendix, includes interviews with 95 parents (in 55 families), 26 children with cancer, and 23 siblings. A search of prior literature in these areas suggests that this is a relatively large number of families, and of parents, at least for a study using intensive interviews and questionnaires.

Personal interviews were conducted with these family members, separately, in their own homes. The general questions in the interview with
parents of living children covered topics such as:

The nature and process of the diagnosis;
The course of illness and treatment;
Family members' responses to the illness;
Reactions of friends and neighbors;
Toughest times and problems during the illness;
Positive events or outcomes for the family or the patient;
Images of the child's future;
Changes in the family and in family members' roles;
Relations with the school and with the hospital;
Use of professional and lay help.

Interviews with parents of deceased children focused upon additional
issues, such as preparation for and experience with death and dying.

The average interview took about an hour and one-half to complete,
with several lasting three hours or more. When the interview was completed, all parents were asked to complete a short questionnaire and
return it in a self-addressed, stamped envelope. The questionnaire repeated some of the issues raised in the interview, and it also asked for
more information on responses to the illness, demographic information,
and reactions to the interview itself. Eighty-six (91%) of the 95 adults
interviewed returned the questionnaire.

We did not begin this study by translating the concepts of stress,
coping, and social support into formal hypotheses and traditional variables and measures. Rather, we used these concepts as orienting points
and proceeded from a phenomenological and inductive basis to understand families' experiences as they themselves reported them. Then we
codified and interpreted these families' subjective reports from a more
analytic and objective stance, using aspects of both a deductive and an
inductive approach.

Our first step in gathering data was to embed ourselves, as far as
possible, in the reality of childhood cancer.[7] We broadened our experience through informal conversations and observations with families of
children with cancer and with health care practitioners. The development of questions and instruments with which to gather data from the
study sample was the next step. Recording and analyzing the reports
of many families with childhood cancer gradually led to an understanding and conceptualization of their experience.[8] In developing such conceptualization we sought to combine the traditionally "objective" work
style of social scientists with the intensely personal reflections pres-

ented in parents' comments and narratives and in our own experience. These parents, "common sense scholars" themselves, have contributed much of the wisdom in this volume. Formal data analysis was undertaken by means of rigorous qualitative and quantitative procedures.

The last step was to connect these conceptual understandings, these attempts to create meaning out of our own and others' experiences, to prior medical and social science theory and scholarship. As the step most distant from the subjective reality of families, it is the most fragile and abstract link in the inquiry chain, fraught with potential lack of meaning or errors in interpretation. This step also has the greatest potential for broadening our understanding of these issues, for advancing scholarly knowledge, and for informing us of needed changes in the character and delivery of medical and social services to families. More elaborate technical details of the research design used here, including samples and instruments, are contained in the Appendix.

Throughout this volume, we present the results of this research in the form of personal anecdotes and reflections, as well as in statistical tabulations and comparisons. Both styles are helpful in advancing our understanding of the experiences of children and their families and in improving the delivery of health care. Statistics and scientific data alone will not convince parents or professionals of the need for improvement, but they can help. And accounts of the heartfelt experiences of parents and youngsters will not of themselves settle the need for and direction of change, but they, too, can help. These multiple forms of data and analysis can help all of us involved with the care of children with cancer – children, parents, other family members, friends and neighbors, medical staffs, social service staffs, educators – think anew about the psychosocial care of youngsters and their families.

CHAPTER NOTES

1. Different category systems, and different data sources, provide slightly different incidence rates. The rates indicated in Table 1.1 are computed from Sutow, Tables 1.1 and 1.2 (1984, pp. 2–5).

2. Interested readers may supplement this brief and nontechnical introduction to pediatric cancers and treatments by consulting a variety of recent texts: Levine (1982), Sutow, Fernbach, and Vietti (1984), Tebbi (1982).

3. A series of reports on these late effects of treatment include: D'Angio (1980), Eiser (1978), Holmes and Holmes (1975), Li, Cassady, and Jaffe (1975), Li and Stone (1976), Robison et al. (1984) and Simone et al. (1978). Jaffe (1984) and Oliff and Levine (1982) provide excellent summaries of studies examining the impacts of varied treatments on a range of organs and organ systems.

4. See, for example, Duffner, Cohen, and Flannery (1982), Griffel (1977), and Meadows, Hopson, Lustbader, and Evans (1979).

5. Even these figures are outdated, because of time lags in publishing most recently available data. For incomplete, but later results, see Miller and McKay (1984), Ries, Pollack, and Young (1983), and interim reports of the Childhood Cancer Study Group (nonpublished material). The American Cancer Society reports 50% to 75% survival rates for childhood ALL in some medical centers (*Cancer Facts and Figures*, 1984). However, it should be noted that all these reports refer to two- to five-year survival rates, and not to long-term cure.

6. See, for example, Adams (1979), Adams and Deveau (1984), Kellerman (1980), Koocher and O'Malley (1981), Schulman and Kupst (1980), Spinetta and Spinetta (1981).

7. Mark Chesler is a social psychologist who is the parent of two children, one of whom was diagnosed at age 11+ with cancer and is in long-term remission. He has been an active member of a self-help group for families of children with cancer and has met with parents, families, and professionals in medical centers and communities across the nation. Oscar Barbarin is a clinical psychologist who also is the parent of two children, one of whom has asthma. He has met with and counseled parents of children with cancer and other serious illness for a number of years. Thus, direct "insider" experience and closely related "outsider" experience have been combined.

8. This style of scientific work generates theory that is derived from and firmly grounded in the data of people's direct experience; thus the label "grounded theory" (Glaser & Strauss, 1967).

CHAPTER 2

Medical Stress

Families of children with cancer are challenged by a number of un-anticipated and powerful stresses. The patient, parents, and all family members must meet this challenge and deal with many new and difficult situations. For most families the course of childhood cancer is a series of *medical* events or benchmarks that signal important movement toward or away from recovery. Families' accounts of their experiences with the illness are often structured around these disease-related markers. Even though the course of the illness varies from child to child, there are patterns and stresses that typify most families' experience of childhood cancer.

STRESS

The concept of stress has a long, complex history, and the term has been used to describe many different events or feelings. Some authors suggest that stressful events include only objective situations which anyone might perceive as disruptive – death of an intimate, a disabling accident or illness, loss of employment, or bankruptcy. Others argue that stress describes subjective experiences which create the feeling of pressure or disruption, whether or not they appear that way to external observers.[1] Both approaches have value. The objective approach draws attention to the universal aspects of serious illness; the subjective approach emphasizes individuals' unique reactions. We utilize both approaches, taking the course of the child's illness and health status as markers of objective stress, and parents' reports of their experiences and feelings as indicators of subjective stress.

Researchers assessing the impact of major life stresses also distinguish two different classes of crises. One category is developmental or normal crises, stresses that can be expected to occur in the lives of most persons and families. Examples include childbirth, entry of children to school, major promotions, household moves from one city to another, children leaving home, and even loss of an aging parent. Although these events are stressful, they are all sequential parts of the developmental process. The fact that they can be anticipated means people can prepare to cope with them and reduce their impact, and their normalcy permits people to feel relatively comfortable with them.

A second category of major life events includes unexpected crises, stresses not anticipated as part of the normal flow of life. Examples include the early death of a spouse, a flood or other natural disaster, a major traffic accident, and the serious illness or death of a child.[2] The nonnormal and atypical character of these crises often heightens stress, especially since few other people in the local community may have had such experiences.

Not all these stresses have tragic or negative outcomes. For many people such stress is a positive challenge, an opportunity for learning, for growth, for renewed faith and meaning, and for a better life. Resolution can be toward growth, not just toward stasis or a return to prior normalcy. In the process of dealing with crises, many people have discovered previously untapped internal strength and new sources of courage and caring.[3]

Although it is undoubtedly true that what is stressful for one person or group may not be so for another, chronic and serious illness is likely to have serious impact on all persons closely related to the ill person. This has led Cassileth and Hamilton (1979) to describe cancer as a "family disease":

> *A cancer diagnosis in any member of the family imposes change, disrupts the family's homeostatic balance, and unsettles the operational guidelines for interpersonal behavior. (p. 234)*

Cancer is a family disease because it has an impact on all members of the family and creates stress for all of them, not just for the ill person. If this is true for cancer in general, it is all the more likely to be true for childhood cancer. The child is the most vulnerable and cherished family member, and childhood illness threatens parents' basic hopes and sense of competence. Unexpected crisis and tragedy that affects the life or welfare of a child is most unsettling and disruptive for other family members.

MEDICAL STRESS OF CHILDHOOD CANCER

Throughout our interviews, questionnaires, and stress charts[4] the most common and potent stresses that parents note include diagnosis, surgery, treatment side effects, and relapse. Prediagnostic symptoms, chemotherapy and radiation, and continuing checkups are mentioned less often and as less powerful. Although it was possible for parents to indicate nonmedical events, medical issues dominate their responses. For instance, in responding to questionnaire items about which events caused "very strong" stress, parents give highest priority to the following items:

The fact my child has cancer (80%);
Fear of my child's death (61%);
My child's reaction to treatment (57%);
Fear of my child's relapse (52%).

Clearly, these disease- and treatment-related issues are direct and major stresses – immediate and concrete challenges to parents.

Detailed analyses of the stress charts give additional insights. Figures 2.1 and 2.2 present composite stress charts that summarize the events parents mention most commonly and the mean height or potency of the stresses they indicate.[5] Because the experiences of families of living and families of deceased children are so different, separate composite charts are presented for these two groups.

Figure 2.1 indicates that parents of living children experience the greatest stress (frequency and potency) at diagnosis. The universal phenomena of treatment and treatment side effects (especially surgery, when it occurred) also are reported as potent. Relapse, although less common, is also potent. Figure 2.2 shows that for parents of deceased children, relapse always occurs and it takes on great importance; it is the beginning of the turn in the road. Hope, kindled by remission, is severely challenged by the relapse. Even though these parents also mention diagnosis most often, it is not as potent as other stresses, notably relapse, deterioration or the terminal illness phase, and death. Reminders of life and death such as birthdays, anniversaries, and important family events also are mentioned often by parents of deceased children.

This sequence of stressful events reflects what Ross has called the "changing critical phases" of childhood cancer (1978), or what Adams has called the typical "illness cycle" (1979, pp. 17–21). Ross's (1978) phases include before the diagnosis, diagnostic period, remission, re-

HERE IS A CHART, A TIMELINE, THAT CAN BE USED TO DESCRIBE THE TIME THAT HAS ELAPSED FROM BEFORE YOU LEARNED THE DIAGNOSIS UNTIL NOW.

1. MARK ON THIS LINE THE CRITICAL EVENTS OR STAGES IN YOUR EXPERIENCE WITH YOUR CHILD'S CANCER. INDICATE THE APPROXIMATE DATE OF EACH.

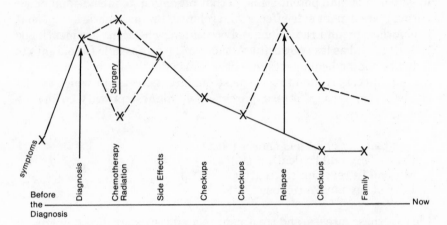

2. WHICH OF THESE EVENTS OR STAGES WERE MOST STRESSFUL? DRAW AN ARROW FOR EACH EVENT, INDICATING WITH A HIGH LINE THE HIGHEST STRESS TIMES OR EVENTS, AND WITH A LOW LINE THE LESSER STRESS TIMES OR EVENTS.

Figure 2.1. Composite stress chart of parents of living children

HERE IS A CHART, A TIMELINE, THAT CAN BE USED TO DESCRIBE THE TIME THAT HAS ELAPSED FROM BEFORE YOU LEARNED THE DIAGNOSIS UNTIL NOW.

1. MARK ON THIS LINE THE CRITICAL EVENTS OR STAGES IN YOUR EXPERIENCE WITH YOUR CHILD'S CANCER. INDICATE THE APPROXIMATE DATE OF EACH.

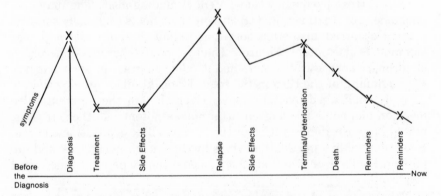

2. WHICH OF THESE EVENTS OR STAGES WERE MOST STRESSFUL? DRAW AN ARROW FOR EACH EVENT, INDICATING WITH A HIGH LINE THE HIGHEST STRESS TIMES OR EVENTS, AND WITH A LOW LINE THE LESSER STRESS TIMES OR EVENTS.

Figure 2.2. Composite stress chart of parents of deceased children

lapse, and death and mourning. Adams (1979) provides somewhat more detail in his discussion of an illness cycle that includes diagnosis, nearing remission, during remission, relapse, second relapse, death, after death, and long-term survival. Other observers, noting a rhythm to families' stress at different stages of an illness, or different stages of adjustment to illness, suggest providing different kinds of help or social services at different points of such a stressline.[6] Each of these major events or stages has its own impact.

Early Symptoms

The concern over unclear early symptoms often pales beside the emergent reality of childhood cancer. But the prediagnostic period is stressful nevertheless. Several parents indicated just how difficult it was to marshall the energy to seek an accurate diagnosis, to convince themselves or their physicians that their child's situation was serious, or to wind their way through contradictory diagnoses and inadequate treatment systems.

> *My mother had noticed that her eye glowed like a cat's eye. We took her to the doctor and he told us several times that it was an infection. I really didn't have confidence in that doctor, but it was six months before we saw another one. By then she had formed a bubble around her eye and the opthalmologist said that the eye definitely had to come out.*

> *I was taking him to the doctor for tummy aches, and the pediatrician kept telling me that children his age have a lot of tummy aches and not to worry about it, it will go away. Well, I kept dragging him back and dragging him back, because things like cobblestones under the stroller or crawling on the floor was hurting him. Finally a lump appeared on his back but the doctor said, "Don't worry about that. It's probably just a fatty cyst." Then he sent us to a hospital and the surgeons there "pooh-poohed it" and promised to biopsy it in another two weeks, as a matter of routine. But it didn't turn out to be routine.*

> *At the first hospital where we stayed for two weeks they said there was nothing they could do for her. They said their hands were tied and she had maybe 10 days–2 weeks to live at most. We went to a larger children's hospital and the doctors there did wonders for her.*

These reports are quite typical of the problems some parents experience in getting an accurate diagnosis and getting to a medical institution that has the capacity to correctly diagnose and treat children's cancer. But these experiences are by no means universal. Many parents report that once symptoms become clear they receive timely, accurate diagnoses and rapid, effective treatment. As a result, their initial stress is minimized.

Diagnosis

The report that diagnosis is the most stressful event for many parents, and at least a potent event for all others, is consistent with other theoretical and empirical investigations of childhood cancer.[7] Diagnosis is a process or series of events beginning with the detection of physical abnormality or impaired functions, continuing through medical tests and consultations, and culminating in a conference or physician communication. Somewhere during this period of time, whether in a single instant or a period of hours or days, life is ripped from its normal context. Parents' prior reality is shattered; they enter a new reality, with new definitions of themselves and others. At some level of consciousness they know they are embarking on a long, difficult struggle. Even though they have hope for a good outcome, and perhaps a rapid return to a "normal" existence, they know their lives will never be exactly what they were before.

An indication of the stress and shock of diagnosis, a sense of parents' pain, fear, and even unreality, is quite clear in their reports:

I cried a lot. We were all scared. It was like being in a deep black hole.

I felt like my heart had been torn right out of me. I was terribly despondent at first. I was bitter and asked myself why it had happened. It was very rough to take.

For a while I didn't deal with it; nothing they told me sunk in. They had to tell me three times before I was grasping it. They told me things and two minutes later I couldn't tell you what they told me in terms of medicine, treatment and stuff.

I left the room, I ran. I don't know where I went. I know I ended up on the 7th floor. I know that I was trying to dial numbers and couldn't see the phone. I know I must have called four people before I was aware of what I was doing. I was so totally alone I didn't know how to function. I was going up and down the stairs of the hospital. It certainly was the worst day of my life. I thought the day that my Dad fell dead was the worst experience of my life, but this was the worst.

The dominant themes of shock, fear, disbelief, and occasionally anger that run through many parents' comments about diagnosis are confirmed by other studies and reports:

The next thing Sherry remembered Dr. Nelson saying was, "I was so surprised when I opened her up and saw the invasion by the tumor. I was so surprised I couldn't believe it."... He had removed what he could but he was not able to get very much. He told them that the immediate concern was whether or not she would survive the surgery.... They had been waiting most of the day for Teddi to come through the surgery, to get through that part of it. They thought it was going to be the final step — not the first step. Never in all their imaginings did they consider Teddi's imminent death. ... Meanwhile, Gary had turned around and Skip could see that his eyes were red... As they passed through the automatic doors Gary began to sob. "Why? Why my baby? Why my baby?" (Buttino, 1983, pp. 24–25)

Some parents not only received the diagnosis that their child had cancer, but that the odds of survival were very low or that their child only had a short time to live. Medical predictions of imminent death or of a short life span are rarer now than they used to be, but that offers little solace to parents who do face such bad news.

Treatments and Side Effects

Treatment varies for children with different kinds of cancer, and also for children with different severity or complications of their disease. In those cases in which parents have or feel they have a choice of therapy, they often agonize over the decision. Some continue to reflect on these choices long after the decision has been made.

Chemotherapy was hard because I wasn't sure it was necessary.

We didn't know whether to decide to amputate or have radioactive therapy, and even now we don't know if we made the right choice. There were choices and we're still living with them.

In most cases, however, there are few choices. Standard protocols exist for most childhood cancers, and treatment at any major medical center or children's cancer hospital is relatively standardized.

Painful treatments create stress for parents. Seeing their child undergoing radiation or chemotherapy is difficult, since the radiation machines often frighten children and chemotherapy infusions often are lengthy and painful. In addition, parents and children have to deal with the common side effects of these treatments: nausea and vomiting; loss of hair; loss of appetite and weight; extreme fatigue; crankiness and irritability. Less common but typical side effects include extreme joint pain, weakness that makes children bedridden, serious internal sores, prolonged bleeding from IV sites, and general infection. Even when parents anticipate that the treatments will make their child well in the long run, witnessing such pain and suffering is often disheartening.

The medication made him cranky and that was hard for me to tolerate.

It was tough seeing her go through chemotherapy... throwing up... being in constant pain.

Radiation was the most horrible experience; it was worse than the cancer, far worse. He couldn't have reacted worse, the treatment and complications and all lasted 72 days. I know that we almost lost him twice. We had to put him on the machines to pump life back into him because he had dehydrated so badly and lost so much weight. I didn't know what to do. I would put water on his arms because his skin would scratch off. I would put water on his face. I took a popsicle and pushed it in and out of his mouth. I didn't know how to make him come back to life. He developed thrush, like babies do, because he was so dry and developed bacteria in his mouth. Then he couldn't swallow a thing and his throat closed. He lost his hair and his will to live, and we thought we had made a big mistake. But the minute they left him alone that boy came back. His body is making it up.

One example of the reality of chemotherapy, and its impact on mother and son, is provided by a young cancer patient's own description (Craig, 1983):

A 19-year-old man sits before her (a nurse) in shirt sleeves, his right cuff rolled up past his elbow. She takes the longer of the two rubber straps and wraps it around the young man's scalp line, tying it into a slipknot on his forehead. "This will help minimize hair loss," she tells him. From the corner of the room, there is a gasp. A mother who doesn't see a man, but her baby, her first born, breathes with him in nervous anticipation. The nurse ties the second tourniquet tight above his elbow. He makes a fist and she pokes his forearm gently, feeling for an adequate vein, one that hasn't been hardened from the trauma that comes with cancer chemotherapy. The mother tries to stifle another gasp as her son

*squints with the insertion of the first needle, a connecting tube
called a butterfly for its two orange handles. The nurse tapes down
the handles and the intravenous treatment begins. The first drug
to flow through the tube is Oncovin. Its acrid odor triggers nausea
in the man, causing him to salivate heavily. The nurse reminds
him, "If you feel queasy, take deep breaths through your mouth."
He does and feels settled. The second syringe contains only fifty
c.c. of liquid—about three tablespoons—but it looks like a quart.
It is a solution of nitrogen mustard, developed in gas form for
chemical warfare in World War I, and just the thought of having
it pumped into his veins adds to the man's nausea. The mother
leans forward. Lines are deeply defined in the flesh around her
mouth. Her face is drawn and sallow. The ordeal, the detection and
treatment of Stage IV Hodgkin's disease in her son, has aged her
beyond 43 years. . . . He runs to the sink, and the deep retching in
his stomach explodes. The eight-hour aftermath of his life-prolong-
ing treatment has begun. The nurse returns with a cup of cool
water. He takes a sip and vomits again. After the initial nausea
passes, mother and son walk arm-in-arm to the receptionist who
sets a date for the next treatment. The man's face shows no relief,
for he knows that the physical side effects of the therapy will mar
his entire day, and the emotional scars will be with him for a
lifetime. (p. 2)*

A list of the common treatment side effects, and special signs that
parents must become accustomed to watch for, are often provided by
physicians or by parent groups, as in the following list prepared for a
parent handbook (Schweers, Farnes & Foreman, 1977):

Special Signs to Watch for

*A few side effects require immediate cessation of medication and
consultation with the physician:*

a. Mouth ulcers or severe diarrhea while on methotrexate;
b. Jaundice while on any medication;
c. Allergic reactions: Hives, swelling of eyelids, hands, feet;
d. Excessive bruising or bleeding from low platelets due to drugs;
*e. Hemorrhagic cystitis or blood in urine with pain while on cyclo-
phosphamide;*
*f. Shortness of breath while on daunomycin, adriamycin, or metho-
trexate;*
*g. Excessive thirst or urination while on prednisone or dexameth-
asone;*
*h. Extreme weakness developing after discontinuing a cortisone-
like medication (prednisone, dexamethasone). When a patient takes*

these drugs for a few weeks, his adrenal gland slows down its production of cortisone. After stopping the medication it takes some time for the gland to become normally active. This side effect is rarely seen, as physicians generally recommend a gradual reduction in dosage over several days ("tapering"), allowing the gland to "wake up." If a child is in a serious accident or must undergo surgery within a couple of months of discontinuing cortisone-like drugs, it may be advisable to restart the drug for a short period. The body needs increased cortisone levels during stress and the gland may still be somewhat sluggish.

Since each drug or treatment has its own peculiar effects, more detailed lists are available for particular chemotherapeutic regimes. Becoming knowledgeable and alert about side effects is a major and difficult adjustment for parents and child alike.[8]

As Figure 2.1 indicates, parents of children who had surgery often feel that surgery is even more stressful than chemotherapy. Four aspects are involved: (1) major surgical procedures always carry the risk of death on the operating table, a death that will end parents' hopes of long-term recovery; (2) the immediate aftermath of surgery usually includes pain, heightened vulnerability, and hospitalization; (3) surgery involves physical alteration of the body that mother and father, as man and woman, created, nurtured, and cherish; (4) surgery, especially for bone cancers or osteogenic sarcomas, may be a visible reminder of the struggle with childhood cancer, and perhaps even a permanent disability.

The amputation was the toughest decision to make.

Surgery was the toughest. We feared she wouldn't live through the operation. Then, because it was brain surgery, we feared brain damage. The surgery took longer than expected because they got started late, but they didn't tell us that, so we got real upset at how long it was taking.

Betsy Griffin writes of her own experience with her son's illness, and in particular amputation, in the following terms (1982):

I wanted to go to Dwayne, tell him how deeply sorry I felt, do something for him — anything to make him feel better — somehow stop his pain! I wanted to say the magic word and give him his right arm and shoulder back, have a miracle touch that would take us back to when he was a healthy, robust little boy playing football and tracking mud into the house. But, I knew all that was impossible and that I was doing all I could. (p. 4)

Checkups During Remission

The feelings of confusion and emotional pain arising at diagnosis continue throughout treatment. They may abate over time and be moderated by positive experience and apparent recovery, but they resurface again and again throughout the course of treatment. After all, childhood cancer is not a one-time event; it is a chronically life-threatening disease. Every cold or sore that does not heal quickly, every prolonged headache or stomachache, and every sustained bout of fatigue or flulike discomfort may carry a dangerous message. Since cancer is diagnosed at a microscopic level, the significance of even minor symptoms must be confirmed or disconfirmed by a trip to the clinic or hospital. In the meantime parents and child live on pins and needles of hope and fear.[9]

> *We had a scare recently that just brought back all those memories again. She started having some asymmetrical breast development and was complaining about her breasts being painful. I checked her and it did feel as if there was some type of lump in her breast. So I called the doctor and spent a night up all night just terrified. It was really frightening and I had a hard time getting myself back together again after that. I took her down and had her examined and all it was was asymmetrical breast development and that's that. But it really was terrifying for me.*

> *I worry when he says, "Mom, my stomach hurts." And I worry what's going on there, "Oh, no!" But as time goes on you learn what to worry about and what not to. It could be the flu or something.*

By the same token, negative changes in the child's health are not always observable. An apparently healthy and recovering or recovered child may be discovered in microscopic examination to be in very serious condition. Thus, each return to the hospital for a checkup presents parents with a threat.

> *I think of the possibility of a relapse every month at blood count time and every three months at bone marrow time.*

> *Regular CAT scans worry me, because they show potential progress of the disease. Each subsequent scan has been stressful, but they're getting less stressful, because they're coming out well. It was hard for me to wait for the results from the tests because they could show evidence of the disease.*

Over time parents learn to live with these fears, learn "what to worry about and what not to." However, these reports indicate that much of the stress reported as occurring at diagnosis is sustained even when things are going well. Continuing uncertainty, alertness, and adaptation to new treatments become a constant stress.

Ross (1978) notes that during this stage, particularly if the remission is extended and uncomplicated, the family may "forget" about the illness and return to an equilibrium. The illness is never completely forgotten, of course, and the new equilibrium is not quite like life before the diagnosis, but the lengthy process of adaptation and normalization may have begun.

Relapse

Despite the best efforts of the medical staff, a substantial proportion of children being treated for childhood cancer come out of remission and suffer a relapse, as the disease reasserts itself. We have discussed the fears of relapse revealed in parents' reported concerns about colds, sniffles, and checkups even when there are no apparent symptoms of the cancer. For parents of children who do relapse, this fear is now a reality – a severe blow.[10] Hope, and perhaps tranquillity, built up during remission is threatened or even dashed, and at best a new and long period of treatment again lies ahead.

> *The relapse was worse than the diagnosis.*

> *I knew relapse was a possibility so the shock was not as great as the diagnosis, but many of the original feelings and shock are there. But I think you get over it quicker. It was most dramatic in the beginning but it is basically the same thing all over again.*

> *It made me tired to think about starting all over again. It was an exasperating thought. It bothered me more than the original diagnosis because this time I knew what we were going to have to go through.*

The prospect of repeated remissions and relapses is especially discouraging, since it typically is associated with decreased confidence in a cure. As Sourkes notes (1982), it creates a roller coaster of emotions for all involved:

> *Both patient and family have to prepare for loss with each announcement of relapse, only to rearrange for life when remission is attained. The sense of exhaustion that accompanies this process is inordinate. The family begins to feel as if someone is "crying wolf." (p. 72)*

For parents of children who have died, the relapse, in retrospect, takes on additional meaning. It was not only a new shock, but the beginning of the downward course of the life of their child. The second or third relapse even more clearly presages a period of deterioration and perhaps the terminal phase in their child's life.

I felt despair at the second tumor. The first time you really don't know how serious it is. But on the second occasion it sounded like this was an accelerating condition. Now we are facing definitely an uphill battle and his chances for survival suddenly plummeted. After the second occasion it was a matter of desperation.

Metastasis was the worst time. When it spread to his lungs we knew this was real bad news.

The Terminal Phase . . . and Death

A number of parents of children who died indicate that the beginning of the terminal phase, or the point at which it became clear that death was a certainty, was the hardest part of their encounter with childhood cancer.

The last period before she died was the toughest. I didn't work at all so I could spend time with her.

When he deteriorated from a perfectly normal child to an infant was the toughest.

Other parents note that, without question, the death of their child was the most difficult event or stage of the illness.

Of course the hardest time was his death.

The hardest time was when we took her to the hospital for the last time and they told us it would be the last time.

Mary Cornils describes her reaction to her daughter's death from cancer in the following eloquent and moving terms (1981):

Carol, my youngest daughter, was 16 years old when we found out what was causing her pain and making her feel lethargic — an unusual type of cancer, rarely diagnosed in persons under the age of 40. The next 14 months were times of alternating bewilderment, anger, hope, and despair. For eight months everything looked good, and then the dreaded metastases showed up on her lung x-ray. Her chemotherapy was changed; a more aggressive protocol begun. But, it was the beginning of the end, and we all knew it. For six more months she fought a courageous battle and we prayed for a miracle, but it was not to be. On April 17, 1977, early on a Sunday morning she said her last goodbyes and left this earth forever.

I was filled with heartache and overwhelmed by sadness. My lovely daughter, so full of joy, love and hope, would not have the opportunity to graduate from . . . high school with her friends. She would never attend the university . . . where she had been accepted. . . . She would never marry and have the children she wanted so dearly. I was angry that she had been so cruelly robbed of the chance to grow to womanhood and the fulfillment of her dreams. And I felt cheated myself, for Carol had always given so much more to me and the others whose lives she touched than she had ever received in return. (p. 5)

Cornils summarizes the views of many parents, physicians, and researchers, as she notes that, "The death of a child is one of the most devastating, if not the most devastating, things that can happen to a family" (1981, p. 5). In addition to the direct pain of loss, many parents report that they experience a terrible sense of aloneness and isolation from their families and friends. In discussing the death of children with cystic fibrosis, Burton (1975) points out that this isolation is greater because infant and child mortality has become relatively rare in the developed nations. Most friends and family members have no experience with the death of a child, and are ignorant about the ways and means of providing support to newly bereaved parents.

Some parents say that death, itself, is not the worst part of their experience.[11] Death from childhood cancer is generally not a sudden event; it is well anticipated in most cases. And, as some parents note, when it comes it may release the child from pain and suffering.

Death was not so hard because she'd been sick so long. It was a relief that she wouldn't suffer anymore.

Death was not the worst time. It was anticipated. And it would relieve him from a lot of pain at the end.

Of course, no amount of anticipatory mourning ever fully prepares a parent for the death of a child, and no parent wishes death for his or her child. As parents report, however, death not only releases their child from pain, it also releases them from the pain of helplessly watching their child suffer. Although death is not the end of pain and sadness, it often marks the beginning of a time when sickness and hospitalization no longer dominate the family's life.

Going Off Treatment

The most positive outcome of treatment for childhood cancer is for the child to be in long-term (optimally first) remission, to complete the course of treatment, and to go off all drugs and radiation therapy. However, even the cessation of therapy and the cautious pronouncement of "cure" carries a risk (5–10%) of future relapse, of a second later cancer or of late side effects of treatment.[12] Checkups continue, as do some of the stresses associated with remission. Koocher (1984b) reports the existence of heightened fears around "lump anniversaries," and many adolescents report greater fears of relapse when they are under stress from schoolwork or difficult social relations.

Not much has been written about the stress of going off treatment, simply because this is a relatively new development for a significant number of youngsters with cancer. But successful checkups and a "cure" can be stressful in themselves. Parents who have been alert for returning symptoms for several years must now learn to relax that watchfulness. Attention must be given to other personal or family issues that may have been put on hold. Family members who invested tremendous energy fearing and preparing for the child's death may subtly or unconsciously resent that their worrying was for naught.[13] They may demand a payback from the child (good behavior, continued health) for their emotional investment.

As the "crutch" of treatment is cast off, the child and family go into the future on their own. They typically develop concerns about how they will fare without the disease-fighting drugs and treatments. Parents and physicians are reluctant to use the word "cure" until several years have passed after the end of treatment. Parents of children who are off all treatment and are doing well often stumble over reporting whether their child "has" or "had" cancer. As the fear of relapse fades, more typical worries about the child's psychological and social development, school achievement, career plans, and other issues of normal family life come to the fore.

Whereas some youngsters and their parents have fears about going off treatment, others overreact in the opposite direction, assuming that if they have "beaten the big C" they can take all manners of risks. Many acting-out or experimental behaviors that were denied or shelved for the years of treatment may now become quite attractive as well as feasible for the child, especially for adolescents. Thus, the normal developmental stresses of family life reassert themselves. Most unfortunately, several recent reports suggest that survivors of childhood cancer can expect to encounter substantial employment and insurance discrimination in the years ahead (Feldman, 1980; Teta et al., 1984).[14] Society will continue to create stress for the child with cancer, even after the medical danger fades.

Thus the adaptations required by recovery or cure may be as stressful as were the prior adaptations that had been built in response to the medical threat.

THE IMPACT ON DIFFERENT FAMILIES

Identification of these major stresses or stressful events helps describe parents' reality as they deal with childhood cancer. One critical issue affecting parental stress levels is how the course of the disease and its treatment differs for different children. Parents who have to deal with very different objective circumstances experience different levels of stress. As the differences between the composite stress charts in Figures 2.1 and 2.2 indicate, not all parents or families experience the same stresses, or experience them in the same way. For instance, Figures 2.3 and 2.4 present two markedly different individual stress charts. In Figure 2.3 a father notes 12 different events, none of them very powerful (height off the horizontal); if we assign numerical values for how high each stress is we can compute this person's total stress score (sum of each event × total height of each line drawn) as 30. The father reporting in Figure 2.4 notes nine different events, many of them quite powerful, totaling to a score of 85. What accounts for these differences? The father in Figure 2.3 has a child diagnosed with Wilms' tumor, a

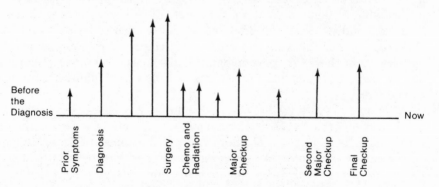

Figure 2.3. Father of living child

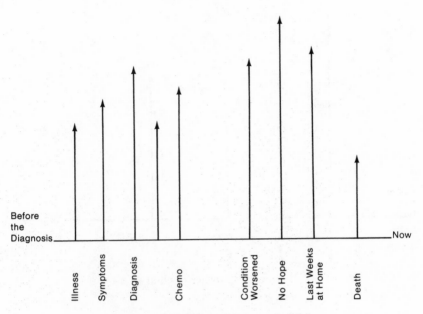

Figure 2.4. Father of deceased child

disease that has a relatively high rate of successful treatment. After initial surgery and other treatment the child progressed steadily, remaining in good health with few side effects and surviving in excellent shape. The child of the father in Figure 2.4 died; the child was diagnosed at a young age with neuroblastoma and experienced a series of relapses prior to his death. The two figures confirm that the family with a child who died from cancer is in a different situation than the family of a child who is living with cancer. There is also considerable variation within the category of families of children living with cancer . . . according to the nature of the disease, the vigor and trauma of treatment (surgery or not, for instance), and the occurrence of a relapse.[15]

This explanation is not sufficient to explain all the variations in parental reports of medical stress. Even when objective medical circumstances are quite similar, different people report widely varying levels of stress. This is illustrated in a comparison of stress charts from a mother and a father in the same family. As parents of the same child, their objective medical situations are similar. However, they interpret or react to these circumstances differently. Figure 2.5 is from the mother and Figure 2.6 is from the father of a young child with neuroblastoma. The child went through a minimum of aggressive therapy and is doing very well. Although both parents mention relatively few stress-

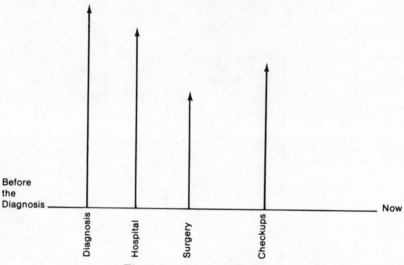

Figure 2.5. Mother of child A

ful events (four and three), and both their total stress scores are low (26 and 09), they report a marked difference in their stress levels. Similarly, a comparison of Figures 2.7 and 2.8, from parents of a child who died from leukemia after several relapses, shows important differences. The father (Figure 2.8) mentions six events, all named, and has a total stress score of 19 – less than that of the father of the living child represented in Figure 2.3. The mother's chart (Figure 2.7) shows many more events, often unnamed and some occurring after the death of the child, and has

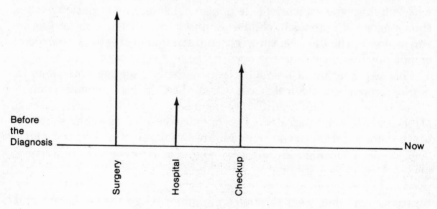

Figure 2.6. Father of child A

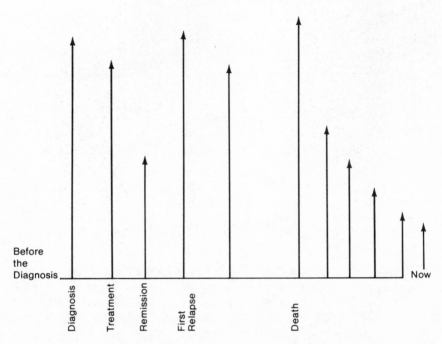

Figure 2.7. Mother of child B

a stress score of 85. What explains these differences in reactions when parents experienced the same illness and objective medical conditions?

Obviously, even the same stresses mean different things to different people. Based upon their prior personal experiences and psychological style, each person has a unique perspective. People of different gender, with different personal coping styles, with various experiences with cancer, and with different needs for support, stability, and autonomy, will encounter different subjective realities in the attempt to deal with childhood cancer.[16] Families in different social situations may experience similar stressors in different ways and also may experience quite different stresses.

Demographics/Resources as Mediators of Stress

Different personal and family backgrounds, and therefore varying perspectives and available resources, place families in quite different circumstances. Any attempt to describe the experience of childhood cancer as common or universal overlooks these differences.

Parents' stress chart scores and questionnaire responses (see the list

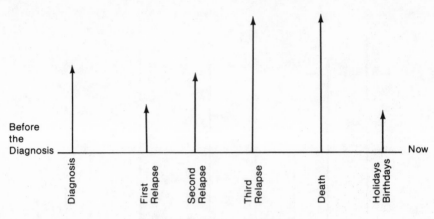

Figure 2.8. Father of child B

of events that cause stress, page 19) reveal that the objective health status of the child has a significant impact on parental stress. Table 2.1 confirms that parents of deceased children more often report higher amounts of disease-related stress than do parents of living children, in both the questionnaire and the interview. Table 2.1 also indicates that parents whose children experienced a relapse, but who are in remission

Table 2.1
Measures of Parents' Medically Related Stress,
By Life Status of the Child

Parent Group	Number of Stressful Events (Interview-Chart)	Power (height) of All Events (Interview-Chart)	Stress from Child's Disease (Questionnaire)
Parents of living children who are in remission	6.4 ($N=54$)	35.5 ($N=54$)	9.6 ($N=54$)
Parents of living children who have relapsed	6.4 ($N=10$)	34.7 ($N=10$)	10.1 ($N=12$)
Parents of deceased children	9.1 ($N=20$)	47.8 ($N=20$)	11.0 ($N=17$)
	$F=2.54$ $p<.08$	$F=NS$	$F=2.57$ $p<.08$

once again, do not report significantly greater stress than parents of children who have remained in remission.

An examination of the relationship between parental stress and a variety of background factors indicates that the child's specific diagnosis does not have a significant relationship to parental stress. However, the child's age at the time of diagnosis relates significantly to parental reports of stress. Parents of living children who were diagnosed when they were between four and seven years of age report less stress than do parents of children diagnosed at less than four years of age or more than seven years. Parents of a child who is diagnosed at a very young age may feel especially strongly about their child's vulnerability and inability to deal with or understand this assault on the body. Stress may be particularly great when parents' strong protective feelings cannot shield their very young child from severe illness. Youngsters in the four- to seven-year age group are somewhat able to care for themselves and to engage in conversation and collaboration that can lessen the strain of parental adjustment. The unexpected burdens on parents of older children may be related to the disease's disruptions of the roles and activities of these children. At six or seven years of age children begin to move out of their parents' immediate domain, to enter school, neighborhood playgrounds, and so on. There they often encounter social anxiety and rejection. The impact of a serious illness may create a significant change in parents' roles in relationship to these somewhat independent children.

The study also explores the impact of parents' different social situations, with few significant findings. For instance, parents' gender, age, and religion do not have a significant relationship to their reports of medical stress. Neither does socioeconomic status (level of income and education). Thus, stress emanating from the course of the disease appears to cut across a variety of background factors with a force that diminishes the normal power of social and economic distinctions.

The findings reported in this chapter sketch important themes in the lives of parents of children with cancer. First, it is clear that the medical facts of cancer are enormously stressful for parents. Diagnosis is a major shock. Treatments and their side effects create continuing stress. Even when things appear to be going well, stress levels may be high. Moreover, these medical stresses are not transitory; they are chronic and continue over a long period, often for years. They continue after a child's recovery or after a child's death. The stresses of uncertainty of the illness, and thus the continuing threat to the child's life, to the child's safety and comfort, and to the family's comfort and peace of mind, are cumulative.

Second, the experience of stress varies according to some important factors in the child's life. The actual progress of the disease, in terms of the child's life or death, is a major factor affecting parental stress levels. The child's age also has an impact on parents' stress.

Third, and contrary to expectations, not many parent/family social or lifestyle differences affect parental stress. Parents' gender, income, education, and religion do not result in different reports. The commonality of the experience of childhood cancer appears to cut across status levels; one does not escape the impact through accumulated wealth or wisdom. Just as cancer, in both children and adults, strikes regardless of race, social status, and sex, the stresses of childhood cancer show no respect for typical social distinctions.

CHAPTER NOTES

1. In the latter tradition, Lazarus and Launier (1978) and Antonovsky (1980) argue that stress is dependent upon the meaning a stimulus or event has for the person. Similarly, Dohrenwend argues that " . . . individuals' perceptions of the stressfulness of particular life events are the best predictors of whether their life events will be followed by illness (distress) or not" (1974, p. 325).

2. Pearlin and Lieberman refer to the serious illness of a child as a nonnormative event, in that it generates an "unexpected" crisis (1979). In a similar vein, Futterman and Hoffman (1973) refer to the "situational crisis" of childhood cancer, to differentiate it from the normal developmental tasks or crises of most children and families.

3. A similar perspective on positive adaptations to stress is emphasized by Adams (1979), Desmond (1980), Futterman and Hoffman (1973), Hymovich (1976), Kellerman (1980), Sussman, Hollenbeck, Nannis, and Strope (1980). Desmond, in particular, objects to the literature's bias in "viewing the experience of strong and distressing emotions as maladaptive rather than adaptive behavior" (1980, p. 123). No one wishes to romanticize these tragedies and struggles, but we do want to emphasize concern with the actions of normal and able persons to a series of abnormal situations and with the potential for positive outcomes.

4. In individual interviews we asked family members to describe the toughest times during the illness. On the questionnaire, after the interview was completed, parents rated 16 major stressors (3=very strong, 1=not strong). Four of these 16 stressors were specifically related to medical events: the diagnosis, side effects of treatment, relapse, and death. Even when the families had not experienced relapse or death, their threat was ominous and real and could not be ignored. In addition, stress charts were created by asking each parent to list the stressful events they experienced, from the time of diagnosis to the time of the interview, and to indicate the degree of stress at each point. Parents were given a sheet of paper with a line drawn at the bottom: on one end of the line were the words "before the diagnosis" and on the other end of the line, the word "now." At the top of the sheet were the following directions:

> Here is a chart, a time line that can be used to describe the time that has elapsed from before you learned the diagnosis until now. Do two things: (1) mark on this line the critical events or stages in your experience with your child's cancer, indicating the approximate date of each; (2) indicate which of these events or stages were the most stressful by drawing an arrow for each event indicating with a high line the highest stress times or events and with a low line the lower stress time or events.

5. Parents' drawings of stress charts were coded for the kinds of events they mentioned, as well as for the vertical height of each line they drew. Events with the highest average lines (height in the entire sample divided by number of times mentioned) are reported in Figures 2.1 and 2.2. However, to distinguish between those events mentioned by almost all parents (diagnosis, side effects, checkups) and those mentioned by relatively few (surgery, relapse), we have used dotted lines for the latter.

6. See, for example, Kaplan, Smith, Grobstein, and Fishman (1973), Obetz et al. (1980), and Ross (1978).

7. Binger et al. (1969), Knapp and Hansen (1973), Adams (1979), Hamburg and Adams (1967), McCollum and Schwartz (1972), Koch, Hermann, and Donaldson (1974), and Ross (1978) all have discussed the shock associated with the initial diagnosis of childhood cancer. McCollum (1975) identifies such shock as applying to many serious childhood illnesses, such as deafness (Meadow, 1968), mental retardation (Jacobs, 1982), diabetes (Hamburg & Inoff, 1983), cystic fibrosis (Burton, 1975), and various forms of birth defects and disabilities (Davis, Eckert, Golden, and McMillan, 1981; Featherstone, 1981).

8. Scholarly discussions of current treatment regimens for childhood cancer indicate the potent side effects of surgery, radiation, and chemotherapy, and clearly suggest how they might be stressful for any patient or parent (Hughes, 1976; Katz, 1980). Aside from the direct physical impacts of these treatments, Clapp (1976) and Koocher and Sallan (1978) discuss how their (sometimes lasting) side effects may threaten children's social and psychological well-being.

9. As de Traubenberg notes with regard to childhood heart disease, "the fear of a disaster and the specter of a fatal seizure are always present, overshadowing every other consideration" (1973, p. 81).

10. *Coping with Cancer* (1980), Futterman and Hoffman (1973), and Ross (1978) note the ways in which relapse may be even more stressful than diagnosis; parents and child literally must "start all over again." The utility of denial as a defense loses effectiveness and the fear of the child's death again becomes potent.

11. Lascari and Stehbens (1973) report that the parents of deceased children whom they interviewed were divided evenly as to whether diagnosis or death was the most difficult period.

12. See the discussion and references in Chapter 1, note 3.

13. Sourkes (1982) notes that although such feelings may be understandable, they are seldom articulated openly and may be a source of enormous guilt and confusion.

14. As of this writing, congressional hearings are underway regarding federal legislation to protect the civil rights of (ex)cancer patients.

15. For a discussion of these and other objective medical factors that may account for differences in parental stress, see: Hamovitch (1964), Pless and Pinkerton (1975), and Adams (1979).

16. Several anthologies of research on stressful life events discuss the role of these social and psychological filters, resources, etc. See, for instance, Dohrenwend and Dohrenwend (1974) and Datan and Ginsberg (1975).

CHAPTER 3

Personal and Social Stresses

The psychosocial challenge of childhood cancer has its origin not in the disease itself, but in the personal and social contexts within which the illness occurs. Childhood cancer raises personal emotional issues with which parents must deal and significantly affects parents' and children's networks of social relationships. A paradox of serious and chronic childhood illness is that parents' attempts to meet the challenge posed by the disease may create other stresses with which they must then deal. Another paradox is that each of the persons or social forces who might be a source of support for parents may also be a source of added stress. The stresses emanating from these emotional reactions and social relationships are discussed in this chapter. Parents' use of coping mechanisms is discussed in Chapters 5 and 6, and their use of social support systems is discussed in Chapters 9 and 10.

KINDS OF PSYCHOSOCIAL STRESS

Interviews with parents of children with cancer reveal a series of personal and social stresses that are set in motion by this serious and chronic childhood illness. They include:

Portions of this chapter first appeared in: Chesler, M., & Yoak, M. Self-help groups for families of children with cancer: Patterns of stress and social support. From H. Roback (Ed.), *Helping Patients and Their Families Cope with Medical Problems*. San Francisco: Jossey-Bass, 1984. Reprinted by permission.

Intellectual stress, which is created by massive amounts of technical information about the disease and treatments and by the unfamiliar culture of the medical system;

Instrumental stress, which is created by the myriad of new daily practical tasks involved in maintaining a home, family, and work life in the midst of the medical crisis;

Interpersonal stress, which is created by the escalating needs of all family members and the changing sets of relations with old and new friends and with service providers;

Emotional stress, which is created by the psychological and often physical consequences of fear, distress, and loss of sleep and energy;

Existential stress, which is created by confusion about the meaning and order of life challenged by "unjust" pain and terror for a child.

Intellectual Stress

What is difficult and even shocking for parents of children with cancer is the sudden presentation of a great deal of new medical information. Few parents understand how cancer works and what cellular transformations are involved as the disease arises and progresses. They may be overwhelmed by an array of new disease and treatment terms, such as acute lymphoblastic leukemia, rhabdomyosarcoma, or intrathecal methotrexate. As they learn the names of lifesaving drugs they also need to gain familiarity with standard dosages, timing of treatments, and side effects.

The shock and surprise that parents report experiencing at diagnosis is partly a product of their ignorance of cancer and their lack of immediate understanding of the meaning of the diagnosis and prognosis.

We did ask some questions but it was just so much at a time. I don't really know if we asked the right questions, although the staff would answer whatever we asked them. Sometimes you feel silly asking a doctor over and over again, but it just doesn't sink in.

Not much information about that type of tumor was easily available. Most of the information we got was from the doctors and was verbal. But too much was happening for me to remember really all the verbal information. It would have been helpful to have written information to consult when we were ready to absorb it.

It would have been very helpful if we had been given a complete picture as soon as possible. We needed information on what to

*expect, the percentage of children that are cured, whether our
daughter would live, etc. I needed to feel informed as quickly as
possible.*

Not all parents want "a complete picture as soon as possible." For some
parents, that would be too much information, and it might increase their
stress even more. Some parents are glad to receive information a little
at a time, "when we were ready to absorb it."

If parents are to be involved in the long-term care of chronically and
seriously ill children, they must have adequate and detailed information
about symptoms, danger signals, and treatment procedures and options. The task of gathering and understanding information may be
critical to the child's survival, as well as to parents' own emotional
stability and integrity. The need for information becomes even more
critical when the child leaves the hospital and returns home. As treatment continues on an outpatient basis, parents experience the stress
of wondering if the child is taking the right medication, at the right time,
and in the right way. The stress of wondering if they are handling
treatments and side effects properly is escalated by the stakes involved –
the child's comfort and even life may hang in the balance.

Parents are often confused by the geographic and operational maze
of a hospital. Especially when the treatment facility is part of a major
medical center, as opposed to a small community hospital, parents must
learn the location of the oncology/hematology clinic, the outpatient
service, the billing office, and so on. In dealing with the hospital bureaucracy, parents often find it difficult to discover "who is who," and to
understand the subtle but powerful relationship between jacket length
and color and the power and status of clerks, nurses, interns, residents,
fellows, junior staff officers, house doctors, and clinic chiefs. Short-term
rotations in teaching hospitals add to the difficulty. Parents may be
uncertain about who is really responsible for the medical care of their
child.

Parents experiencing these intellectual stresses sometimes encounter
a medical staff that exacerbates their feelings of inadequacy or ignorance. Stress is increased when medical information is withheld or when
it is presented in ways that are confusing to persons without medical
training. The particular vocabulary, jargon, and even style of the medical staff often make it more difficult to understand what is happening,
as one parent notes:

*Cancer is a disease, like many others, but I really think the doctors
are hyped about it more than anyone else. I think it's a language
situation. I don't know why it's so damn hard for the doctors to*

speak like they are talking to their next door neighbors about the dandelions in the yard or whatever, but when they put their white coats on, they adopt an attitude.

Understanding this technical information, as well as the medical culture within which they must now operate, is still not enough. Many parents who have a working knowledge of these issues find themselves at a loss when they have to explain what is happening to their family members and friends. They often do not know how to answer others' questions. Sometimes they are worn out, moving back and forth as message carriers between the medical staff and others in their environment who also need the information.

Instrumental Stress

As the child with cancer is treated and perhaps hospitalized for chemotherapy or surgery, parents face many concrete problems. They must establish new patterns of family life that permit them to care for the ill child, to care for other family members, to continue their jobs, to manage transportation to the hospital, and to ensure that household duties are accomplished. Cooking, cleaning, mowing the lawn, shoveling snow, and fixing burnt-out light bulbs may all become problems. Several mothers report difficulties in juggling their practical daily routines and roles.

My toughest problem was trying to be a mother to my children at home and trying to take care of her in the hospital. I don't want her or the children at home to feel as if I am deserting them.

It was hard having to be with him in the hospital so much. There were so many things to do at home and yet I had to be in the hospital. I didn't feel that I could leave him for long periods.

Many parents also found it difficult to maintain their normal working roles. Tucker (1982) reports this about the father of a leukemic child, Ellie:

At work, [he] had been preoccupied and depressed, and it was only the fear of losing his job that had forced him out of his daze and back to work. He could not even take a day off to rest his nerves. ... (p. 204)

This stress seems especially potent for parents who find it personally fulfilling or financially necessary to work outside the home. Burton (1975) also reports this problem for parents of children with cystic fibrosis, noting that 40% of the fathers she interviewed "felt that their work had been interfered with or negatively influenced by the child's illness."

For some parents these stresses are compounded by their distance from the hospital and by the time and energy it takes to bring their child in for treatment.

Our biggest problem was our geographic situation and the travel.

The separation from the rest of the family has been the hardest for me. I handled it well the first time, but I told my husband that I couldn't take him to New York the next time. I was driving back from the hospital one evening near Christmas and the weather was horrible. When I arrived home I told my husband either we move nearer the hospital or I'm going to stay there.

In some medical centers parents who must travel long distances to the hospital stay at a local Ronald McDonald House at minimal cost.[1]

Monitoring and taking an active role in the daily care of their child in the hospital and at home may create additional stress for parents.

Doctors keep changing, and many come in without having even bothered to sit down and read the records, and don't know what is going on. You have to keep constantly telling them things over and over. You feel you have to be there or she won't get taken care of.

He had a diaper rash and because he had no resistance to anything it turned into a big wound. It took us weeks to clear that up and it was very tough, because he had to be hospitalized for a long time. I was taking classes in a different city at that time and he had to be in isolation, and I had to go on back to the hospital every day to help deal with it. After he got out of the hospital my wife and I, everyday, had to clean that thing out. It was tough on him and it was tough on us.

As children with cancer are treated on an outpatient basis, only occasionally coming to a clinic, parents become front-line caretakers. Then they must become proficient in providing practical medical care that traditionally has been reserved for professionals (Futterman & Hoffman, 1973).

Current regimens for the treatment of childhood cancer do not leave many reasonable decisions in parents' hands. "Proven" treatment modes, which have provided medical advances, lay out standard courses of initial treatment. But parents often need to select a treatment facility and may be asked to participate in research studies or experimental

treatment programs before they have mastered the intellectual challenges posed by their child's diagnosis. And later, if the child's situation
deteriorates, parents become involved in making instrumental choices
about whether or when to cease treatment or where and how their child
may die.

Parents who must deal with the medical system on a long-term basis
typically become involved with complex details of medical records,
hospital billing procedures, and insurance forms. This often produces
the double stress of frustration and confusion and overwhelming financial impact. Some parents report making major changes in their
living styles in order to cope with new financial demands.

> *We had to sell our house because he went through most of my
> health insurance policy in six months. So my sister said we could
> come live with her family until we got started again. We did, but
> it was really hard along with all the other emotional stresses we
> were going through. Recently, my husband's been laid off again,
> and we're going through the financial strain again.*
>
> *The bills are bad. I work, but I'm still in debt.*

The nonmedical costs of childhood cancer to the family may be truly
enormous. Lansky et al. (1979), in one of the few detailed studies available, estimate that noninsured expenses involved in caring for a child
with cancer, such as food, travel, and loss of pay, amount to 25% of
weekly income.

The direct financial costs are only one issue, however; in American
society, money affects people's lives in a variety of subtle ways. Financial resources establish a context for living and for dealing with a myriad
of problems. Low-income families are exposed to unfavorable living conditions and varied social stresses that affect their medical histories.[2]
Childhood cancer exacerbates an already unequal life situation and com-
plicates many of the practical problems of daily living. In some extreme
cases, families without broad medical insurance coverage literally cannot pay for the medical treatment of their child; in the absence of hospital willingness to absorb such costs, some of these children do not
receive adequate treatment – the ultimate concrete stress.

Interpersonal Stress

Relating to the child, dealing with his or her adjustment to the disease and treatment, and to the many new or altered life situations it
brings, may create stressful family situations (Kaplan, Smith, Grobstein,
& Fishman, 1973). Although most parents report that their spouse is

very supportive, the process of adjustment to a child's illness may create interpersonal stress within the marriage. Mothers and fathers who have very different contacts with doctors and other sources of medical information may experience an imbalance in normal family expertise and roles. Parents who are quite depressed or angry may be unable to create intimate time and space with their partners, which considerably stretches the marital bond.

Nancy Roach, the mother of a dying child with leukemia, provides a poignant example of how stress may be felt in the marital relationship (1974):

> *Marital stress brought with it an even greater complexity of feelings. . . . There were many times during the four and a half years of Erin's illness that we were left without the time or energy to see or respond to each other's needs. Sometimes our misplaced anger was vented on one another. . . . Communication was a problem. Initially, we found sharing our feelings extremely difficult. We were both protecting very sensitive areas within ourselves. We had to learn to communicate effectively if we were to pull together in our efforts to support Erin and each other. (p. 72)*

When married couples experience such pain or loneliness in their own relationship, they may feel even less able to deal with their child's illness.

It is typical for siblings to develop feelings of concern about their brother's or sister's illness, to question why this person was selected for this fate, and to experience jealousy or anger about changes in the way time and attention are given to them.[3] In some families, siblings serve as safety valves, acting out or blowing off steam when internal family tension becomes too great. In other instances they act as reality challengers, indicating to parents when they really are paying too much attention to the ill child. If the stress of childhood cancer disturbs the family's prior patterns, it can threaten the interpersonal relationships between the ill child and his or her siblings, and between parents and all their children.

One critical interpersonal stress that parents of a chronically ill child must face is "going public," sharing the new reality, and as much of its meaning as they wish, with their extended family and friends. This is a self-redefining act; in its accomplishment parents inform themselves and others of a major change in their lives. Confusion about the social rules governing the behavior of seriously ill children, concern about how others will react, and a desire to give the right impression to others all create awkward social situations. Society often attaches a stigma to the mysterious and terrifying workings of cancer (Sontag, 1979). As Goffman (1968) notes, people who are close to a stigmatized person often are treated by others as being stigmatized themselves. Such treatment may include isolation, pity, and uneasiness or awkwardness in social relations. Some parents choose to deny or be silent about their child's illness in order to avoid further social stress.

As parents turn their attention to the other people and relationships in their lives, each is a potential stress; sometimes others' reactions increase the stress parents already experience.[4] Thus, despite many reports of increased closeness to friends, parents also report stress and distress associated with their friends' responses and reactions to their child's illness.

You go back to work and everything's pretty calm for a while. And people at work don't know what to say. So they're afraid to say anything.

Some of the people who we thought would be our best friends never showed up for at least a couple of months after. That was particularly tough at the time, because they couldn't handle it themselves.

In addition to managing relationships with friends and co-workers, parents also must deal with representatives of other social institutions. Parents of school-age children may have difficulty in building communication between the medical staff and school personnel as their child reenters the educational environment (Barbarin & Chesler, 1983). If principals, teachers, and parents of classmates are frightened or awkward in dealing with the child with cancer in school, classmates are also likely to be uncomfortable.

Emotional Stress

The diagnostic encounter almost always has an overwhelming emotional impact. After this initial period, and even as the child recovers, parents continue to worry about the uncertain progress of the disease. Stein and Jessop (1984) note with regard to a variety of childhood illnesses: "What does seem to be related to social and psychological outcomes for the child and family is the uncertainty or ambiguity of the condition" (p. 192). A tragic outcome may be more bearable when it is clear, and when the time and place of its occurrence is known. Ironically, the very advances in medical technology that have improved the life chances and extended the life spans of children with cancer may add to parents' emotional stress (Comaroff & McGuire, 1981). When a diag-

nosis of cancer meant certain death, parents knew the probable outcome, knew that their child's life span was brief, and could begin anticipatory grieving. Now, no one knows at diagnosis what the child's real
chances and life span will be, only that the child is severely threatened.
One parent reports eloquently on the emotional stress of an unknown
future:

> *For us, the unknown is much more difficult to deal with. When
> unknown factors are in our lives, that becomes very stressful.
> When we can confront those difficulties and resolve them—we
> work much better. When we see a problem coming, face the prob-
> lem, and get it over with, resolve it, we can go on living. I don't
> think any of us deals well with going on for long periods of time
> with unknown factors.*

Constant alertness for small signs of recurrent disease and constant
worry about side effects tax the mind, heart, and body. Many parents
report signs of personal and psychosomatic illness in their own aches
and pains, sleeplessness, fatigue, weight loss or weight gain. Some
become easily irritable, provoked by otherwise minor events; others
become depressed and anxious.

> *I had quite a problem with my stomach. It bothered me. In fact,
> I was close to having ulcers afterwards, but I had always had some
> problems with a nervous stomach. When he was in the hospital,
> I had quite a time with my stomach . . . nervous problems I think.*
>
> *I was very hurt and hopeless and I didn't know what to do. I had
> a lot of depression and anger during certain periods, and a lot of
> frustration. I lost a lot of sleep and didn't eat for the longest time.*
>
> *During her illness, my problem was patience. I was very impatient.
> I got upset with her even though I knew she was in a lot of pain,
> but I wanted her to keep it to herself. The medication made her
> cranky and that was hard for me to tolerate. I was upset because
> she hurt. I didn't want her to hurt but I didn't want her to tell me
> about it either.*

A hurt child creates a hurting parent. Few parents can tolerate the
stress of seeing their child in pain, especially when they feel there is
nothing they can do about it. Several parents report the particularly
poignant emotional stress of feeling helpless in the face of their child's
real suffering.

In my mind the toughest thing was the amount of pain he had. He had severe pain after surgery and the medication did not do the job.

When he was in the hospital and cried, "Do something Daddy," I felt horribly frustrated.

The feeling of helplessness made everything worse. Mothers can usually make anything better but I could not do anything for my dying daughter.

Since parents are front-line caregivers, they know that their own reactions are transmitted to their child and that management of their own internal feelings is critical. Knowledge of the importance of managing their own feelings of pain and helplessness can be an added stress.

Existential Stress

Many parents find it stressful to fit the experience of childhood cancer into their prior understanding of the nature and purpose of life. Serious and chronic childhood illness is a challenge to the ways in which most people understand and organize their views of the world (Spinetta, Swarner, & Sheposh, 1981). Death is conceived as the fate of the elderly, perhaps the evil or warlike, but certainly not the young and innocent. The threat to the life of one's child may disrupt one's image of normal existence and one's faith in an orderly and just world. Kushner (1981) discusses this issue at length from a religious point of view. Sourkes (1982) captures the metaphysical and emotional dilemma:

A child or adolescent diagnosed with a life-threatening illness throws an assumed sequence out of order. A time of role reversal is expected, when children will care for dying parents. When parents instead find themselves watching their child face death, a sense of tragic absurdity prevails. Not only is time shortened, but its order is shattered. (p. 27)

As one considers the threat to the child's existence, and to the universe as previously understood, some things may begin to be seen in a new light. Tucker (1982) discusses the experience of a father of a leukemic child, in the midst of such an existential confrontation:

Passing through Times Square he looked out at the human detritus of society: whores, pimps, bums, junkies, dope dealers, pornographers. . . . It angered Brian that these people were alive and

*thriving while his little girl, who had never harmed a soul, was
dying. . . . It seemed as if there was something very wrong with the
world, a vast conspiracy to replace all things good, pure, and beautiful with those corrupt, degraded, and perverse. Why the hell were
all these evil people making it, he wondered, when so many good
people were dying? (p. 63)*

Indeed, it challenges our sense of right and wrong *When Bad Things
Happen to Good People* (Kushner, 1981).

In the face of such challenge, many parents ask why this happened
to them and to their child. At one level this question may represent a
serious intellectual search, but more often it represents a cry of pain
and anguish, of confusion and outrage.

*I asked myself "why" immediately. Then I started looking at dif-
ferent possibilities. Did we do something wrong at home? I tried
to figure out if I had done something wrong, I had a flashback on
my life. I asked, why is God letting this happen to me?*

*I asked, Why me? Why him? Why us? What did we do wrong?
What did I do wrong? Am I being punished? Is he being punished?
For what? What did he do? He didn't do anything, he's just a kid.
How come? What is the reason for all this? There is no reason. I
sat out there last summer in the swing in the middle of the night
wondering all about God and religion and the church with no real
answer.*

*The biggest thing of course is, "Why me? Why does this have to
happen to me?" The answer is, "There is no answer." It's almost
like Bingo, with a different winner every night and a different loser.
If you know how to take care of yourself, everything else falls into
place. I've been to Vietnam and saw people shot. To be able to get
through that situation I had to rationalize, and I came out pretty
sane, no drug problems. This, too, is just a game you have to play.
There are no answers, so you make your own answers.*

Some parents' answers to the why of childhood cancer are environmental or hereditary causes, although they seldom describe these with
much clarity or confidence. Others feel the cause is an act of God or fate:

*We feel that our lives are controlled by God, and that he allowed
this for a learning process.*

*For a while I thought the Man upstairs was punishing me for
something I've done.*

Some people give up trying to discover meaning in what appears to be a meaningless event or situation.

The attempt to make sense of an experience that challenges the normal sense of the world requires grappling with the meaning of one's own existence. Resolution of these issues within the realms of normal experience seems quite difficult and often challenges prior religious or spiritual commitments. Some parents report altering their religious beliefs and practices. Others report considering major changes in their career patterns, personal priorities, and goals for the future.

Table 3.1 illustrates the five different kinds of stress, with examples within each category.

Table 3.1
Stress Reported by Parents of Children with Cancer

Categories of Stress	Relevant Stresses
Intellectual	Confusion Ignorance of medical terms Ignorance about where things are in the hospital Ignorance about who the physicians are Lack of clarity about how to explain the illness to others
Instrumental	Disorder and chaos at home Financial pressures Lack of time and transport to the hospital Need to monitor treatments
Interpersonal	Needs of other family members Friends' needs and reactions Relations with the medical staff Behaving in public as the parent of an ill child . . . and stigma
Emotional	Shock Lack of sleep and nutrition Feelings of defeat, anger, fear, powerlessness Physical or psychosomatic reactions
Existential	Confusion about "why this happened to me" Uncertainty about the future Uncertainty about God, fate, and a "just world"

STRESS OF SOCIAL CONTEXTS AND RELATIONSHIPS

Stresses experienced by parents of children with cancer are often rooted in relationships with people with whom they interact regularly. These other people may be *direct* stressors if they place inappropriate pressures or demands on parents or fail to provide legitimately requested assistance. For instance, a spouse may require the other parent to come home from the hospital and cease caretaking the ill child, a grandparent may refuse to provide assistance, or a friend may blame the parents for the child's illness. People may be *indirect* stressors if they even unwittingly become an additional source of concern for parents who wish to be primarily or solely concerned with their ill child. For example, a parent may be concerned that his/her own parents may become sick from worry or that siblings may react poorly.

In addition to asking parents about their interactions with various people, we also provided them with a list of potential stressors and asked them to rate the potency of each for them. Table 3.2 lists these items and the percentage of parents rating each as a moderate or strong source of stress. In Chapter 2 we reported parents' responses to items related to the illness and disease/treatment process, labeled "stress from the child's illness." Parents more often report this disease-related cluster of stresses as potent and substantial than the items relating to personal and social concerns. Stresses relating to "the child's social adjustment" and "personal ability to cope" are reported as being the next most substantial. Concerns about "nuclear family relations" and about "extended family/friends relations" are less potent.

Why are medical stresses substantially more potent than stresses from family and social relationships? The nature of the disease and its treatments, and parents' concern for the physical welfare of their ill child, are so overwhelming that they dwarf all other issues. Other issues take a back seat until the medical crisis is resolved. Several observers of stress in families of ill children support such an interpretation and have labeled it "pile-up" (McCubbin & Patterson, 1982). Personal and psychosocial stress is a low family priority because the child's medical condition and survival are more immediate and compelling. In time these "piled-up" issues may be acknowledged and dealt with, although generally not until the child's condition is relatively stable.[5] Moreover, the difference between disease-related stress and psychosocial stress is only relative. Parents' descriptions of psychosocial stress make it clear that these issues are also characterized by anxiety and anguish. Parents are not *not distressed* by these concerns, but only *less distressed* in

Table 3.2
Percentage of Parents Who Indicate Moderate to Strong Stress
from Various Factors

Stress Factors	Percentage of Parents	
	Strong	Moderate to Strong
Stress from child's illness		
the fact my child has cancer	80	96
my fear of my child's death	61	76
my child's reaction to the drugs	57	88
fear my child might have a relapse	52	78
Stress from child's social adjustment		
fear child will learn seriousness of disease	32	51
fear of "spoiling" the child	7	38
Stress from personal ability to cope		
concern if something happened to me	28	60
fear of a nervous breakdown	10	24
Stress from nuclear family relations		
marital problems	7	30
sibling problems	7	27
worry about effect on other children	16	51
fear other children will get sick	18	52
Stress from extended family/friends relations		
relations with my parents (grandparents)	4	16
relations with friends and neighbors	5	26

comparison to the uncertainty and sense of tragedy associated with the illness itself.

Since one critical task that parents of chronically ill children must face is "going public," we asked parents of living children with cancer "Who was hardest to tell" about the disease? See Table 3.3 for parents' responses.

Spouse

Parents seldom experienced difficulty telling their spouses about the illness, because both parents generally were on hand during the diagnostic conference. But regardless of the specific individual role they assume vis-à-vis the medical system and the ill child, they now have a new situation to deal with together. Whereas parents generally report that their spouse is the most helpful person in their attempt to deal with

Table 3.3
Who Was Hardest to Tell About the Disease?

Hardest Person to Tell	Percent of Parents Responding
Everybody	17
Spouse	9
Child (with cancer)	13
Siblings	15
Grandparents	39
Other relatives	7

the experience of childhood cancer, many also report added stress from their spouse's reactions to the disease and its treatment:

> *My husband insisted it be kept a secret. It was two weeks before he could pronounce the diagnosis. Since my husband saw death as imminent, I had to persuade him not to be so pessimistic.*

> *My wife went crazy and I had a daughter to take care of, plus the child who was sick. I suppose I accepted the traditional role of being the strong guy. I think I tend to be an optimist and my wife tends to be a pessimist. She assumed the worst and I assumed the best.*

> *The relationship between me and my wife got very strained. We finally pinned it down to remorse come late. I guess I missed my son and took it out on my wife.*

Although some early research predicted high rates of marital separation in families of children with cancer, more recent reports indicate that despite stress, divorce and marital failure are not common. They are not common in this sample.[6]

The Child with Cancer

It is sometimes hard to tell a child with cancer about the illness because parents are concerned about the child's reaction – not an unreasonable concern given what parents share about their own reactions.[7] When asked about their child's reactions, 29% of parents say their child responded positively. What constitutes a positive reaction? A number of parents report that their youngster accepted the diagnosis with optimism and hope and showed courage and strength. Thirty-five percent say their child had a mild negative reaction, and 14% reported a strong negative reaction (the remaining 22% report no reaction). Negative reactions include varying degrees of passive resignation, regression, and increased immaturity, or anger at feeling cheated. Any of these responses, especially anger and denial, or hope and faith, may be more or less healthy or adaptive at various stages of the disease-coping process. And any of them may be more or less effective for different youngsters, regardless of their stressful meaning and impact on parents.

The majority of parents who indicate in Table 3.3 that their child was the hardest person to communicate with about the diagnosis were parents of adolescents. Younger children were evidently easier to tell, or perhaps they never were told.[8]

However positive the child's adjustment to the disease, treatment, and new or altered life situations, the child's reaction often creates stress for parents. Parents report the following stresses as they try to deal with their child with cancer:

Trying to avoid overprotection, and coping with life as usual without panic or stress.

Because he has been sick for such a long time, some of this development of responsibility is lagging behind. It was an achievement just for him to go to school when he was so sick. So now that he's well, he isn't interested in chores such as cleaning his room, helping in the house and garden, and things like that. Now that he's well we want him to do these things and he refuses. These skills and attitudes are built into the other children a step at a time, but they are missing in him, and it's hard for me to be patient, and build them in now, little by little.

Children with cancer do not exist in a vacuum; nor can the family protect them from other events in the world of children.

I think the hardest time was when he first had the surgery on his leg — he had his cast on for quite a while. When I sent him to school, the school complained about an odor coming from the cast. The bus driver came out right flat and told me: "Hey, give your kid a bath, he stinks. You better do something or I ain't picking him up anymore."

I was watching him play through the window one day and he went up to ask if he could play, and the other children told him no. That's when I become very emotional and upset. . . . I really went into a rage and shook this little boy and yelled at him. Then the little boy apologized and I had to grab myself and think that this little boy never knew anyone that was different. I ended up apologizing to them.

As some parents report, in addition to reacting to the child's condition, they are upset by how the external world (peers, playmates, neighbors, and school personnel) affects the ill child.[9]

Siblings

Parents also report that the reactions of the ill child's siblings often are quite stressful. They note that siblings feel left out of new family developments and changing roles and may become deeply upset.[10]

> *My oldest son spaced out. At first he felt concern but then he began feeling jealous and left out.*
>
> *When I got home I told my older daughter, and she just screamed and really carried on. I still can't think about it.*
>
> *Our only real problem is that I think it's hurt his sister emotionally. She always feels like she's competing . . . they're real close in age.*

Siblings who experience these feelings express them in ways that draw parents' attention and concern. In some families these concerns are quite minimal, as siblings move in to play major housekeeping and child-care roles, taking some of the pressure off parents. Typically, older siblings are especially helpful, whereas younger siblings are a major cause of worry (Burton, 1975). In addition to intrafamily dynamics, siblings experience stress from the world outside the home. As they go to school or play with their friends, many siblings report being torn between their loyalty to the ill child and the desire to avoid stigma. As siblings encounter and report these issues, parents find them to be new sources of stress.

Grandparents and Extended Family

The persons parents most often report as hardest to communicate with are the child's grandparents, the parents' own parents. Why is this? First, grandparents often live outside the immediate family neighborhood and can seldom be told face-to-face; very delicate and shocking information has to be relayed over the telephone.[11] Second, grandparents share many of the same concerns as parents do about the child's life and welfare. They, too, perhaps from the unique perspective of their advanced years, feel that the natural order of life and death is being reversed. Third, grandparents are also concerned about the trauma and struggle that their own children – the child's parents – are experiencing.

When grandparents respond by needing help and attention, instead of providing it, they further stress the family's resources.[12]

Parents express their concern and feelings of stress about their own parents' or in-laws' reactions to the diagnosis.

My father-in-law was the hardest to tell. He thought our daughter would die the minute he heard it. He was already in mourning. He couldn't look at her without crying. Even today if they talk about it very long he has to leave the room because he starts to cry.

My father. It hit him harder because of his age. He felt, "Why him and not me?"

My mother was dying of cancer at the time. When they told her about my son it crushed her. She had accepted her own cancer because she was older, but that her grandson had cancer just about killed her.

My mother is from the old school and felt that God was punishing us. She wanted to know what we had done. Now she has come around 200%. I called my in-laws and after about five days I realized that my mother-in-law was not accepting what I was saying. I talked to my sister-in-law and she said that what I told her was nothing at all like what my mother-in-law relayed to them.

Stress emanating from parents' relations with the child's grandparents is partly rooted in the pain that the illness creates for the grandparents and partly in the negative ways some grandparents relate to the parents. Only 19% of the parents indicate that the grandparents were truly open and helpful over the course of the child's illness. Another 65% report that grandparents were deeply shocked and hurt, some even to the point of illness; these people could not be helpful. Finally, 16% of the parents report that grandparents preached at them, criticized them, or just withdrew and created distance between themselves and the ill child and family. Interestingly, parents whose own parents live nearer to them (within 50 miles) report significantly greater stress in these relations than do parents whose parents live further away; parents who live closer to their own parents also report receiving more support from them. Closeness may make it possible for this source of both stress and support to impact more intimately and more often on the parents.

Parents report that other relatives, typically their own brothers and sisters, also sometimes behave in ways that are stressful.

The family wouldn't accept it; not the immediate family but other relatives on either side. They wouldn't talk about it, which was hard on me.

I'm not from a very close family so my family couldn't help me out.

There also are reports of great assistance from all these relatives.

Friends

Some parents report stress associated with friends' responses and reactions. When close friends, in particular, behave in ways that are not helpful, or worse, parents often feel that they are indeed alone and forsaken. As Burton notes (1975), the experience of serious childhood illness itself is often isolating for parents, as they feel no one else knows or can appreciate what is happening to them. Friends who inadvertently confirm these feelings add to the stress and trauma of the entire illness experience. Parents' relationships with their own friends are examined in greater detail in Chapter 9.

DIFFERENCES IN THE EXPERIENCE OF SOCIAL STRESS

Not all parents and families experience these personal and social stresses in the same way or to the same degree. In an attempt to understand the relationship between such stress and different life situations, we examined a variety of personal and family background factors.

The general health status of the child (remission, relapse, or deceased) has a positive relationship to parents' level of stress from the disease (Chapter 2). However, health status does not relate significantly to any of the major social stresses discussed in this chapter. Neither does the child's specific diagnosis.

The child's age at diagnosis is related significantly to two classes of social stress: stress in the nuclear family ($F=3.24$, $p. <.05$) and concern about the child's social adjustment ($F=5.16$, $p. <.01$). In both instances parents report greater stress when the ill child is older (over seven years) at diagnosis. Earlier in this chapter we noted that parents of older children report it is more difficult to share the diagnosis with their child; these two sets of findings seem quite consistent. Older youngsters are more likely to comprehend the seriousness of the diagnosis and to be distressed by it; their distress undoubtedly reverberates onto their parents. Moreover, children diagnosed at a later age are already enmeshed in a network of social relations, and parents' concerns about children's social adjustment may increase as children age, especially if they engage in socially challenging or distressing behavior.

Although this parental sample is mostly composed of married persons (82%), unmarried parents consistently report fewer social and personal stresses. In particular, they report significantly less concern about their personal ability to cope ($F=3.3$, $p. <.05$) and less stress from nuclear family relationships ($F=4.35$, $p. <.05$). Contrary to some expectations that the burden of responding to an ill child is greater for single parents, these single parents are relieved from the burdens of coping with spouses and worry less about their own ability to handle the situation. To the extent that marital relationships are stressful before an illness of this sort, they are likely to escalate as a function of the illness. (Whether single parents also cope better or find other critical social supports is explored in Chapter 6.)

Parents of living children who reside further away from the hospital (more than 25 miles) report significantly greater stress in their personal ability to cope with the issues than parents living closer to the hospital ($\chi^2=5.4$, $df=2$, $p. <.05$). These parents do not differ with regard to the other sources of social stress (child's social adjustment, nuclear family relations, extended relations), but the problems of travel obviously exact a special kind of personal wear and tear. In addition to the problems of travel time and energy, parents who travel further to this major treatment center might have children with more serious or complex illnesses or illness reactions, or illnesses requiring the availability of highly specialized personnel and facilities. Indeed, parents traveling further distances also report significantly greater medical stress – concern about a relapse and about fear of their child's death – than parents who live closer to the hospital.

Parents' stress from these social and personal factors also were examined in terms of the family's socioeconomic status, and the results for different income levels are presented in Table 3.4. Parents' reports of stresses related to the child's social adjustment differ significantly by income level, but not by education; persons with higher incomes report less stress from these factors than do families with lower incomes. Parents' reports of stress from personal concerns about their coping abilities and from stresses located outside the immediate family are significantly differentiated by both education and income. Families with higher income and education report less stress from these factors than do lower-status families. Neither education nor income distinguish parents' reports of stress from their most intimate social relations, those from within the nuclear family.

Why might income level be associated with different family experiences with stress? Or, why does stress impact differently on families in different socioeconomic situations? Poorer people may be more likely to feel the impact of many stresses than are wealthier people; that is,

Table 3.4
Parents' Reports of Psychosocial Stress Differentiated by Family Income Level

| Family Income | Form and Level of Psychosocial Stress (Percent) | | | | | | | |
| | Child Social Adjustment | | Personal Ability to Cope | | Nuclear Family Relations | | Extended Family/Friends Relations | |
	High Stress	Low Stress	High Stress	Low Stress	High Stress	Low Stress	High Stress	Low Stress
Under $15,000 (N=15)	67%	33%	67%	33%	40%	60%	40%	60%
Between $15–25,000 (N=32)	47	53	36	64	38	62	13	87
Over $25,000 (N=34)	32	68	32	68	42	58	11	89
	$\chi^2=5.2$, p.<.07		$\chi^2=5.6$, p.<.06		$\chi^2=.12$ NS		$\chi^2=7.2$ p.<.03	

stress is more likely to have greater subjective impact on them and on their ability to maintain a normal life. Perhaps poorer people have fewer resources to utilize in coping with high stress, or perhaps they have fewer ways of buffering themselves from such stress. An example of a buffering resource is a bank account. The financial impact of unemployment on a family with a low bank account is likely to be great. A family with a substantial bank account has a greater buffer between itself and deprivation. The same analogy may fit our emotional bank accounts. Poorer people may have smaller emotional and social bank accounts than wealthier people.

At the extremes, income may make a difference in a family's ability to afford various necessities, particularly if added medical expenses or insurance inadequacies thrust an economically marginal family into financial crisis.[13] Reports from parents bear out this relationship between financial resources and the economic crisis of chronic medical care. Sixty-two percent of the parents report the financial impact of the illness upon the family as "none" or "slight." Those parents (38%) who report the impact as "somewhat serious" or "serious" are disproportionately concentrated in lower-income groups ($\chi^2 = 7.8$, $df = 2$, $p. < .05$). Indeed, a few parents in the lower-income group report that they had to make major changes in their living style to cope with the financial demands of a child with cancer. Such major changes in turn may threaten parents' personal stability and ways of relating to friends and family members.

Lower-income families may be less able to afford second opinions on diagnosis or treatment regimens, to travel to specialized treatment sites, and to hire social workers and psychologists if their services are not included. More affluent families also are better able to absorb or avoid the financial stresses associated with nonmedical costs of hospital parking, motels when the child is an inpatient, meals in the hospital cafeteria, unpaid leave from work, relaxing vacations, sitters for children at home, and so on. Thus, wealthier people may be better able to reduce the emotional and instrumental stresses that disrupt their personal lives.

Parents whose economic status or educational experience makes them normally concerned about whether their child can be upwardly mobile in a heavily tracked and stratified society may become especially concerned or anxious when their child is stricken with the added burden of cancer. Parents who assume, and whose status can more or less guarantee, an affluent life for their child may not feel that the cancer seriously jeopardizes this status. Thus, parents in higher-income brackets may worry less about their child's current and future social adjustment.

Families of different economic statuses also may not report stress in the same ways. Considerable research suggests that different cultural and ethnic groups respond to pain and illness in different ways; the same may be true of people in different social classes and statuses (Antonovsky, 1980). With particular regard to children, Campbell reports a "stiff upper lip, business as usual approach to illness on the part of children whose parents are in the higher levels of the status structure" (1978, p. 46). If this is true of children, it may also be true of the parents they learned it from, helping to explain why higher-status parents report less personal and social stress.[14]

A BRIEF SUMMARY

Parents experience several different kinds of stress. Some are rooted in aspects of the disease and in its treatment; they are connected directly to the course of illness and to the possibilities of life and death. Other stresses are rooted in the social and personal environment in which parents exist.

Parents' reports of their experiences emphasize that the impact of childhood cancer on a family continues over time. Although the shock and sudden changes that accompany diagnosis may make that the most stressful time for most parents, continuing treatments and checkups (even when the outcomes are positive) are also stressful. Moreover, the social stresses associated with the disease and its impact on family life persist. The difficulty of telling others, of sharing one's new status as parents of a seriously and chronically ill child, recurs in different times and places. Even parents of children who have died report continuing stress related to anniversaries, memories, new family patterns, and reorganized social relationships. Whereas these stresses may be moderated by successful treatment of the disease, or exacerbated by relapse and/or death, they continue to have long-term impact on parents' feelings, orientations to their children, and ways of managing their personal and social tasks.

Parents in different medical or social situations do experience and/or report some stresses quite differently. The fact of cancer in a child and the progress of the disease have a major impact across a variety of social situations and socioeconomic statuses. The powerful realities of life and death, of relapse or remission, cut across many social distinctions, rendering all families vulnerable to medical stress. However, the child's age and the family's socioeconomic status do appear to mediate the *social stresses* of childhood cancer, and these strains fall especially heavily upon parents who already have had less opportunity for worldly success.

CHAPTER NOTES

1. Ronald McDonald Houses, or other institutions not partially sponsored by the McDonald's Corporation, offer low-cost temporary lodging close to the medical center. Typically constructed by means of community fund-raising programs, these facilities help ease the stresses of travel, finance, and separation for families of hospitalized children.

2. See, for example, Dohrenwend (1970), Myers, Lindenthat, and Pepper (1974), and Pearlin and Schooler (1978).

3. See, for example, Gogan, Koocher, Foster, and O'Malley (1977), Sourkes (1980), and Spinetta, Spinetta, Kung, and Schwartz (1976). Sibling issues, and how families cope with them, are discussed in greater detail in Chapter 6.

4. See, for example, Cassileth and Hamilton (1979), Hymovich (1976), Kaplan, Smith, Grobstein, and Fishman (1973), Katz (1980), Voysey (1972), and Wortman and Dunkel-Schetter (1979).

5. It is also possible that personal and social stresses are rated as less potent because of the methods used to collect these data and to talk to these parents. The research was announced as a study of families of children with cancer, and parents were told that we were interested in studying how they dealt with the illness situation. The research was not presented as a study in family or social relations, and parents may not have attended carefully to these more general interview questions. Some parents may also have decided (more or less consciously) to present themselves as managing well the nonmedical aspects of family and social life, attempting to avoid the stigma so often associated with families of ill children. As they struggle to maintain a normal life, they may discuss their situation as they would *like* it to be and as they would like others to see it.

6. Chapter 6 contains an extended discussion of marital relationships and coping patterns.

7. O'Malley, Koocher, Foster, and Slavin (1979) indicate that the diagnostic period is a critical stage for the child with cancer, as well as for the parents: "The way patients reacted to learning their diagnosis (relief or shock) is related to their later adjustment" (p. 165).

8. Share (1972) presents an incisive review of medical and psychological perspectives on this aspect of family communication patterns, and Bluebond-Langer (1978) sensitively records patterns of concealment and "mutual pretense" between dying young leukemic patients and their parents and doctors. Spinetta (1978, 1980) also discusses a number of important issues in family communication about childhood cancer, especially concerning "how to tell" the child about the seriousness of the illness. These issues are dealt with in greater detail in Chapter 7.

9. Katz (1980) discusses the importance of peers' reactions to the child with cancer and the child's potential reintegration into normal social relations. Wortman and Dunkel-Schetter's (1979) examination of the negative stereotypes many adults hold about people with cancer is, no doubt, relevant to youth as well.

10. Spinetta and his colleagues (1976) have done especially fruitful and illuminating work in this area, including preparing materials for parents that stress the need to manage siblings' feelings in a forthright fashion. Spinetta's work, Sourkes' (1980) review of this literature, and work by Gogan et al. (1977) are very useful and are considered in detail in Chapter 6.

11. Some families orchestrated creative responses to this problem by calling family meetings, making sure grandparents' friends or relatives were told first and were on hand when the call came, and having the child talk on the phone to reassure the grandparents.

12. McCollum (1975) points to this "reversal of roles," when potential helpers end up requiring substantial help. Although there are few systematic studies of relations with grandparents, Binger et al. (1969) report that half of their sample of parents report that one or both sets of grandparents were a burden or a hindrance during the course of the child's fatal illness. In many other families grandparents offered considerable support.

13. For instance, a bone marrow transplant generally costs over $100,000, and some medical centers require proof of insurance, mortgage transfer, or evidence of other assets before beginning treatment. Not all insurance companies will pay for such "experimental" treatment.

14. It is unclear from these data whether parents from families with lower levels of income and education experience more personal and social stress or simply report more. This is a constant dilemma in interpreting self-report data.

CHAPTER 4

Relationships with the Medical Care Organization

The medical system's growing sophistication and effectiveness in treating children's cancer have been accompanied by parental interest in participating in this process. In part, parental interest is stimulated by increased information about treatment choices and the serious side effects of drugs, radiation, and surgery. Interest also is stimulated by the chronicity of the illness: As childhood cancer has become a long-term illness, with most of the outpatient care provided and monitored by parents, parents become partners in the treatment process.

The relationship between medical professionals and parents concerned with childhood cancer is delicate. It begins in moments of great tension and anxiety and proceeds through a period of uncertainty and physical as well as emotional pain. Regardless of the eventual outcome, parents and professionals are bonded by the child's illness, caught in an ongoing relationship defined by the child's progress. The quality of this relationship is crucial to the comfort of both the family and the professional. The medical staff's actions may contribute to the family's stress or may be supportive in lessening its impact. A poor relationship can make doctors' and nurses' work even tougher; a good relationship can provide medical team members rewarding moments of intimacy and collaboration.

Portions of this chapter first appeared in: Chesler, M. & Barbarin, O. Relating to the medical staff: How parents of children with cancer see the issues. *Health and Social Work*, 1984, 9(1), 49–65; and Barbarin, O. & Chesler M. The medical context of parental coping with childhood cancer. *American Journal of Community Psychology*, 1986, *14*(2), 221–235. Reprinted by permission.

A good relationship with the staff is an important aspect of any-body's medical care and influences the ways in which patients and family members cope with illness.[1] Relationships among medical staff members, patients, and patients' families are likely to be even more important when the patient is a child. A child is a uniquely vulnerable patient. Parents often are involved directly as caretakers and protectors in helping the child cope with illness, treatment, and their psychosocial consequences.

Parents of children with serious chronic illnesses often deal with medical staffs in stabilized or institutionalized relationships. The child often adopts the role of "sick person," is removed from the direct care and control of the family for extended periods, receives specialized care the family is unable to provide at home, and experiences disruption of normal functioning (e.g., household chores, school attendance). The parent comes to know, interact with, and depend upon the staff over a long period, must rearrange household or work tasks to accommodate the disease's medical regimen, and often becomes a fixture in the clinic or hospital. The doctors or nurses become well acquainted with the child and parent, may care for the child and family deeply, and often deal with issues only tangentially related to the illness. In patient-parent-staff in-teraction within highly institutionalized settings, such as specialty clin-ics or hospitals, issues that may be transitory and easily overlooked in short-term illnesses become strong determinants of future interaction patterns for children, their families, and medical care providers.

Detailed information on parents' relations with the medical care sys-tem is not available from most psychosocial research on childhood can-cer. Generally researchers treat the medical staff as the constant factor in a world determined by children's illnesses, parents' responses, family relations, and the like. They seldom look at this relationship as a chal-lenging one, or at the staff as having independent impact on individual patients and families. Psychosocial researchers, who usually work for or with the medical staff, seldom analyze critically and publicly the systems of which they are a part, and the ways those systems deal with patients and their families. Our study probes beyond parents' generally respectful and positive views of the medical staff to analyze issues that are typical of many parent-staff relationships.

PARENTS' VIEWS OF THE MEDICAL STAFF

Overall, parents express a great deal of positive regard for the medi-cal staff members with whom they deal. Seventy-four percent of the parents evaluate their experiences with doctors and nurses as positive or very positive. Fifty-three percent report receiving very or quite help-ful assistance from doctors, and 69% report that nurses are very or quite helpful. Moreover, the entire sample of parents reports a shift in their views of doctors and the medical profession as a result of their ex-perience: 51% report having more respect for the medical system and feeling better about doctors than before their child was diagnosed. An overwhelming reason for this increased respect is that parents know that most staff members care. They also know that the staff tries very hard to heal their children. Parents express their positive regard:

> *I think the staff is doing all that they can. Everyone was very concerned and tried to comfort us.*

> *The doctors hold a very soft spot in my heart. They saved my daughter's life.*

Even if a child dies, the parents' feelings that the staff cared, and tried, are a source of personal comfort and a basis for continuing respect for the medical system.

Despite these generally positive trends, no one would deny the ex-istence of problems, or the need for improvements. Twenty-five percent of the parents reported finding doctors only a little helpful or not help-ful, and 17% reported receiving only minimal help from the nursing staff. And despite the overall report of increased positive respect, not all parents report newly positive feelings toward the medical system. Table 4.1 indicates that whereas 41% of the parents of living children report experiencing no problems with the medical staff, 39% report three or more problems. An understanding of the specific staff behaviors that foster problems or good relationships can assist in the development of more positive interactions.

Table 4.1
Parents of Living Children Reporting
"Problems" with the Medical Staff

Number of Problems Reported by Parents	Number of Parents (N=74)	Percent of Parents (100%)
No reported problems	30	41
1–2 problems	15	20
3–4 problems	20	27
More than 4 problems	9	12

Parents identify seven major dimensions of their interactions with the medical staff, indicating both the content of problems and the characteristics of a high-quality relationship.

1. Staff transmission of information to parents;
2. Straightforward and honest two-way communication;
3. Personal regard and interaction between parent and staff;
4. Staff's responsiveness to and empathy with the child;
5. A sense of parental efficacy in the relationship and in the treatment – staff acceptance and encouragement of parental competence;
6. The ability to resolve occasional conflicts or disagreements; and
7. Perception of staff competence.

Transmission of Information

A number of scholars suggest that many parents respond to the intellectual stress of childhood cancer by seeking information and understanding of the disease and its treatments.[2] Futterman and Hoffman report that some parents "use intellectual mastery to gain some sense of control, as though knowledge actually were power" (1973, p. 133). Parents of a newly diagnosed child with cancer are required to make a rapid transition into a different culture, with different rules and language. Different styles of communication may not be easy for health care professionals and parents to overcome.[3] Mulhern, Crisco, and Camitta (1981) indicate how common it is for physicians and parents to have different perceptions of diagnosis-related information.

Several parents report that the shock and confusion of the diagnosis made it difficult for them to absorb medical information at first.

> *Nothing they told me sunk in. They had to tell me three times before I grasped it. They told me things and two minutes later I couldn't tell you what they told me, in terms of medicine, treatment, and stuff.*

Years later, however, parents can remember the initial diagnostic conference in great detail. Halpern (1984) regards the effectiveness of physician-patient communication at this point in time as having enormous implications for a future relationship, as well as for family adaptation.

Some parents express their need for information directly to the medical staff and, as these comments indicate, feel that the response is quite adequate.

What impressed me most was the time they took to answer my dumb, stupid questions. Whatever it might be, they took that time.

There was no printed information available on Wilms' tumor for lay people. But on my request one doctor told a nurse to Xerox the information available in the Pediatric Oncology book for me. The nurse did it and I received great information. The doctor was a great help.

Other parents, faced with the same need, do not feel that their concerns are met appropriately.

When I brought a book on hematology and wanted to discuss something in it with a nurse, she tended to discourage rather than encourage my reading from other sources. None of them could understand why I wanted second opinions on some of the treatments.

Radiology was not willing to answer any questions.

When staff members feel pressed by the time and energy demands of their roles, and perhaps challenged by parents' questions or concerns, parents are shut off from key sources of information and aid.

Not all parents want a lot of medical information. Some feel overwhelmed, others choose not to use intellectual mastery as a coping device, and still others report they wouldn't know what they would do with the information if they had it. For those who do want information, however, it is an important part of their attempt to deal with their child's illness, and an important aspect of their relationship with the medical staff.

Honesty and Clarity of Communication

The amount of medical information physicians and nurses share is not the only issue parents identify in characterizing effective communication. The extent to which the staff is open and clear in communicating about nonmedical matters, such as personal, familial, and school issues also is important. Parents often seek information about the management of daily nonmedical problems, such as whether the child can go to a movie, play with friends, be disciplined, and so on. Parents describe the degree of accurate and forthright information they received, as opposed to false assurances.[4]

> *The doctors weren't straightforward. Even at diagnosis they said,*
> *"We've found a few bad cells." They didn't tell us that she had the*
> *worst kind of cancer tumor. They didn't tell us it had a very poor*
> *diagnosis. The doctors didn't tell us it was a very aggressive type*
> *of cancer. Maybe if they had told us, we'd have been angry and*
> *rejected it anyway, but we weren't given the chance.*

> *In another city, I felt like the doctors were not honest with us at*
> *the beginning. They didn't tell us about the side effects of chemo-*
> *therapy.*

Sometimes it is difficult for parents to ask staff members all the questions they have, especially when the questions focus on nonmedical
issues. Aside from feeling worried, ignorant, and intimidated, the parents' sense of parental competence may be eroded if they repeatedly
need to seek expert opinion in the day-to-day care of their ill child. As
a result, many parents stop looking for open staff communication and
stop asking their deeply felt questions.

Parents generally are able to identify some doctors who communicate
quite effectively and some who do not.

> *Some doctors don't communicate enough . . . some don't care and*
> *some are too busy. Especially the ones who care are too busy.*

> *I really appreciate the one doctor, because he could talk with us.*
> *There were other doctors whom I appreciate for the brains that*
> *they do have but I don't feel they have the ability to communicate*
> *with the common person.*

In addition to noting individual differences among staff members,
parents observe how the organizational structure and staffing patterns
of the hospital impede effective communication.

> *There was a communication gap between the doctors and us par-*
> *ents. The hematology staff would tell the residents who would tell*
> *the medical students who would tell the residents again. By fun-*
> *neling the information through in this way . . . there is a chance it*
> *will get muddled. Therefore, more direct communication in the*
> *relationship between parents and doctor would be helpful.*

In this case, when questions were asked, different staff members had
different answers, based upon individual reactions and not upon an
integrated staff approach to the child and family. If the medical staff
does not communicate openly and fully within its own ranks, there is
little likelihood the staff can be clear with parents.

Quality of Interpersonal Contact

Another dimension affecting staff-parent relationships is the quality of social and emotional contact between parents and physicians. To the extent these contacts are characterized by mutual respect and caring, or by tension and suspicion, the relationship is ultimately satisfying or a source of continuing stress and dissatisfaction.

Some parents identify the importance of warm, caring, and sensitive doctors.

> *The doctor was very helpful. He let us handle the situation the way we wanted to, when it was apparent that my daughter would die. He also came to our home for the week before she died. I am very grateful for this.*

> *The doctors were horrible, they were cold. There was one good one who really cared. He came to the funeral.*

> *I didn't care for the doctor that explained the treatment for his type of cancer. I didn't care for him at all. He treated me like a shop rat and my wife like a dumb hillbilly.*

When the quality of the interpersonal relationship is judged as poor, the family typically perceives staff rudeness and lack of sensitivity to their emotional stress. In some cases, parents describe doctors as being uncouth, lacking tact, and being unsympathetic, cold, and distancing. In other cases, there is simply an absence of mutual respect and trust between parents and doctors.

Other research on the doctor-patient relationship affirms that many doctors have difficulty expressing care and warmth in such situations (Cassileth & Hamilton, 1979).

> *The standard medical school orientation thus does little to help students deal with patients' conjoint needs for expert technological care and personal supportive relationships. (p. 311)*

With regard to the particularly potent issues of childhood illness, the physician's typical (and perhaps self-protective) pattern of emotional distance may clash with parents' emotional needs (Meadow, 1968).

Parents may try to maximize the positive aspects of their relationship with the staff by putting on a good front. By being "up," parents may appear more personally attractive and pleasant and avoid staff pity or discomfort. Sabbeth (1984, p. 47) suggests parents think that "if they look all right then the doctor will be pleased, rather than disappointed or angry, and thus will provide better care for the child." Whether or not it produces better care, a positive stance may be an incentive for more positive staff-parent contact.

These interactions do not occur in a vacuum, but in the context of a large medical bureaucracy. Parents report that at times the medical care organization marches right over their needs and feelings.

> *One nurse turned the light out in the room while I was kneeling and praying because she said I'd bother the children. However, every child was sound asleep. I don't think she had a right to insist I turn the light out immediately. I was so upset that I cried for hours. She disrupted the only comfort I had found—praying.*

Impersonal rules and regulations do not just occur on hospital wards. It is not unusual for children and their parents to wait two to three hours for treatment in outpatient clinics and treatment rooms. As Wilson (1982) points out, such bureaucratic disdain for children's comfort is matched by the drabness, lack of toys and reading material, and interpersonal isolation of many clinics and waiting rooms.

Given the operational needs of a large bureaucracy, and typical professional-client role definitions and constraints, it is not surprising that some parents do not experience interpersonal or emotional support and help from medical professionals.[5] The costs of such practices may be quite high. Comments from parents who have left this country to seek alternative treatments for their children often highlight the personal caring and attention they and their children received at foreign (Mexican) clinics. Regardless of the medical effectiveness of laetrile and other therapies, some very dissatisfied and frustrated parents react strongly to the impersonality of care provided in some American institutions.[6]

Responsiveness to the Child

Of all the factors in parent-child-staff interactions, the source of parents' strongest feelings (both positive and negative) relate to the ways physicians and nurses deal with their children. Staff who behave in an engaging, warm, caring way with the child usually are able to establish a meaningful relationship with the family.[7] The crucial determinants of this relationship are the amount of staff attentiveness; concern about pain and other side effects of treatment; monitoring of the children's IVs, bandages, and drug reactions; and expression of positive feeling. Two parents reflect on these issues:

He had a lot of pain and they wouldn't believe it was anything. Finally, a new X-ray showed a return of the tumor so they gave him more medication. I am very resentful that they didn't believe him.

On many occasions his tests were delayed. I understand a large hospital and staff, but a three-year-old cannot understand why he can't have a cold drink for hours on end. His cries for water still haunt me. There is no reason for this type of treatment.

These parents feel that their children suffered physically and emotionally because of lack of attention and concern from the staff.

However, parents do not expect the staff to cater to every whim and fancy of the child. In fact, some parents report respect for the ability of physicians and nurses to strike a balance between empathy with the child's condition and the control of the child's behavior. One parent says in praise of doctors:

They're great—they don't take nothing from the kids either.

On occasion, parents interpret the staff's lack of attentiveness to their child's needs as indifference and personalize this to the point that overt conflict develops. When medical personnel make side comments that indicate insensitivity, it drives this point home for parents.

The radiation people told my son he might be sterile. My son thought they meant he couldn't have sex.

The radiology technician said to me, in front of my young son, "He will be like a woman now." My son was very upset, and wanted to know what he meant.

Beyond normal standards of sensitivity and courtesy, Featherstone notes that, "Parents appreciate it when outsiders respect their child, too. . . . Evidence that the professions LIKE their child softens the blow" (1981, p. 183). Howarth (1974) also argues that doctors dealing with terminally ill children need to generate personal rapport that "goes beyond the usual sympathetic and kindly manner which most people have for sick children, and implies that the doctor develops a respect for the child as a person, a knowledge of his temperamental characteristics, and his reaction to previous experiences" (p. 135). This is a tall order, indeed, but one that may ease parents' and children's emotional stress.

Parental Efficacy

The typically passive and powerless position of patients undoubtedly influences parents' concern about their own involvement in the care of their children. Antonovsky (1980) raises several important questions about the model of medical practice that concentrates so much power in physicians and unnecessarily strips patients of some of their most important resources – self-esteem, coherence, assertive posture toward the illness, and so on.[8] If problems of patient loss of control and learned helplessness are typical of doctor-patient relationships, they are even more problematic for parents who are worried about their fragile and vulnerable children. Parents wish to maintain their parental role, expecting and needing to be actively involved in protecting and caring for their children.

Several authors argue that active parental participation in the care of children with cancer may help relieve parents' feelings of guilt, helplessness, and impending loss. A number of other practitioners and scholars observe that parents can and do make a positive contribution to the medical care of their children. Moreover, they may help ease the staff's burden and prevent them from making medical mistakes. Good medical and psychosocial care, and not just concern for upset parents, is the key factor.[9]

Many parents feel that the medical care organization exhibits ambivalence, if not resistance, to active parent involvement in their children's treatment. One parent captured this tension between her own needs and the apparent reaction of the medical care organization:

> *The nurses didn't seem to want me around and they didn't wish to talk to me. They also didn't give me enough control or let me care for my daughter myself.*

Not all parents have such desires or experiences. And not all parents are sufficiently able to care for their seriously ill children that a nurse or other professional should give them all the control they want. Whereas most parents acknowledge the high degree of competence, training, and professionalism in the medical care organization, they also are aware that there are choice points or decisions that cannot be based solely on technical skill and knowledge, but which depend on personal values and judgments and on parental love and concern.

In some large hospitals, with complex staff relationships, parents play a liaison role between different medical personnel. A number of parents emphasize that they are, after all, experts about their own children. Thus, parents often have knowledge that may not be utilized fully by the child's medical caretakers.

I have only come across one or two doctors I didn't care for. They didn't seem concerned with what I had to say or that I knew anything. I knew which leg was best for I.V., and most doctors welcomed my knowledge. But this one doctor poked and probed until my daughter was screaming. He wouldn't listen to me. He finally ended up with the I.V. where I told him to put it, and it went all right.

Another family of a child with cancer was over one day and I told them about my son's strange behavior and pains. They said it happened to their child too, and that it was one of the drugs. Then we knew what to do. I backed the doctors against the wall, and they backed off the dosage. And then he was much better. . . . I don't want to tell the doctors what to do but I know there have been some cases where doctors have made bad misjudgments. I feel like the parent should be included in the deciding of the dosages. I know that the doctors have their training, but I live with my child every day. I know him. Every child is unique.

In one elaborate vignette, a parent shares her experience of powerlessness in the face of what she feels was professional insensitivity. Unless addressed, such powerlessness can result in guilt about abandoning her child to strange and apparently nonresponsive staff members.

The hospital wouldn't let me go into the treatment room with my child. I thought that that was wrong. Here you are, a little three-year-old child with six doctors holding you down, doing something that hurts, and you don't understand it. I think that this is very frightening to a child. The doctors brush it off and say he is going to have to be mature and take this like an adult. I don't feel that way. I feel a three-year-old child can't be that mature and if parents want to (and the parents can handle it), they should go in with the child. They should be able to. We argued about this lots of times. I finally told them that if I can't go in, my child's not going in either. In a strange way the child may begin resenting the parent for handing him over to the doctors to hurt him. I think a child and adult can face anything if they know what to expect. Since I am able to go in I have been a real help to the doctors. I know how to hold him. He doesn't kick. He doesn't do anything with me there. It gives him confidence.

Another parent describes his attitude about involvement in treatment:

> *I say that I am not being totally objective, but they were just so*
> *calculated about giving him more and more radiation. It looked to*
> *me like he was dying. And finally I told them that they were going*
> *to split the vote, every time they would make a decision, I would*
> *get one-half the vote and they weren't to do a single thing until I*
> *agreed upon it because I began to find out that their mistakes had*
> *died. I wasn't going to let my boy be one of them. I have some*
> *problems, but I would say that for every patient who goes to the*
> *hospital to stay awake. They're not God, and you should demand*
> *to know what's going on. I don't think one should be aggressive,*
> *especially in the hospital setting, because they are trying. But you*
> *have to be assertive. I think that if you are very clear with them,*
> *they do hear you.*

Certainly the staff hears. Persistent assertive behavior does get results for parents who want to be active in the care of their child.

Ability to Resolve Conflict

Conflict may push parents and medical staff over the brink of a delicate relationship. It creates tension and unpleasantness that is difficult for all parties to tolerate. Conflicts arise when parents do not consider the staff to be sensitive and responsive to their needs and priorities, or when parents and staff members do not understand or trust one another.

In any large organization, especially where different groups are interdependent, conflicts are bound to exist. Conflicts occur within families, and within or between departments of government and corporations. It follows naturally that conflicts should also occur between the doctors and nurses who are service providers and the patients and parents who are service consumers. The critical issue that parents raise is not conflict itself, but the way in which conflict is handled. Are all conflicts to be resolved in the way doctors, nurses, or even interns decide? Are the parents' wishes to be favored? Or can compromises occur that suit various groups' needs and preferences? The differences in status and knowledge of doctors and parents often provide little basis or precedence for effective conflict resolution.

> *I said put it down in the record that that doctor is not going to*
> *touch our child again. Another doctor became quite incensed over*

my comments. He got quite upset about that. He came down to our room and called me a "rabble-rouser," and said if I did not allow whomever was there to work on our child she would not be treated at the hospital. They said if we didn't like it we could take her someplace else. I think at that point we made some comments about contacting our attorney, because we weren't going to put up with that. Since then we have talked about it and there have been no more problems.

Another parent, faced with similar concerns, reports satisfaction with the outcome.

I went directly to the head doctor and told her about it. She took care of it.

These are delicate matters. For the physician or the nurse, pride in one's work and reputation may be at stake. Parents may be reluctant to voice their opinions because of fears that their behavior may not be seen as appropriate, because they are intimidated by the status and knowledge of doctors, or because they fear subtle retaliation from the medical staff who may hold the power of life and death over their child. One parent reports such high stakes:

Some can't handle dying kids. If I confronted the nurses with how I feel about some of them, my child would suffer.

Many parents experience similar fears, often at an unconscious level. Regardless of the reality of retaliatory actions, parents' anxieties and their consequent "good" behavior often reflect their feelings of powerlessness vis-à-vis the medical staff. From such a low-power position, it is hard to resolve conflicts in a mutually satisfactory manner.

If conflicts can be raised and negotiated with mutual respect and shared concern, creative resolutions may occur. If, because of parent ignorance or fear of retaliation, or because of staff defensiveness and anger about interference, conflicts are driven underground, they are likely to fester and explode in more destructive forms later. If all conflicts are managed by the rules inherent in an asymmetrical power relationship between practitioner and patient/parent, a parent's sole option may be to reduce that asymmetry. That may seem like a personal attack to professionals, when it really is a response to an organizational conflict.

Staff Competence

A final factor that parents report as contributing to the quality of parent-medical relationships is their perception that the medical staff is competent.[10] Parents sometimes raise critical questions about the competence of the medical staffs that they meet at outlying hospitals. They report that their own pediatricians, although close and caring, sometimes are quite overwhelmed by the special character of the disease and its diagnostic and treatment problems. However, parents agree almost universally that the hospital staff is competent beyond question.

Parents also generally accept the hospital's role as a teaching institution and the need for medical students, interns, and residents to learn from treating their children. They do object, however, to abuses of this learning situation, to rudeness and miscalculation by young medical practitioners learning their trade in this very delicate and tense situation. When young doctors try to tough it out, to hide their inexperience behind bluff and brusque behavior, parents become quite upset. Despite the obvious and understandable disadvantages of medical care at a high-technology, tertiary care, research/training institution, most parents willingly accept these problems. They feel it is part of the package of special expertise to which they owe their children's potential for life.

Not all of these problems are reported by all parents; some are more common than others. Table 4.2 shows the proportion of parents of living

Table 4.2
Parents' Reports of "Problems" in Various Dimensions of
Their Relations with Medical Staff

Dimension of Staff Relationship	Number of Parents Reporting Problems* (N=44)	Percent of Parents Reporting Problems* (100%)
Information transmission	12	27
Communication	16	36
Interpersonal contact	21	48
Empathy with the child	18	41
Acceptance of parental efficacy	19	43
Conflict resolution	23	52
Staff competence	19	43

*Number and percent of parents reporting any problems (N=44; see Table 4.1), who report this problem.

children who report problems in each of the medical-relationship dimensions. Resolving conflicts is the most widely reported problem, followed closely by problems in interpersonal contact.[11]

DIFFERENT EXPERIENCES WITH THE MEDICAL STAFF

Data presented in Table 4.3 indicate a significant relationship between parents' (of living children) problems with the medical staff and various background characteristics (parental degree of education, child's age at diagnosis, and child's relapse). Neither the child's age at the time of the study nor the parents' gender have any bearing on reports of problems. Although the number of youngsters in each diagnostic category is too small to permit firm conclusions, the specific type of childhood cancer does not, by itself, account for variations in parental prob-

Table 4.3

Background Characteristics of Living Children Related to
Parents' Reports of Problems with the Medical Staff

Characteristics	Parents Who Had Problems $(N=44)$*	Parents Who Did Not Have Problems $(N=30)$*
Age of child at diagnosis		
Under 4 years	13	11
4–7 years	13	14
Over 7 years	18	5
$\chi^2=6.4$, $df=2$, $p.<.05$		
Child has experienced a relapse		
Yes	12	1
No	30	28
$\chi^2=7.2$, $df=1$, $p.<.01$		
Parental level of education		
Some high school	3	4
High school graduate	7	10
Some college	10	10
College graduate	10	0
Postcollege study	10	3
$\chi^2=15.5$, $df=4$, $p.<.01$		
χ^2 (college graduate vs. noncollege graduate)$=10.8$, $df=1$, $p.<.01$		

*The Ns in each analysis vary slightly because of parents' failure to provide data on all background characteristics.

lems with the staff. Parents of children with neuroblastoma (a cancer with a poor record of successful treatment) report few problems with the staff, whereas parents of children with bone cancer (another cancer with a relatively poor success record) report many problems. Thus, the prognosis associated with different diagnoses is not a key factor. Since the children with neuroblastoma were diagnosed at the youngest mean age of any disease, and those with bone cancer were diagnosed at the oldest mean age, disease-related differences probably reflect the age-related effects demonstrated in Table 4.3.[12]

Why are parents' education, the child's age at diagnosis, and the occurrence of a relapse significantly associated with more problems in parent-staff relationships?

The connection between higher educational background and more problems with the medical staff is quite provocative. Perhaps it reflects the societal trend for people with higher educational status to be more critical of all human service institutions (such as schools and municipal governments). Perhaps this critical, assertive stance irritates professionals, who then respond in ways that exacerbate problems in these interactions.

The finding that parents of children diagnosed at an older age report more medical staff problems may be explained by older youngsters' greater awareness of their health status and their subsequent anxieties in dealing with the disease and the staff. Older youngsters also may be more active patients, engaging the staff in a variety of ways, including typical adolescent power struggles. Younger children are more likely to be passive patients. Although they are not necessarily compliant, their resistance to painful procedures is less of a social interaction than a similar struggle between the staff and older patients. Previous analyses (Chapters 2 and 3) indicate that parents of older youngsters also report more psychosocial and more medically related stress. Thus, parents' reports of more medical staff problems may be part of a broader picture of the especially intense psychosocial struggle of older children and their parents.

Children who have suffered at least one relapse have a more difficult disease course; the duration and difficulty of treatment are increased, as is the emotional stress. Moreover, their prognosis is less positive than that of children who remain disease-free. Extended and more complex treatment and increased emotional strain on parents and staff alike may explain why these parents report more problems in interacting with the staff. Parents' problems in staff relationships can be especially potent if their child's relapse is interpreted as evidence of failure by the medical staff.

We asked parents of both deceased and living children to rate the quality of their relationship with the staff. Table 4.4 indicates that parents of deceased children report receiving less support from medical personnel (doctors and nurses), and they less often change their views of the staff in a positive direction than do parents of living children.[13] It is possible that parents of deceased children may assess the medical staff as having failed their child, and thus see death and failure of treatment as indications of a lack of help. Moreover, parents of deceased children may have significantly greater needs for support; they certainly report greater stress from the disease and treatments (see Chapter 2). Thus, even if these parents received the same amount of help and support as parents of living children did, their greater need might lead to an assessment of lesser support.

Parents of children who died report some especially painful problems with the staff, involving decisions regarding the cessation of treatment.

We wanted her taken off the machines, which they wouldn't do. When she died they tried reviving her. We asked them not to. Her doctor was not around, and the ones working on her were interns. If we had known she was dying we would have kept her home and

Table 4.4
Comparison of Reports of Parents of Living Children and Parents of Deceased Children on Relations with the Medical Staff

	Percent of Parents of Living Children ($N=67$)	Percent of Parents of Deceased Children ($N=18$)
Parents reporting more positive views of the staff	57	28
Parents reporting more negative or no change in views of the staff	43	72
$\chi^2=4.8$, $df=1$, $p. <.05$		
Parents reporting a great deal of support from the physician	58	33
Parents reporting some or a little support from the physician	42	67
$\chi^2=3.5$, $df=1$, $p. <.05$		

*let her die peacefully. We wanted to be alone with her and they
wouldn't allow it.*

*She was not allowed to die peacefully. After she died they tried to
resuscitate her, and we had to call an intern at his home to make
them stop. Why would they want to bring a body full of cancer back
to life? It was as if they were proceeding right from the textbook.
They ignored our wishes completely and made us leave the room.*

Physicians may contribute to parental dissatisfaction as their own discomfort and confusion escalate when young patients take a turn for the
worse. Levine (1975) discusses the hero element present in many physicians' self-concepts and the sense of guilt associated with "failure of
treatment." Both Vaux (1977) and Binger et al. (1969) report parents'
feelings that the medical staff withdraws as death approaches and as
decisions about how to handle death become prominent.

The medical staff may feel a sense of personal loss at the death of
a child; no amount of professionalization or rationalization fully compensates for what some doctors have referred to as the "loss of several
of my young friends every year." Medical professionals also may be
uncertain about how to act and often are cautious about intruding
during the terminal phases of a child's illness. If, on the one hand,
parents fear the loss of their medical teammates as death approaches,
and, on the other hand, medical personnel become increasingly protective of their own feelings and cautious about encroaching on family
privacy, there is a "Catch 22" situation. How does one answer residents
and interns who ask: "Should we go to the funeral?" There is no way to
answer in the abstract; the answer must come out of the actual fami-
ly-professional relationship. If a caring relationship exists, and doctors
and nurses wish to attend a child's funeral, we know that parents are
extraordinarily grateful for this human act. It is remembered and re-
marked upon long afterwards. If a caring relationship does not exist,
or if doctors and nurses are acutely uncomfortable, why should they go
to the funeral? They have enough to do, and perhaps need to protect
themselves against their own sense of loss, overcommitment, and burn-
out.[14]

When parents who have cared for a chronically ill child for several
years no longer have this child to care for, they are no longer integrated
into the life of a hospital and medical care team. Especially when they
had a positive relationship with the staff, they may miss their co-workers,
who cared for them as well as for their child. The staff may miss them
as well.

IMPLICATIONS OF RELATIONSHIPS FOR PARENTS

Several aspects of these findings deserve special attention. First, parents in this sample are not patients, but rather the guardians and advocates of patients. Like patients, parents are dependent on the medical system; they are somewhat powerless, vicariously part of the "sick role," and caught in the stigma of cancer. When patients are too young, too weak, too dependent, or too ignorant to advocate their own interests, parents are there to do it for them. As parents, they may be more likely to be active consumers than they would be if they were patients themselves.

Second, these parents/patients are involved with a *chronic* disease process. The extended period of treatment is a factor that Szasz and Hollander (1956) suggest should help move the practitioner-patient relationship from a deeply asymmetrical "active-passive" pattern to something more like a "guidance-cooperation" or even "mutual participation" model. Moreover, the fact that parents monitor much of the long-term care educates them to a more knowledgeable and active role. If the staff does not acknowledge or respond to this changing situation, conflict will follow.

Third, the parents in this study repeatedly stress their concerns about the quality of their children's lives, whether living with cancer, living beyond cancer, or dying from cancer. These concerns press physicians beyond their technical expertise and require them to deal with social, philosophical, and moral issues. Moreover, the emphasis parents place on quality of life accentuates aspects of interpersonal relations with medical practitioners.

Fourth, parents are not always acquiescent; they do not readily accept an asymmetrical power relationship with doctors. They may at first, when they are numbed by the diagnosis and the initial stages of "crisis-coping," or they may decide to appear compliant (indeed, some suggest it is quite politic to do so) in order to avoid conflict and potential retaliation. However, they do evaluate and make demands on physicians,[15] and many parents seek an active form of partnership. Parents' increasing sophistication as medical consumers has contributed to their move from clients to consumers, and even to consumer advocates.[16]

Parental satisfaction with the quality of medical care, and with the relationship they have with the medical staff, may influence their choices of practitioners and facilities. Parents of children with cancer who are in continuous long-term care at secondary or tertiary medical care centers interact with many doctors, nurses, residents, interns, technicians, and social workers. They seldom are bound to a single practitioner.

Some parents and patients may shop around the hospital for the practitioners with whom they relate most satisfactorily; a young patient
may insist on having a preferred doctor or nurse perform procedures.
Most children with cancer and their families realistically cannot shop
around for institutional sites of treatment, however; but of course, some
do. Some patients and parents ask for second opinions and seek hospitals whose facilities or treatment programs or interpersonal style they
prefer. They may even (in rare but highly publicized instances) reject
the traditional medical model and seek radically alternative therapies.

It might be helpful to compare parents' list of dimensions of a good
relationship with a similar list generated by doctors and nurses, outlin-
ing ways that they feel parents could help to develop a more effective
partnership. A professional's list might include:

Trust in physician and nurse medical competence;
Consideration for health care staff's time/energy problems;
Acceptance of professionals as human rather than Godlike;
Willingness to be active without being intrusive;
Questioning without being abrasive;
Conviction that the medical staff is working in the best interest of
    the child.

We welcome a parallel investigation of physicians' and nurses' views of
their experiences with families of chronically ill children. If they, too,
were to specify characteristics of an effective working relationship, both
service providers and service consumers might know better how to
understand and deal with one another.

In Chapters 2 and 3 we indicated that children with cancer and their
parents simultaneously face a variety of stresses and consequent coping
tasks. Their choices of coping strategies, and the effectiveness of their
responses, do not occur in a vacuum. The quality and character of their
relationships with the medical staff and institutions may have a potent
impact on how they try to manage the psychosocial stresses described
in Chapter 3.

Each type of stress may interact with, or be influenced by, specific
dimensions of the relationship between parents and the medical staff,
as suggested in Table 4.5. Parents' need for intellectual mastery may
be expressed in their desire for a relationship in which understandable
and complete details about the disease and its treatment are openly and
honestly transmitted. Parents' need for instrumental competence may
be expressed in taking an active role in treatment, monitoring side
effects, and influencing the staff's thinking in areas in which parents
are knowledgeable. The mastery of practical tasks also may involve

Table 4.5

Interaction Between Parental Stresses and Relevant Issues
in Parent-Staff Relationships

Stresses	Relevant Issues in Parent-Staff Relations
Intellectual Confusion Ignorance of medical terms Ignorance about where things are in the hospital Ignorance about who the physicians are Lack of clarity about how to explain the illness to others	Transmission of information Communication
Instrumental Disorder and chaos at home Financial pressures Lack of time and transport to the hospital Need to monitor treatments	Transmission of information Staff competence Conflict resolution Acceptance of parental efficacy
Interpersonal Needs of other family members Friends' needs and reactions Relations with the medical staff Behaving in public as the parent of an ill child . . . and stigma	Interpersonal contact Empathy with the child Conflict resolution
Emotional Shock Lack of sleep and nutrition Feelings of defeat, anger, fear, powerlessness Physical or psychosomatic reactions	Conflict resolution Empathy with the child Acceptance of parental efficacy
Existential Confusion about "why this happened to me" Uncertainty about the future Uncertainty about God, fate, and a "just world"	Acceptance of parental efficacy

facing staff-patient-parent conflicts before they escalate. Parents' need for both interpersonal trust and emotional support may focus on a desire for mutually considerate and respectful interactions with the medical staff. Parents' emotional integrity and sense of control over their own fate, and over a world gone out of control, may be enhanced by an active role in the care of their child.

IMPLICATIONS OF RELATIONSHIPS FOR PROFESSIONALS

These findings have important implications for pediatric health professionals, suggesting roles and activities beyond those presented in most of the literature. Prior discussions of the roles of pediatric oncology social workers, although useful, emphasize direct work with patients and families, such as providing information and counseling, or even short-term therapy, to individual family members – to parents, to the ill child or to siblings. Discussion groups, support groups, or group counseling activities also are described and recommended.[17] Rarely do scholars or practitioners examine or propose social workers' roles in assisting the medical staff with the issues raised by pediatric cancer. If they do, they emphasize interpreting individual families' needs to the medical staff, informing the staff of general research on families' needs, and assisting the staff to understand and ventilate their own feelings.[18] Our research suggests the need for mediating functions that address the relationship *between* the family and the medical staff. Beyond informing or assisting the staff, there is a need for problem-solving activities to deal with the institutionalized staff-parent relationship. It is not just the patient or parent, nor just the medical staff, that needs assistance; the *interactive system of staff-parent relationships* requires attention. Some newly relevant social worker roles may be useful.

> Informing parents of the pressures operative on the staff and assisting them to understand staff behaviors;
> Counseling staff members about the impact of their behavior on parents;
> Engaging in problem-solving activities that go beyond responding to individual interactions, to address the structural or institutional forces that create these problems or issues in parent-staff relations;
> Negotiating or mediating staff-family conflicts.

We have argued that the mutual construction of a good relationship between patients and their doctors is much more critical when these relationships occur in a long-term and highly interdependent situation, the illness is chronic and serious, the patient is a more powerless and vulnerable child, and parents' roles and feelings are confused and chaotic. In attempting to create a sustained high-quality relationship, parents and professionals wrestle with their expectations of self and others, with a decision of how active to be in trying to meet their own needs, and with their perceptions of children's needs. To the extent that parents experience difficulty with any aspect of the relationship, it may lessen their satisfaction with and commitment to the medical system. It also may cause distress and may lessen their ability to cope with the disease, its treatment, and corollary social stresses. Ultimately, these relationships may have a great impact not only on parental coping style and effectiveness but also on the effective treatment and even on the life of the child with cancer.

ACTION STEPS FOR PARENTS

On the basis of the research and experience reported here, we recommend the following action steps for parents.

1. Learn all you can about your child's diagnosis and treatment. Keep a log or journal of medications and schedules. Make a list of your own questions for the staff. Ask your questions. If a staff member won't or can't answer your questions, find one who will or can. Remember, if it concerns the health and welfare of your child and family, no question is insignificant.
2. Be assertive – but not aggressive. If staff members make you feel dumb, tell them so, and ask them not to do so. Keep alert when your child is in the hospital, and help the staff monitor your child's medications. Be sure to tell your doctor/nurse anything about your child that might make treatment easier. Help your child develop his/her own relationship with the staff. Find out how you can stay with your child in the treatment room and in the hospital if you wish to.
3. Monitor your feelings of fear and anger. Such feelings are natural and common, and their expression is often appropriate. However, care should be taken not to direct these feelings inappropriately at staff members. If it is clear that staff members' actions truly deserve your anger, such expression may be desirable and even helpful to all involved.
4. Look around for some staff members with whom you can feel comfortable. Remember that the staff cares about you and your child – even if they don't show it. Remember that staff members also have feelings – of hope and despair, of fear, of pride. Find out

whether the hospital has a patient relations office or a patient representative/advocate.

5. Talk with other parents whose children have a similar diagnosis or ask the staff to put you in touch with parents in a similar situation. Find out how they dealt with the staff.

CHAPTER NOTES

1. DiMatteo and Hays (1980), Becker and Maiman (1980), and Stone (1979) discuss the relations between physician-patient (adult) rapport and patient compliance with treatment and satisfaction.

2. See the discussion in Chapter 3 and Futterman and Hoffman (1973), Lazarus (1966), Friedman et al. (1963), Hamovitch (1964), McCollum and Schwartz (1972), Lascari and Stehbens (1973), and Adams (1979). Hamburg and Adams note that in their study of parents of (fatally ill) leukemic children, "There appears to be an intense need to know a great deal about the disease" (1967, p. 279). Parents sought some of the information in order to understand and reduce their own sense of guilt and responsibility for the disease. Other information was sought to buttress conversations with doctors and to explore alternative cures, since "parents felt there was a significant limitation on how much could be accurately retained after talking with a doctor" (p. 280).

3. Several authors have noted that it is not only parents (and patients) who find the time of diagnosis and "telling" very stressful. Health care professionals also experience discomfort, pain, and sadness during these times, and a variety of doctor-parent or doctor-patient interactions are strongly influenced by the professionals' tension and strain. See, for instance, Cassileth and Hamilton (1979), McFate (1979), Richmond and Waisman (1955), and Vaux (1977).

4. Binger et al. (1969) report that parents of leukemic children singled out the honesty and frankness of the physicians as a key factor in their ability to hear and adjust to the initial diagnosis.

5. One framework for understanding such behavior is provided by Rutherford's (1977) discussion of "self-serving" and "patient-serving" aspects of institutional care for sick children. Another approach is provided by Harris's (1978) distinction between organizations' "patient orientation" or "professional orientation." He defines patient orientation as "the extent to which the health organization is aware of, has concern for, and is responsive to the patient as a 'whole' person" (p. 383).

6. Wortman and Dunkel-Schetter note that adult cancer "patients may feel that it is inappropriate to express emotional concerns to their doctors, both because they feel doctors are too busy for such conversation and because they believe the doctor will react negatively if they express their feelings" (1979, p. 130). DiMatteo (1979), in reviewing several studies on patient rapport, comments on a study by Cobb, in which cancer patients "rejected the medical establishment and sought help from nonmedical healers because of a lack of understanding and reassurance from their physicians, and a lack of sufficient information about what was being done for them" (p. 19).

7. Of course, it is not just parents who judge the staff's caring and commitment; children with cancer often make their own judgments, and thereby may influence their parents. Vernick (1973) suggests that children with serious illnesses are both concerned and sophisticated about the medical staff's relationships with them. In his view, children "evaluate staff members in terms of their professional skills as well as their ability to communicate meaningfully with the children. Staff members who can get across to small patients are a minority in any hospital" (p. 111).

8. Taylor (1979) reviews a number of studies of the "passive role" expected of hospitalized patients in particular, suggesting that the "loss of control" these patients experience may have negative effects for themselves and for the medical care organization.

9. Adams (1979) describes a hospital in which parents were encouraged to participate in the care of their child as critical preparation for the time (extended, we hope) when the child is at home or returning to a normal life. Richmond and Waisman (1955), Hamovitch (1964), and Futterman and Hoffman (1973) also argue for such participation. The other side is that physicians and nurses sometimes see assertive parents as overcontrolling, overprotecting, and interfering (Futterman & Hoffman, 1973), or as sacrificing other family responsibilities and members (Richmond & Waisman, 1955).

10. Mechanic (1978) notes how difficult it is for patients to judge adequately the technical competence of a physician. The cues typically used are social in nature, very much like those included in our prior dimensions of interpersonal relations and attentiveness to the child.

11. Most of the seven dimensions appear quite consistent with the characteristics of good relationships or good doctors as identified by Mechanic (1964) and DiMatteo and Hays (1980). However, it also appears that two unique dimensions arise in this sample: the need to resolve conflicts, and a concern for efficacy and involvement in decision making about the treatment process. Perhaps both represent issues unique to parents rather than to patients, or to parents of children with a serious and chronic illness rather than of children with a transitory illness.

12. It would be interesting to test this proposition by means of a multivariate analysis of the relationships among disease category, age, and parents' reports of problems with the staff, but a much larger sample would be needed.

13. Binger et al. report that "the parents with the most negative attitudes toward the professional staff were those whose children had had the shortest course of illness" (1969, p. 415). He only studied parents of children who had died from cancer, but the same trend should apply to comparisons between parents of living and deceased children.

14. However, a number of analysts have argued that it is precisely professionals' inability to grieve (whether at funerals or not) and to share their feelings of stress and failure and loss with patients that escalates the loneliness and frustration causing burnout (Maslach, 1976). Hurt shared is hurt cared for, and this is as true for doctors and nurses as it is for friends and family members.

15. While they are making demands, it does not appear to us that parents are challenging the current structure of professional practice in the sense that Haug and Lavin (1978) or Haug and Sussman (1969) describe; there is no "revolt of the client" here.

16. This is by no means a local trend, nor is its focus limited to local issues. In communities across the country, parents of children with cancer have organized to articulate and press their concerns. At the national, and even international level, several coalition organizations (including the Candlelighters Childhood Cancer Foundation) have presented parents' concerns to medical organizations, health care agencies, and legislative bodies.

17. See, for example, Adams (1978), Binger et al. (1969), Kartha and Ertel (1976), Knapp and Hansen (1973), Orbach, Sutherland, and Bozeman (1955), Ross (1978, 1979), and Stolberg and Cunningham (1980).

18. See McCollum and Schwartz (1972) and Stuetzer (1980).

CHAPTER 5

Parent Coping Strategies

Individuals and families vary considerably in the ways they respond to the challenge of childhood cancer. Some are severely traumatized and impaired physically and emotionally. Others handle similar stress with equanimity, continue to fulfill their responsibilities, and conduct their relationships with little noticeable change. Still others change and grow in ways that lead them to function more lovingly and efficiently than they had before the illness. Psychological styles or social skills that existed prior to the illness lead to the use of different coping styles and resources.

How parents interpret and react to these events is as important as the events themselves in determining coping responses. In comparing the subjective interpretation of stressful events of parents in the same family (see Chapter 2, Figures 2.5-2.8), "what happened to the child" is constant, but parents' views of their experiences vary considerably. Parents who experience the diagnosis as a challenge to their lifestyle and to their child's future may rise to that challenge, formulate plans, and direct their energy into positive actions. Parents who experience the diagnosis as a threat to their hopes and dreams, to their child's life may respond with anxiety, fear, avoidance, and defensive action. Parents who experience the diagnosis as evidence of a loss of the child's life or of a peaceful and sheltered life may find it more difficult to generate energy to deal with the situation. It is in this sense that Futterman and

Portions of this chapter first appeared in: Barbarin, O. & Chesler, M. Coping as interpersonal strategy: Families with childhood cancer. *Family Systems Medicine*, 1984, 2(3), 279-289. Reprinted by permission.

Hoffman (1973) warn of the negative consequences of anticipatory or premature grieving, noting that parents who treat the diagnosis of cancer as a death warrant, and who immediately begin to grieve for their child, create for themselves and their child the environment of psychological death – a loss of hope and coping energy. Since there are such widely different ways of experiencing the diagnosis of childhood cancer and the treatment-related and psychosocial events that follow, it seems quite important to explore in more detail just how parents do cope.

CONCEPTIONS OF COPING

Coping refers to people's efforts to meet the challenge presented by stressful life situations. Some scholars view coping as part of personality, as a relatively coherent and fixed style of thinking and behaving. Accordingly, a person's coping style is consistent across stressful events and situations, and people can be identified as active or passive, flexible or rigid, effective or poor copers.[1]

Other scholars emphasize the demands of stressful environments or situations. Abramson, Seligman, and Teasdale (1978) suggest that when individuals experience a threat over which they have little control, they come to believe they are powerless to resist its impact. Although they may initially try to alter the situation, if they are unsuccessful or if the situation does not change, they become depressed and behave with resignation, emotional despondence, and passivity. A subtle variation of this view (Kübler-Ross, 1969; Schontz, 1965) argues that persons under severe stress naturally, and perhaps inevitably, pass through a series of coping stages. The demands of the stressful situation produce similar responses regardless of personality characteristics.

An interactional view emphasizes the interplay between the demands of the situation and individual styles. The purpose of any particular coping strategy is to prevent stressful events from having a physically or psychologically destructive impact. In childhood cancer, it is impossible to alter the fact of the cancer, but it may well be possible to reduce psychological problems that flow from such a diagnosis. In addition to reducing some stresses, the adoption of certain coping patterns may buffer the individual from the full impact of other stresses.[2]

In our view coping is not only interactional, but also largely a conscious process through which individuals guide or select responses to identifiable stresses. Since individuals can understand how they cope, reflect on the consequences of their behavior, and evaluate its effectiveness, much can be gained from talking directly with parents of children with cancer.

WAYS PARENTS COPE WITH CHILDHOOD CANCER

Much of what has been learned about how parents cope with childhood cancer is similar for other chronic and serious childhood illnesses.[3] Featherstone reports how important it was for a mother coping with a disabled child to realize that her son's "limitations need not wholly define life" (1981, p. 107). Many parents would echo this general definition of coping as the ability to carry on a relatively normal family life in the midst of dealing with their child's illness.

Tucker (1982) reflects another theme of parental coping, in a dialogue between Sally, the mother of a leukemic child, and a close friend, Cindy:

> *"My God,"* she murmured. *"I could never handle that." "Cindy, nobody asks you if you can handle it,"* Sally replied wearily. *"You just handle it." (p. 94)*

It is "handled." Most parents meet the challenge by doing whatever must be done.

Another common theme is expressed by parents as taking "one day at a time" or "each day as it comes." Both Featherstone (1981), discussing life with a disabled child, and Burton (1975), discussing parents of children with cystic fibrosis, also report this strategy. These parents refuse to plan (or worry) too far in advance.

When asked to describe how they deal specifically with stressful experiences, parents provided substantial detail about their feelings and behaviors. We derive eight different categories of coping strategies from their reports: denial, optimism, acceptance, maintenance of emotional balance, reliance on religion, search for information, problem solving, and search for help from others. The use of any particular coping strategy, at any particular time, is a somewhat deliberate (although not always conscious and planned) choice; when the demands of the situation change, parents utilize different strategies.

Denial

Denial is the use of beliefs and behaviors that do not demand attention or focus upon the seriousness of the child's situation. It includes occasionally refusing to accept negative implications of the illness, behaving as though the cancer did not exist, or withdrawing from situations reminiscent of the illness. Some parents report utilizing denial to shut the dreadful reality of cancer out of their minds.

It was two weeks before my husband could pronounce the word leukemia. I denied the diagnosis and what it meant.

I deny the possibility of a relapse. I refuse to believe it's possible.

I denied the issue. I went to a meeting of a group of parents of children with cancer and said to myself, "I don't belong here. I don't like your meetings. I think you're all so trite. You're talking about too serious things."

I try to keep my mind off it. I don't watch TV shows or anything pertaining to it. I shut them right off. For instance, my brother called and started telling me about "Brian's Song." He'd seen it and it made him cry, and he asked if I had watched it. I said, "No." He said, "Don't you want to hear about it?," and I said, "No." So he shut up. Why hurt yourself by watching that garbage?

The first mother, who "denied the diagnosis and what it meant," reflects an extreme form of denial that is a common, but short-lived, reaction to the terrible shock of cancer diagnosis. She could not sustain this style in the face of her need to help her child deal with the cancer. The second quote, from a father, does not deny the illness, but expresses an unwillingness to think about the return of the disease. If the child's treatment is successful, this father may never have to deal with a relapse, and denial may save him considerable emotional energy. The third and fourth examples are also of mild forms of denial, reflecting parents' unwillingness to place themselves in positions in which they must be reminded of painful and difficult issues. By denying an interest in or the relevance of these voluntary circumstances (going to a group meeting or watching a television program) they save themselves discomfort and emotional pain.

In discussing her initial attempts to cope with her daughter's leukemia, Roach (1974) illustrates the dynamics of denial:

Understanding that Erin had leukemia was one thing; full realization and acceptance of the fact, we discovered, was quite another. Our denial of the total implications of the disease could be recognized in many ways. Initially Bob managed to keep himself very busy and distracted. I launched into my art work with greater determination than ever. On one occasion Erin's doctor introduced us to another mother and her son saying, "You share a common problem." I found I did not want to see another child showing evidence of leukemia. This was too much reality for me. I found another way I could escape the emotional acceptance of the disease was to become involved in the clinical aspects. I was recognizing leukemia, but not facing its full implications.

Erin's 15-month first remission prolonged this self-deceit. She looked and seemed so well, we entertained the thought that perhaps some mistake had been made. Maybe there had been a wrong diagnosis. (p. 19)

By utilizing denial and avoiding overattentiveness to the illness, parents may reduce its impact on their lives, permit themselves to deal with other family issues, and normalize the home environment. Denial also may lessen the intense preoccupation with small details, and may minimize the terror that can accompany a daily and ongoing threat to the life of a loved and vulnerable child. Adams and Deveau (1984) note, "Parents who cope well tell us that they 'don't constantly think about the disease' and need 'time off'" (p. 77).

Lazarus (1981a) suggests that denial is especially useful when "direct action is irrelevant to the adaptational outcome" (p. 62). This certainly is the case with the eventual outcomes of childhood cancer . . . there is nothing much that a parent can do to affect these facts of life. If worrying about the child's death or relapse accomplishes nothing positive, denial of the possibility of relapse or death, as long as it does not interfere with treatment, may release parents' energies for other activity. When immediate problem-solving behaviors can be employed to ease the psychosocial stresses of childhood cancer, denial might not be an effective long-term strategy. Denial may even be dangerous if parents "forget" that their child requires certain medications or checkups or if they overlook obvious psychological problems. Reminders of the seriousness of the illness and the necessity of medication and attention, even for the apparently well ill child, are essential. Finally, Lazarus (1981a) notes that continuing parental denial of a child's possible death may leave one unprepared for his/her actual death. Denial, like other coping strategies, is situation-linked; it may be fruitful at certain times, but damaging at others.

Optimism

A coping style sometimes closely aligned with denial is optimism. In many cases of childhood cancer there is now more realistic cause for optimism than in the past. Regardless of the odds of survival in any particular case, many parents report using optimism as a way of dealing with the stressful impact of the disease, treatments, and side effects. These parents view the illness in its most favorable light, with an emphasis on those aspects that offer the most hope. They also treat negative indicators as insignificant.

After the initial shock and everything we looked to the brighter side. Now we're not that scared of it.

We're not that afraid of it because of the confidence of the people in the hospital, the doctors and everyone. I think positively. I think in terms of her growing up and going to school and getting better and doing the things that a normal child would do. We're preparing for her future.

Adams and Deveau (1984) and Koocher (1984a) discuss the importance of parents' strong sense of hope. Without hope in the child's survival, or at least remission, parents may find it difficult to agree to toxic and often painful treatments. Moreover, "without hope, parents tend to overprotect and overindulge their children to the point where children feel that their parents have totally given up on them" (Adams & Deveau, 1984, p. 78). Burton (1975) notes that parents of children with cystic fibrosis also confront a very pessimistic medical situation. Those parents who feel they dealt well with its negative long-term prognosis "deliberately cultivated more positive attitudes," reminded themselves of continuing improvements in medication and treatment, and took great pleasure in small victories (p. 225).

Optimism, like denial or any other coping strategy, has its limits and may be used in different degrees at various times. During a prolonged remission, with a good prognosis, optimism is relatively easy to sustain. In the midst of a relapse, or at the earliest stages of diagnostic shock, it is more difficult to retain an optimistic outlook.

Acceptance

Another coping strategy that some parents adopt is acceptance of their child's situation and their own stressful condition. Acceptance is characterized by the reaction to a stressful situation as inevitable and unalterable. It is typified in the statement: "What will happen will happen. I can't do much about it . . . but I will survive it." Fatalism is moderated by the courageous conviction that survival comes not by resistance or denial, but by acknowledging reality and getting on with the rest of one's life.

I've always said that "if it's gonna happen it's gonna happen."

Everybody expected me to cry. They said I should cry and let it out, and I just said, "Why should I cry." I just handled it and accepted it and that was that. I just tried to look at it and deal with it.

Acceptance does not mean surrender, however. Accepting the reality of a serious and chronic childhood illness does not mean that one puts out less effort or simply lets the illness take its course. It does mean recognition that "although we can help, we cannot cure" (Featherstone, 1981, p. 216).

Maintenance of Emotional Balance

Closely related to acceptance is a deliberate effort to create or maintain an emotional balance. Balance is characterized by the use of cognitive or behavioral tactics to attain inner peace and avoid extreme mood swings such as great optimism or great depression. This strategy emphasizes maintenance of emotional control that allows one to continue with life, to fulfill work and family obligations, and to care for the sick child. Parents try to retain or recapture a degree of the prediagnostic normalcy in their personal styles and social relations.

I try to keep my life as normal as possible. I try to see that the hustle and bustle of life is not important. I haven't fully learned this because I still lead a hectic life. However, I'm trying to take each day as it comes, and to experience each day more. I've often practiced hypnotherapy and relaxation techniques, and I really use them on myself. I also use a little rationalization.

Running helped me to relieve a lot of tension and you can then look at things in a different perspective. I took it one day at a time.

As emotion-stabilizing devices, physical relaxation techniques such as exercise, meditation, and hypnosis may be very useful.

Maintaining an emotional balance does not exclude having and expressing strong feelings of anger and sadness. Several researchers suggest that strong and even distressing emotions are reasonable and normal, and should be viewed as "adaptive rather than maladaptive behavior" (Desmond, 1980, p. 123).[4] Both Adams and Deveau (1984) and Featherstone (1981), writing about two very different childhood illnesses, note how common it is for parents to experience a great deal of anger. In fact, the recognition and effective expression of anger may moderate or mediate its impact. Several specific techniques for dealing with anger are shared by a parent of a child with cancer (Klagstad, 1982):

Anger almost always seems to have exclamation points after it. But why do we get angry and at whom?

Sometimes it's at the cancer because it's a "sneaky" disease that doesn't want to leave and feeds off our children.

Sometimes we are angry at our spouses because they don't understand where we are and often we cannot understand them.

Sometimes we get angry at our children who are ill. It's hard to say, but it is true. The demands on time, effort and money seem to be never ending.

And crises, big and little, happen frequently.

And sometimes we are angry with other people. "Oh, they can cure that now" seems to be the favorite phrase, but all too often they don't understand what that cure has cost the child and the family.

So what can we do about our anger? It can consume us to the point that we can no longer function as adults.

First, we can think through our anger to see if we can do something about it. If we are angry with our spouses, then we need to sit down and discuss our feelings with them. It's not always easy, but it's very important.

If we are angry with our children then we need to take a break, get out of the house and see a movie, window shop or take a long walk. Also, explain to our children that our anger is not at them, but at their illness. And, remember to tell your children you love them.

Hope is a great weapon against anger. Hope is a real part of all our children's prognosis. All of us can look forward to cures, longer survival times, and less toxic side effects.

Finally, sometimes the best way to handle anger is to let go and get angry. But, direct that anger into acceptable channels. For example, if you bake, bake bread and knead the heck out of it. Or pound nails or go bowling or something. And finally, you can go into the bathroom, shut the door and scream. Just let your family know what you are doing.

And remember, it's okay to be angry, but it's even better to learn to deal with it. (p. 3)

Just as anger can be overwhelming if not kept in balance, so may sadness, fear, or even joy. Too much sadness may lead to depression and a loss of energy needed for practical and emotional tasks. Whereas some fear is not only normal, but also quite healthy, too much of it may be paralyzing and debilitating, leaving parents unable to carry out some of the simplest tasks involved in caring for their child and family. Joy, at times appropriate in the course of a chronic illness, may lead to an up and down yo-yo effect. The attempt to maintain emotional balance requires parents to struggle for effective and appropriate ways to manage these strong emotions.

Reliance on Religion

A number of parents cope by relying on their religious beliefs and practices. Religion helps some parents derive emotional comfort from their personal relationship with God:

> *I practice my beliefs more. This has led me back to the traditional beliefs that I've always had. I feel that was the only place I could turn to to get help when I really needed it. I made a best friend out of God and I usually just talk with him and ask him not to let me down.*

> *The only thing that can help you here is religious faith, because it is a level of existence that is stronger than anything you can bring into play either physically or intellectually. It's a mystical experience in which you can gain a tremendous amount of strength.*

Religious beliefs provide some parents with a cognitive system for making sense out of the illness (and perhaps the death) experience.

> *I would not have gotten through this without God. I really had to answer for myself what heaven is and I was satisfied that it is not a bad place. My daughter will be reborn and her death was not the end.*

> *Knowing that God is up there makes things easier on my husband. He has totally left the situation up to God and God's judgment. What else can you do? God has control of your life.*

The usefulness of religious beliefs and practices has been affirmed in other recent research on parents' efforts to deal with the stresses of serious childhood illnesses.[5] Edelstyn (1974) notes, "Frequently religious faith is tested, if not broken by the diagnosis" (p. 157). This test may stem from the feeling that childhood cancer is unfair (Kushner, 1981), that it does not fit our sense of a just and an orderly world created by a just and orderly God. Parents' attempts to answer the question of why this happened to them and their child may also utilize a religious perspective. A coherent cosmology or theology may be especially useful for parents' success in coping with the death of a child from cancer (Spinetta, Swarner, & Sheposh, 1981).[6]

Not only do many parents find their religious beliefs helpful in dealing with their child's cancer, but also a substantial proportion (36%) report greater faith in God and more frequent practice and observation as a result of their experiences. About half (53%) of the sample report no change in religious outlook, and only 11% report a decrease in religious belief or practice.

Search for Information

Gathering information is useful in interpreting the significance of the diagnosis, making choices about or monitoring treatments, and anticipating and managing other practical problems. It also helps some parents place their emotional reactions in perspective and reduce uncertainty and fear regarding their child's survival.

I tried to find out everything I could about it.

I read everything I could about it. The things I have read about medical technology and its advances have helped me through the hard times. I keep some of these articles close at hand whenever I feel down.

I am a medical professional but even I thought at the time of diagnosis that it was a death sentence. Then I found out there was a high survival rate, and I read everything I could on this form of cancer.

Roach (1974) reports the value of this coping strategy for herself and her ill child:

Though still overwhelmed by Erin's diagnosis and our own feelings of inadequacy to take care of all the needs of our terribly sick child, we faced our next responsibility – administering her drugs at home. We found it important to first learn as much as we could about the drugs and their function and then to help Erin adjust to them. It was tremendously important for her to first gain confidence in us, then in her doctor and in the other people involved in her care. With candor and confidence established at home, we all felt better equipped to meet what came next. (p. 9)

Featherstone remarks, in the slightly different context of dealing with a handicapped child, that parents can establish a sense of control over a very difficult situation because they "know a good deal more about their child's disabilities" (1981, p. 27). Fears and fantasies can be reduced, and parents may gain confidence in their ability to rear and care for a seriously ill child. Adams and Deveau suggest to parents that "If you and your partner are familiar with the illness and the plan for treatment, your knowledge of what is ahead will probably help both of you" (1984, p. 77).

Problem Solving

Problem solving involves identifying and implementing specific courses of action to deal with stress. It includes the use of behaviorally oriented solutions for specific problems, such as increasing work hours to raise money to meet medical expenses, rearranging schedules to be with the child in the hospital, or planning with teachers for the child's return to school. Some parents emphasize their active effort to solve particular or general problems:

> *I am going to solve that problem, and I will not allow certain things to happen. I don't know how to describe the strength within a human individual except that I said I am stronger than whatever that problem is and I will prevail.*

> *She was in great pain, and I didn't think they cared very much. I began yelling and screaming to get their attention and they finally did something for the pain.*

As one example of active problem solving, Frantz (1983) suggests parents keep a log or a journal of each day's events; this valuable record may be useful later. He especially encourages parents to "keep accurate financial records . . . in case you need to justify your tax return" (p. 78).

Active parental problem solving can be beneficial in different ways. The more a well-informed and active parent can deal with the issues facing the child and family, the more the staff members can fine-tune their own efforts to focus on the immediate medical issues. Becoming actively involved in providing care and in solving problems may help parents adapt to stress. Reflecting upon both her daughter's ordeal with osteogenic sarcoma and her own coping style, one mother reports regret that she did not become active and utilize her own problem-solving resources more (B. Nelcamp, 1980):

I regret that I permitted my grief to become all-encompassing at a time when I needed to think clearly. I regret my lack of participation in the events that happened immediately before and after the diagnosis. I regret being so passive that I let my family and the professionals take over and make the decisions. I hate the memory of being "pushed" and hurried, because there was "not a minute to lose." I wish now that I had been less dependent, asked more questions, been more assertive. (p. 33)

Adams and Deveau note: "Active involvement in the treatment of the child can help you adapt to the illness. . . . When you are involved and busy you have less time to worry and you will gradually become conditioned to the impact of the illness" (1984, p. 77). Thus, coping via active problem solving may bring both external practical and internal emotional benefits.

Search for Help from Others

In reaching out to others for assistance, parents seek help in dealing with a variety of the stresses of childhood cancer. Sometimes the kind of help parents seek, or receive, is aimed primarily at easing their emotional situation: affirmation, caring, love, and a listening ear that permit parents to share their feelings and to deal with emotional concerns. At other times the kind of help that is sought is instrumental or practical in character: assistance on a particular medical or household issue, financial or transportation aid, or simply directions around a strange hospital or community.

Parents report receiving help from a broad spectrum of people, from both family members and friends:

I found that talking to friends and neighbors is extremely important.

Friends and family are very important. I don't know if we could have handled it as well without the support of our friends and family, because you can talk with them and it's not quite as emotional. It's emotional with friends, too, but other people are not quite as involved and sometimes you need to talk with them.

I expected my husband to be strong and he wasn't there when I needed him, he crumpled. It was too much of a burden for me so I turned to my family, I turned to my friends, I turned to my co-workers.

Health care professionals, such as social workers and nurses, also provide help, on either a formal or an informal basis. Some parents find that their emotional needs and stresses require help in the form of professional counseling. To be effective, such help must be extricated from the concerns with psychopathology that underlie much of professional counseling and aimed at supporting psychologically healthy people undergoing abnormal stress loads. A focus on new skills in coping, aid in choosing among different strategies, broadening the insights or interpretations on which coping may be based, and connecting to added material resources all may be appropriate counseling agendas.[7]

Some parents report that their religious associations are particularly important in providing social support.

> *The support from other people in the church helped a lot. They held prayer groups for my child.*

> *My wife goes to the Methodist church. She had a lot of contact with them and the ministers were at the hospital every day. Even people from the Baptist church stopped by to visit my daughter. They were both helpful and supportive and both congregations prayed for us all the time. I'll always be appreciative of that. I really don't think anything else pulled her through it.*

It is not always easy to utilize this coping strategy. Roach (1974) describes the difficulty she faced in getting help from others:

> *We were part of the problem. My pride did not allow me to ask for help when it seemed so obviously needed. I wanted the need to be seen. If I faced the same situation again, I would be open and ask for specific help. This would have been a relief for those who wanted to support but didn't know how, and it would have diminished my feelings of frustration. (p. 26)*

A more detailed discussion of the issues involved in seeking and receiving help is provided in Chapters 9 and 10.

PATTERNS AMONG COPING STRATEGIES

Common themes or patterns link certain coping strategies to others. Some theorists suggest that coping strategies may be grouped into two categories. Internally directed strategies, aimed primarily at managing and controlling one's emotional reactions, include denial, optimism, acceptance, maintenance of emotional balance, and reliance on religious faith. Externally directed strategies, aimed primarily at managing and manipulating events and resources in the social environment outside the person, include information seeking, problem solving and help seeking.[8] Table 5.1 shows the relative frequency of choice of each coping strategy (grouped into external-active and internal-passive categories) by parents of living children with cancer. Parents report a more frequent use of internal or emotionally oriented coping strategies. Acceptance and optimism (both internal) are most common; information seeking and help seeking (both external) are least common.

Parents' descriptive reports also suggest that some coping strategies may be functionally related to others. For example, relying on religious faith may be related to being optimistic and maintaining emotional balance. Maintaining emotional balance and acceptance may combine elements of denial and optimism. Denial assumes that a bad situation is not so bad, acceptance that it may have some good in it, optimism that it will be good, and emotional balance that it is worse if you let it upset you.

Correlations among all eight strategies indicate very few significant relationships, however. Only acceptance is significantly correlated (negatively) with information seeking ($r = -.18$, $p. < .05$) and with problem solving ($r = -.36$, $p. < .01$): The more individuals report using acceptance as a coping strategy, the less they report using information seeking and

Table 5.1
Parental Report of Strategies Used to Cope
with Stress of Childhood Cancer

Coping Strategy	Percent of Parents Reporting This Strategy*
Internally Directed Strategies	
Denial	42
Acceptance	57
Maintenance of emotional balance	47
Optimism	51
Reliance on religion	48
Externally Directed Strategies	
Search for information	31
Problem solving	49
Search for help	16

*Since parents use more than one coping strategy, the figures in these tables add to far more than 100%.

problem solving. Thus, whereas conceptual distinctions among these strategies may at times be elusive and subtle, they are empirically quite distinct.[9]

These coping strategies may be more or less effective in dealing with the different categories of psychosocial stress (delineated in Chapter 3): intellectual, instrumental, interpersonal, emotional, and existential. Table 5.2 charts some of these potential relationships. The passive or emotion-focused coping strategies — denial, optimism, acceptance, religion, and emotional balance — appear most useful in responding to the emotional stresses of childhood cancer. Optimism and denial also may be relevant ways of coping with interpersonal stress; in order to maintain prior social relationships, parents may need to adopt surface images of emotional strength and security.[10] Religious beliefs are relevant to the existential stresses of childhood cancer as well, as a formal path for the exploration of existential and cosmologic questions.

Among the active or problem-focused coping strategies, the search for information is most relevant to intellectual stresses. As practical action is based upon new and valid information, information seeking gives parents a base for planning how they may be helpful to their child, how they can monitor chemotherapeutic dosages, and so on. Problem-solving strategies are most relevant to the practical or instrumental stresses of childhood cancer. The search for help is most potent in responding to instrumental and interpersonal stresses, where aid from family, friends, and other contacts may create new interpersonal resources that can repair strains or replace prior relationships. To the extent that the kinds of help sought relate to informational, practical, or emotional problems, help seeking responds to any of the full range of stresses.

Mothers report relying on religion and search for information more than fathers; fathers report using denial more than mothers. Similar findings are reported in studies of families of children with other chronic illnesses or disabilities. Jacobs's (1982) interviews with mothers and fathers of retarded children reveal that mothers saw fathers as "less able to accept the diagnosis, tried to hide the fact that they had a retarded child from the public" (p. 110). Featherstone (1981) also reports that mothers of handicapped children perceive their husbands more often utilizing denial, both of the illness and of their strong feelings of sadness and pain.

Although variation in the objective medical condition of the child (relapse or not, number of hospitalizations) often is accompanied by different levels of stress, such variation has little relationship to cop-

Table 5.2

Stresses and Coping Strategies for Parents of Children with Cancer

Categories of Stress	Coping Strategies
Intellectual	
Confusion	Search for information
Ignorance of medical terms	Search for help
Ignorance about where things are in the hospital	
Ignorance about who the physicians are	
Lack of clarity about how to explain the illness to others	
Instrumental	
Disorder and chaos at home	Problem solving
Financial pressures	Search for information
Lack of time and transport to the hospital	Search for help
Need to monitor treatments	
Interpersonal	
Needs of other family members	Search for help
Friends' needs and reactions	Optimism
Relations with the medical staff	Denial
Behaving in public as the parent of an ill child . . . and stigma	
Emotional	
Shock	Denial
Lack of sleep and nutrition	Acceptance
Feelings of defeat, anger, fear, powerlessness	Maintenance of emotional balance
	Optimism
Physical or psychosomatic reactions	Reliance on religion
Existential	
Confusion about "why this happened to me"	Reliance on religion
	Acceptance
Uncertainty about the future	Search for information
Uncertainty about God, fate and a "just world"	

ing strategy. Parents' use of specific coping strategies is not strongly related to their reports of medical stress.

Coping strategies are related, however, to parents' reports of the quality of their relationships with the medical staff. Those parents who primarily use acceptance report more positive staff relationships ($r=+.48$, $p. <.01$), but those who utilize problem solving report a more negative relationship with the medical staff ($r=-.24$, $p. <.05$).[11] Perhaps parents with good staff relationships have less need or desire to exert active control over the medical situation: For them effective coping is accepting what can't be changed and trusting in the staff. Parents who experience greater difficulty in their relationship with the medical staff may seek out areas in which they can reestablish control by acting to resolve specific problems. From the staff's perspective, parents' lack of quiet acceptance and use of active problem solving may run counter to a preference for passive patients/parents and may be construed as acting-out behavior that intrudes on the staff's expectations and areas of responsibility.[12]

Parents' level of education also relates significantly with the kinds of coping strategies they report using. Parents with a higher level of education report greater use of problem solving, search for information and optimism, and less use of denial. Moreover, level of education is positively correlated with a composite index of the three active or externally directed coping strategies ($r=+.49$, $p. <.01$). Highly educated parents' more active and attentive approach to the illness and psychosocial issues may explain the relationship between parental education and problems with the medical staff reported in Chapter 4. If medical staffs are generally more comfortable with passive and compliant patients and parents, then more highly educated parents who cope in a more active and assertive manner may be irritants to the staff. Poor relationships also may be more likely to result if medical staff and parent roles overlap, or when medical duties and parental responsibilities overlap. As a result of their social status, highly educated parents may be more used to being active and especially to using information-seeking and problem-solving strategies. The combination of their higher social status and active coping strategy may be threatening to medical staffs. Staffs may view such parents as harder to deal with, harder to control, harder to relate with on a harmonious basis. Because parent-professionals may seek, pay attention to, and know more of the problems endemic to the medical system, they may experience more difficult relations with medical staff.

Brickman et al. (1982) criticize the traditional medical model's asymmetrical relationship between professional caregivers and patients (or parents of patients), in which the helper unilaterally establishes the rules governing behavior and the helpee is expected to adopt a passive role. The way staff members deal with their own stress and their control over patient/parent behavior affects their relationships with parents and may influence parents' choice of coping strategies. Alternatively, parents' adoption of particular coping strategies may affect the ways in which staff members act towards them.

ACTIVE COPING WITH THE MEDICAL SYSTEM

The connection between parents' active coping strategies and the quality of their relationship with the medical staff is often a matter of controversy and warrants further attention. Many parents report that their knowledge and involvement were essential ingredients in ensuring good care, as well as a means to emotional peace and resolution of strong stress. But the suggestion that parents play regular active roles in medical care does not set easily with many medical or psychosocial practitioners. Some professionals are quite cautious about families' actions on behalf of children and view parent activism as an expression of unresolved psychological problems in adjusting to the illness, rather than as a useful act.

They (parents) may also displace and project helpless and angry feelings about their child's condition onto various medical professionals, and blame them for delays and mistakes in treating their child. (Mattsson, 1979, pp. 259–260)

Do parents inappropriately "blame" the medical staff? Do they "displace and project"? Although some criticisms of medical staffs and procedures are ill-founded and inappropriate, other parental criticism and even anger are well-justified and necessary.

To explore active parent coping, and active roles in medical care in particular, we asked parents of children who were living with cancer, "Have there been situations in which you had to intervene to prevent a mistake from occurring in the treatment of your child?"[13] Approximately half (50%) of the parents, and at least one person from 75% of 43 families of living children, report they were involved in some sort of intervention. Parents describe such interventions as efforts to tell or ask the staff about something important, including pressing for information or for response, and sticking up for their own or their children's rights or comforts. The most common interventions reported by parents occurred with regard to the following issues:

1. IV insertions;
2. Dosage of medication and radiation procedures;
3. Continuity of care between services and departments of the medical care system;
4. Interpersonal relations between staff and patient.

Some but not all of these issues have life-threatening consequences. Not all of the examples that parents report are, precisely speaking, mistakes. Some are instances of poorly implemented policies, of errors of omission rather than commission, and of actions that might have been carried out differently or better. It is in the context of what might be improved, not as charges of major mistakes, that we examine the issue of parental intervention or activism.

The issue of the wrong drug or improper dosage is the most visible life-threatening problem. When parents are educated and active monitors of treatment, they know their child's exact drug and dosage schedule. If good and up-to-date medical records are not kept, or if uninformed and rotating interns, residents, or nurses are attending a child, the parent may be the only long-term medical care monitor with accurate and timely information. Medical staff members who are advised by parents on drug dosages may or may not appreciate this action; many parents report staff defensiveness and irritation. In order to ensure corrective action parents may have to insist firmly that their child's dosage be double-checked with the attending physician or chief of service.

IV problems and concerns about the continuity of care are less medically dangerous, but certainly physically and emotionally uncomfortable for both parents and children. Although many parents express understanding and compassion for a staff member's difficulty in inserting an IV into a small child's veins, they have little patience with staff insistence after three, four, or more ineffective sticks. Polite intervention could be a suggestion that the staff member take a break, get a cup of coffee, or let someone else try to find the vein. Less polite or more irritated parents tell staff members to leave the room or get someone more competent. Firm action may release a staff member from an obsessive preoccupation with finding a vein, to the detriment of the child's comfort as well as the staff member's sense of competence.

These examples of intervention represent parental wishes for more efficacious partnerships with the medical staff. Intervention to improve treatment or correct mistakes comes from parents' own access to information and long-term experience with their child and the medical system. The decision to intervene in treatment usually is not lightly made. Even when they are knowledgeable and concerned, parents often are cautious and intimidated. Even when they are sure they are right, parents are fearful about offending professionals, about being told to mind their own business, or about staff retaliation to their child. The fear that staff members whose professional pride is challenged or whose personal dignity is wounded by parental questioning or criticism may not take extra steps to assure the child's survival and/or comfort is a very strong barrier to parental intervention. Nevertheless, parents do intervene; these interventions represent a stance of vigilance and involvement, buttressed by familiarity with medical procedures and their child.

Intervention is not related to overall stress, but is related to experience with the medical staff: parents with more negative views of the staff more often intervene. Parents who intervene also report receiving significantly less support from doctors and nurses. Lack of medical support may be the impetus to intervention; intervention the impetus to less support; or both factors may be present simultaneously. Table 5.3 indicates that mothers intervene slightly more often than fathers, probably because they spend more time at the hospital and have more

Table 5.3
Selected Characteristics of Parents of Living Children Who
Intervened in the Medical Process

Parent Characteristics	% Reporting Intervention
Gender	
Mothers (N=36)	61%
Fathers (N=30)	40%
χ^2=2.9, df=1, $p. < .10$	
Educational Status	
High school or less (N=23)	52%
Some college (N=20)	30%
College graduate (N=22)	73%
χ^2=7.7, df=2, $p. < .05$	
Experiences with the Medical Staff/Services	
Positive (N=35)	40%
Negative (N=12)	75%
χ^2=4.3, df=1, $p. < .05$	
Involvement in Self-help Group	
Yes (N=34)	47%
No (N=29)	24%
χ^2=3.6, df=1, $p. < .05$	

opportunity for intervention. Parents with higher levels of education report intervening more often than parents with lower educational credentials, perhaps because they understand more or because they are used to intervening in many aspects of their child's life. In Chapter 4 we report that higher status is related to more critical views and negative experiences with the medical system, and earlier in this chapter we indicate that more highly educated parents more often adopt active coping strategies. Both status and coping strategies may combine with less positive experiences with the medical system to prepare parents to intervene more often.

Parents in the local self-help group report more intervention than parents who were not involved in that organization. It is unclear whether involvement in the self-help group sensitizes parents into a more active or monitoring role, or whether parents with more active outlooks gravitate to the group. Both may be factors. Parents in the self-help group are also more active in other dimensions of their children's experience, and the group's activities prepare parents for a more informed and active role in their treatment.[14]

Parents who report intervening report less support from their spouses and their other children than parents who do not intervene. Parents who feel less family support may focus their attention (and perhaps anger) on the medical system. On the other hand, the situation prompting intervention, and its aftermath, may be fraught with such tension and conflict that these acts may cause alienation within the family. If both parents witness medical actions that are questionable, or so emotionally painful that they consider acting on them, and then one parent acts and the other does not, the imbalance may be a source of continuing conflict and alienation in the family.

Parents' intervention almost always represents behavior born of feelings of necessity and concern, and with anxiety about strained relations, or even retaliation, from the medical staff. Within the larger context of parental coping with the illness, intervention is the end point on a continuum of active parent response, and the most blatant form of departure from staff norms of compliant patienthood.

STRATEGIES FOR COPING WITH THE DEATH OF A CHILD

Whereas childhood cancer presents many difficult stresses, the child's death is an underlying fear and potential reality for all parents. Coping with a child's death is the culmination of months and years of coping with a variety of other stresses. Since death comes slowly for most children with cancer, parents of children who die generally have been through a series of relapses, continuing and perhaps desperate treatment choices, and the deterioration of their child. By the time death occurs, parents are likely to be emotionally and physically exhausted and may have few coping resources left. Since the death of a child is relatively rare in American society, there are few standard markers by which parents can judge or model their own reactions or behaviors.

Some parents report utilizing denial as a coping strategy even as their child approaches death. Even when they know their child's death is imminent, many parents continue to shut this reality from their mind.

Consciously I denied it. I didn't prepare for it because I was sure that he would live. Any thoughts of my son's death were far in the future.

As the child comes closer to death and more preparatory details must be attended to, denial is less effective. Similarly, optimism vanishes in the latter stages of a child's life. Whereas many parents desperately seek new treatments in the shadows of their child's death, gradual deterioration makes even the staunchest optimists retreat from this strategy. What optimism remains is a uniquely different kind of optimism. Parents report they feel, "Maybe this was for the best," that the child would be "better off" in another life.

Some parents report coping with their child's death with a form of acceptance that relinquishes active preparation and resistance.

I just accepted that it would happen. There was nothing I could do. I couldn't run away from it.

It may help parents to articulate that the child's death brings relief from suffering—from the child's physical suffering and from the parents' emotional distress. Sufficient anticipatory mourning or acceptance prepares the parent for the death of a child, and may also preserve a fragile emotional balance in the midst of trauma. Many parents wonder about the fragility of their emotional balance, and whether or not they will survive the death of their child.

I am afraid if my child dies I will lose it. I am scared I will become an alcoholic, go crazy and that my marriage will break up. It takes a lot of energy for me to relax about that, and to convince myself that that will not happen.

In the attempt to maintain emotional balance, parents alter some of their prior roles. Cook (1984) reports that parents had to rethink "the parental role, which was gradually redefined to include the idea of the 'parent of a dying child'" (p. 84). Adoption of this new and realistic role brings comfort with new behaviors: acceptable sadness, time off from work, anticipatory grief, more family time.

A number of parents make sense of the death of their child and find personal emotional comfort in adherence to religious faith and practices. In research on children who died from cystic fibrosis, Burton reports "Where parents had a strong belief in an after-life, this also helped by enabling them to visualize the child enjoying some alternative to his earthly suffering" (1975, p. 205). Several parents indicate their own comfort in an embracing cosmology or theology:

My daughter will be reborn and her death is not the end.

He will be with Jesus, in a good place, and I will see him again when I die.

Parents also report that their religious congregations often provide emotional support and practical assistance during and after the death of a child.

Some parents prepare for the expected death of their child by gathering information, reading books, or attending lectures on the process of death and bereavement.

I read a lot of books that dealt with death to realize the options we had.

To prepare myself, I read a number of books on death. I also went to a few meetings to talk with other parents of terminally ill children.

Parents now may have the option of whether their child should spend his or her last days and weeks at the hospital or at home.[15] Adams and Deveau (1984) devote careful attention to helping parents sort through their choices, stressing that adequate information about home care for the dying is an essential ingredient in parents' attempts to cope. If the parents or the child elect home care, they will need additional medical and other information to solve a host of new practical problems.

Problem solving as a coping strategy becomes essential as the death of a child nears. In addition to the inner peace that may come from actively dealing with issues, attending to practical matters leaves parents the emotional energy to care for their child.

We made funeral arrangements prior to my child's death because I knew I wouldn't want to do that afterwards. I made lists months in advance of people to call when she died. I also sorted pictures of her long before she died because I knew that I still had her to hug.

I did anything I could for my daughter, bought her everything she wanted, so that I wouldn't feel guilty after she died.

You find all your strength and continue for your child's sake. You have to take care of your child even if you feel like you're exploding inside.

Taking good care of the child and avoiding the possibility of guilt may help parents maintain their emotional balance.

Many parents seek help during this period. Some ask for and receive aid from family members, some from friends, some from other parents of ill children, some from the medical or social service staff, and some from many of these sources at the same time.

I also talked with a couple of mothers who had children who had already died, and I talked openly about it with our family.

Our daughter died at home. We had set up her hospital bed in the family room, at the foot of the Christmas tree and in sight of the television set. My husband and I often sat through the night down there with her, and the dog always lay at the foot of the bed. When she began to get really bad, to be sort of in a coma for a long time, I called two friends, they also were mothers of children with cancer, and asked them to come over and sleep at the house for a few days. I did not want us to be alone with her when the end came. They stayed around the clock, and we slept on and off for the last few days. She died early one morning. I was so glad my friends were there. They helped us by being there, and also by calling the coroner, the funeral home, making us eat, and all the little things you tend to forget.

The coping strategies parents utilize in the face of their child's death are much the same as those utilized by parents who are dealing with a child in remission. They are generic responses, created partly by parents' own personalities and personal styles and partly by the demands of the illness and its psychosocial and medical impact.

JUDGING COPING EFFECTIVENESS

This discussion of parental coping strategies does not indicate which parents cope better than others. Examination of the strategies preferred by different people is not the same as deciding which styles work best – and for whom.[16] Many scholarly discussions of coping effectiveness are clouded by often implicit, unexamined values and inadequate research methods. What is effective coping for some parents may be ineffective for others with different values or experiences. Generally accepted agreement about coping effectiveness centers around grossly inappropriate or dangerous behavior – such as alcoholism, mental illness, child abuse, and dramatic denial. Beyond these obvious outer limits, using standardized measures and labeling coping "good" or "bad" are problematic at best.

The criteria professionals often use to characterize ineffective coping, such as low control of emotions (crying, rage) and the lack of a positive outlook, may at times actually contribute to effective coping. For example, the explicit expression of intense distress may motivate people to attend to their situation and to develop new coping strategies. Even sustained negative outlooks may help some people protect and prepare themselves more realistically for the future.[17]

As an alternative to standardized measures, some research on the effectiveness of coping relies on judges (physicians, nurses, psychologists, social workers, family members, friends) who comprise the social network of the individual. Can these persons provide fair-minded observations of parents' internal states or interactions with their environment? Are the criteria they use to judge behavior congruent with patients' or parents' own preferred standards, lifestyles, or expectations? Most important, if friends prefer parents to be positive and optimistic, if medical personnel prefer parents to be compliant, accepting, and optimistic, can they avoid using such biased criteria in assessing parents' coping effectiveness?[18]

Our evidence challenges the wisdom of using the medical and psychosocial staff, or friends and neighbors, as criterion judges of parents' reactions and behaviors. They are part of the situational stress parents face, not apart from it. Some may judge patients with the strongest egos and best long-range adjustment, who are testy and express their irritation with the medical staff, as not coping well because of their lack of compliance. Others, who define effective coping as the ability to deal directly with the emotional meaning of consequences of stress, encourage free expression of grief and anger, open discussion of fear, and overt display of anxiety. Others for whom effective coping may mean a quick return to apparent normalcy and the triumph of optimism over despair, may encourage anxious or grieving parents to deny their feelings or to strive for emotional balance and control. Given a myriad of external expectations, how can these judges accurately assess a person's coping effectiveness?

We are more concerned with understanding the coping strategies that parents of children with cancer use than with judging their effectiveness. When asked, most parents in our sample feel that they have coped reasonably well: Of 74 parents of living children, only one gives herself a poor rating; 13 (17.6%) give themselves fair ratings; 42 (56.8%) give themselves good ratings; and 18 (24.3%) rate themselves as coping extremely well.[19]

Taylor (1983) notes that when individuals in stressful situations are asked how well they are doing, most report that they cope well. These judgments are not absolute and context-free, but often result from comparisons with others who are less well off, on the basis that their own situations could be worse and that they are "above water!" For individuals under stress, effective coping may mean they are doing "as well as can be expected" even though their lives may still be stressful.[20] Although there are few strong relationships between specific coping strategies and parents' reports of the overall effectiveness of coping, denial of the seriousness of their child's illness and its implications is related to self-rated effectiveness. Moreover, parents feel that simply being able to hold on, to keep on going, to ward off pessimism and a sense of doom are major accomplishments. Different people use different strategies to achieve this end, and no single strategy appears to work well for everyone.

The stress of caring for the child, the strains on family life, and the existence of an uncertain future may all be persistent and relatively impervious to efforts at reduction or buffering. Even the most effective and resolute denials, cognitive manipulations, and efforts to maintain emotional balance may not alter the feelings of embattlement and struggle. More important are the forthright entry into the struggle and a determination to come out relatively whole or even with positive gains.

CHAPTER NOTES

1. In this tradition, "good copers" typically have a favorable view of self, a sense of mastery, a realistic view of the world and approach life with optimism (Jahoda, 1955; White, 1976).

2. The distinction between "reducing" stress and "buffering" stress has been suggested by Lazarus (1981b) and elaborated on by House (1981) and others. Reducing refers to attempts to alter the stressful situation itself, generally by acting on the threat or illness or on the mediators of the impact of the illness. Thus, a parent might reduce some of the stresses of childhood cancer by ensuring that the child takes appropriate medication, asking medical staff members to behave with more concern, and so on. Buffering refers to attempts to diminish the way stress acts on the person, generally by protecting oneself or warding off threats. Thus, a parent might buffer him/herself from the stresses of childhood cancer by meditating, thinking positive thoughts, spending time with loved ones, and so on.

3. With regard to childhood cancer, see especially, Adams and Deveau (1984), Friedman,

Chodoff, Mason, and Hamburg (1963), Futterman and Hoffman (1973), Koocher and O'Malley (1981), Kupst et al. (1982), Spinetta, Swarner, and Sheposh (1981).

4. See, also, Adams (1979), Futterman and Hoffman (1973), Kellerman (1980), and Sussman, Hollenbeck, Nannis, and Strope (1980).

5. Kupst et al. (1982) and Burton (1975).

6. Schiff (1978) observes that "for many people, regardless of their faith, a belief that there was a divine purpose in their child's death is just what they need to sustain them. They can be comfortable thinking that the death was not just an empty, meaningless happening" (p. 109). Other approaches to deal with the "why" question are provided by Kushner (1981) and Massie and Massie (1976).

7. A number of scholars have emphasized the distinction between formal or statutory help and informal or voluntary help, and we have made the distinction between social services and social support (see Figure 1.2). Several researchers and practitioners discuss the ways in which professional psychological or social work counseling may be most useful for parents seeking formal help (Adams, 1979; Kellerman, 1980; Knapp & Hansen, 1973; Ross, 1978).

8. This categorization has been made by Lazarus (1966), Kupst and Schulman (1980), and Miller and Haupt (1984), among others. It has much in common with the earlier distinction between coping strategies that primarily buffer stress and those that primarily reduce it. (See note 2.)

9. It also was relatively simple to identify these distinctions in the interviews. Independent raters were able to agree initially on the coding of parents' responses into distinct strategies 83% of the time, and remaining disagreements were resolved through discussion.

10. Wortman and Dunkel-Schetter (1979) and Sontag (1979) have discussed how important it is for patients to be optimistic in order to sustain friendships and good interpersonal relationships. This phenomenon also may be reflected in certain parents' reports of their desires to be "up" in relating to physicians.

11. These trends are consistent with the findings regarding passive patient and parent roles discussed in Chapter 4 and research by Antonovsky (1980), DiMatteo (1979), Friedson (1970), Stone (1979), and Taylor (1979). However, because these findings are associative (product moment correlations) we do not know the cause or direction of the relationship. A good relationship with the staff may lead to the use of certain strategies or the use of certain strategies may lead to a good relationship; the same duality is true of negative relations and coping strategy.

12. This finding also emphasizes a distinction between the overall amount of stress parents report and the agency from which stress ensues. Amount of general stress has a minimal relation to particular coping strategies, whereas stress associated with staff relations, for instance, does relate significantly with particular strategies.

13. This question was asked only of parents of living children whose interactions with the medical staff were more recent and thus more reliable. Later portions of this chapter suggest that parents of deceased children might have intervened in cessation of treatment.

14. Other data on parents' involvement in a self-help group and the impact of that experience on coping in general are reported in Chapter 10.

15. Excellent discussions of these options are presented in Adams and Deveau (1984) and Moldow and Martinson (1979). Martinson and her colleagues have developed materials for parents that are a great aid to solving the practical problems of caring for a dying child at home.

16. Singer (1984) emphasizes the importance of this "criterion problem" in assessing coping, and Taylor (1984, p. 2313) argues that "what people do in response to a stressor can and must be studied independently of what they do that makes them improve."

17. Although such outlooks can be carried too far, the general theoretical point about anticipatory mourning is made by Futterman and Hoffman (1973).

18. We utilized a panel of external raters composed of undergraduate and graduate students who had conducted the interviews with parents. They read interviews of parents who they had not met and rated the effectiveness of their coping, without further instructions. These judges give highest coping ratings to parents who report least stress and most optimism, just as prior literature suggests. However, a very low correlation of .05 exists between these external ratings (good, fair, poor) and parents' own ratings (very well, good, fair, poor), confirming the lack of fit between external raters of parental coping and parents' own reports.

19. These trends are confirmed in a study by Kupst et al. (1982); using a variety of standardized measures of coping, 72% of the families demonstrate constructive or appropriate coping. Caution must be exercised in interpreting both sets of data, however, since parents may desire to present themselves as "up" to researchers, much as they may do with friends and members of the medical staff (see Chapters 3 and 4).

20. Silberfarb (1982) also emphasizes the distinction between coping (or adaptation) and triumph over the stress. Although it may be impossible to eliminate or even seriously reduce the stresses associated with childhood cancer, it may well be possible to have a high quality life in the midst of such stress. Perhaps this is what many parents mean when they say they are "doing well."

CHAPTER 6

Coping as a Family

This chapter builds on discussions in previous chapters to examine the challenge that illness poses to the entire family. Families are more than the sum of their individual members. They develop coherent patterns by which individuals collaborate to respond emotionally, resolve conflict, and solve problems (Reiss, 1978). Families often allocate particular responsibilities to subgroups of their members, most especially marital and sibling subgroups (Minuchin, 1974).

In the family context, the stresses of childhood cancer are exemplified in three key family coping tasks: managing internal emotional relationships, adapting to many new practical tasks, and managing external relationships. The family's typical ways of operating must accommodate the many new demands that childhood cancer imposes. The illness may alter the family's emotional tone, as pain, fear, and hope take on new importance and meaning; it may alter the family's practical functioning, as members try to care for an ill child and each other; and it may alter the family's status in the community, as the family faces the stigma of childhood cancer and reaches out for help. See Table 6.1 for examples of these stresses and the related coping strategies.

IMPACT ON THE FAMILY

Cancer is a family disease — it challenges the life course not only of the ill person but of the entire family (Cassileth & Hamilton, 1979). One father of a teenager with osteogenic sarcoma sums up its encompassing effect (G. Nelcamp, 1980):

Portions of this chapter first appeared in: Barbarin, O., Hughes, D., & Chesler, M. Stress, coping, and marital functioning among parents of children with cancer. *Journal of Marriage and the Family*, 1985, May, 473–480. Reprinted by permission.

Table 6.1

Stresses and Coping Strategies in Families of Children with Cancer

Family Stresses	Family Coping Strategies

Management of internal emotional relationships
  special status of the patient
  sibling jealousy and concern
  parental pain, exhaustion
  limited spousal time/energy
	Shield others from "bad" feelings and "bad" news
	Have open communication of strong feelings
	Maintain marital intimacy
	Separate from others, keep feelings private, maintain distance
	Coordinate emotional styles
	Talk with siblings about their needs

Adaptation to practical tasks
  overload of new tasks
  limited material resources
  lack of skill in new roles
  care for the ill child
	Maintain prior routines
	Redistribute family chores
	Reallocate spousal division of labor
	Balance time between home and hospital
	Care for ill child as a top priority
	Keep everything "as it was" prior to the illness
	Change family location to ease transportation problems
	Alter employment

Management of external relationships
  reactions of extended family and friends
  access to community services
  financial demands
	Seek help from friends and relatives
	Withdraw from social contact
	Meet with school personnel
	Keep diagnosis from others

Cancer is not a disease of one person, though one person bears the brunt of it; it's a disease that has a tremendous impact on the whole family. (p. 11)

The family is society's primary unit for intimate social interaction, the setting most appropriate for sharing intense feelings. When childhood cancer impacts upon individuals, it is the family in which deepest relationships and fullest expressions of feelings are experienced. The family's ability to help all members feel valued and competent, to meet their needs for affirmation and affection, and to resolve their pain and loneliness may be challenged by the illness.

In order to be effective in processing emotional issues and in accomplishing its other purposes, the family unit must also care for its own maintenance. Family chores, decision making, and those practical tasks that sustain the household still must be accomplished. But childhood cancer also creates a set of new practical tasks (transportation, home care, medical liaison, and the like) that may overload current roles and role distributions. Some families may find it quite difficult to adapt to these changing practical demands because they lack flexibility in (re)allocating personpower and resources. This is especially likely in single parent families or in dual parent families with rigid divisions of labor.

Finally, the family is the setting from which members reach out to other social units, both to gather resources and to contribute to the larger community. Childhood cancer often so strains the family that members have difficulty maintaining prior external social relationships. Moreover, when outside persons or agencies react negatively to the threat of the illness, they make it more difficult for the family to rely upon external sources of support and service.

FAMILY COPING STRATEGIES

The family, as a unit with specific social functions and experiences, deals with stress differently than do its constituent members. The family unit's responses to the challenges and stresses of childhood cancer constitute what we define as family coping.

Managing Internal Emotional Relations

A potential stress for the family involves meeting members' needs for intimacy, empathy, personal affirmation, and support while living through a distressing and potentially debilitating situation. This nurturance of emotional relationships does not happen by accident. Franz (1983) points out:

> *During your child's illness it takes a lot of work — just at the point when you each have less time and energy to work at it. However, since you know what to expect, you can make an effort to be understanding, to plan time together, to talk with each other about your fears, worries, and hopes. Even a small amount of high quality, intimate sharing and acceptance of each other's feelings can work wonders. (p. 15)*

Some parents of children with cancer report that the struggle with the illness leads to improvements in the quality of family life. Such reports are not necessarily self-deceptions or wishful thinking, but may represent families' bona fide success at not merely avoiding disaster but at finding ways to improve family life through effective coping. This does not mean that families do not experience problems. To the contrary, parents report excessive demands on their time and resources that strain family relationships and result in concern about family life (Chapter 3). The potency of these problems may be linked to the ways family members are able to meet their needs by working as a team.

In response to open-ended questions about the impact of the illness, parents indicate overwhelmingly that their families become more cohesive. Sixty percent of the sample indicate that the family is emotionally closer as a result of the illness; 34% indicate that there is no change; and only 5% say that they are further apart. Typically the increased cohesion or closeness in family relations refers to increased emotional attachment to and concern about one another. Many parents express such sentiments using different terms:

It's a closer bond and we're more grateful for the time we have together.

The whole family is closer knit.

At this age children start to move away from their families but we've been supportive—it's brought us closer together at the time when we tend to go our own way.

Of course, this is not always the case, and some parents report that the family has grown further apart.

I don't think our family has grown closer together. The illness has caused problems, it's caused lots of problems.

Family life is strengthened when individuals are able to share and reinforce in each other a sense of hope and confidence about their future. The view of stress as a common problem that can be solved through common effort helps overcome loneliness and may lead to increased interdependence and teamwork.

A second intrafamilial issue is the extent to which members are able to share information and feelings. In some families a wall of silence separates members; so much privacy is maintained that family members have little sense of each other's anguish, despair, or pain.

My husband and I just don't talk about it. He had too hard of a time handling it.

> *Even though she knew her dad cared, he was soft-spoken and just couldn't get his feelings out. It would have been better if he could have talked to her.*

If pain or fear cannot be shared, love may not be shared either. Trusting and sharing feelings promote intimacy and cohesion that strengthen the family's ability to respond to the illness.

Concern about inflicting pain on other family members, and a desire to help them reduce their fear and anxiety, may lead to a lack of communication. Cook (1984) observes that mothers were particularly likely to shield or protect other family members, especially children, from their own terrible feelings and secret concerns. Spouses may also try to shield each other from depressing information or feelings.

A family's communication style also may affect its ability to solve everyday problems. Spinetta, Swarner, and Sheposh (1981) report a positive relationship between a family's favorable long-term adjustment to childhood cancer and its use of an open communication strategy. Open communication promotes joint problem solving or coordination of tasks, so that the activities of individual family members complement one another rather than overlap and duplicate. Moreover, when parents talk openly about their feelings, ill children and their siblings are also likely to join these conversations and, in turn, to promote open communication as a coping strategy for the entire family. The importance of open communication among all family members is expressed by one mother of a child with cancer (Griffin, 1982):

> *If I were asked for just one piece of advice, it would be to keep the family together, even about the child's illness. Explain every detail to each member of the family. Let them know all that's happening. Then, when you and the patient return home, your conversations will not seem to shut out other family members. The sick child is part of the family, and it makes things a lot easier for everyone if the family allows that child's illness to become part of them, in the sense that they share fears, hopes, information, feelings, love and trust. (p. 5)*

Keeping all lines of communication open is not easy and not all parents prefer this family approach.

The management of internal family relations also involves the family's marital and sibling subunits.

The marital subsystem. This subsystem's role is to provide for the intimacy needs of the adult family member(s) for closeness, emotional support, sexual activity and psychological refuge. The marital subsystem is composed of parent figure or figures: the mother and father; a single parent and close friend; foster parents or grandparents. The stress of childhood cancer may divert attention from marital considerations, leaving spouses few opportunities for intimacy, support, and enjoyment. Under the pressure of fear and pain, some spouses may focus their pain or anger on each other.

> *The relationship between me and my wife got very strained. We finally pinned it down to remorse come late. I guess I missed my son and took it out on my wife.*

For a single parent, managing the marital system alone, these issues take a very different shape. Adams and Deveau (1984), among the very few to address issues faced by single parents, note that: "Because you are the key person in your single parent family, tension is more concentrated when you are upset than it would be in most two-parent families" (p. 45). Loneliness, lack of intimate support, and unshared responsibility make for a special kind of burden. Single parents may be spared the stresses of a two-person marital system, but they also lose the extra hands and special comforts of a partner. Two women who separated from their husbands prior to their child's illness regret their current lack of spousal support in the following terms:

> *If I had had a husband with strength and compassion it would have helped.*

> *If my ex-husband had taken more interest and would have shared the load, it would have been helpful.*

Importantly, these mothers are not wishing for just any man, or just any pair of hands, but for a husband with interest, strength, and compassion. In a single-parent family, or even a two-parent family where one parent is absent or distant, an older child, relative, or friend may temporarily be pulled into the subsystem to provide intimacy and support.

Some research reports serious family consequences of chronic childhood illness, such as marital discord, decreased effectiveness of a partner, separation, and divorce. Scholars have observed difficulties expressed in emotional distancing, decreased frequency of sexual intimacy, sexual dysfunction, unresolved personal conflicts or disagreements, and an inability to derive personal satisfaction and comfort from the marriage.[1] However, these studies have methodological flaws that raise serious questions about their conclusions.[2] Moreover, recent studies challenge some of these earlier findings. Lansky et al. (1978) report that families of children with cancer do not show a higher divorce rate than a control population of families with physically healthy children. Koocher and O'Malley (1981) found in their study of parents of long-term survivors of childhood cancer that over time the parents' marriages were stable and the child's illness did not lead to marital disaster. Kalnins's (1983) incisive review of numerous studies of families of chronically and seriously ill children (with leukemia, spina bifida, or cystic fibrosis) emphasizes that although illness has a pervasive effect on family life, " . . . it cannot be concluded that . . . parental separation or divorce is directly related to the stress of caring for the child with a life-threatening illness" (p. 26). Thus, the assumption that caring for such children is a negative experience leading to a divorce not only lacks support, but also it is further refuted by reports of parents in many studies that the illness has brought them closer together.

Although marital relations are not usually weakened or destroyed by the stresses of childhood cancer, preillness difficulties are often exacerbated (Cook, 1984). When parents have coped with normal life stresses by means of distance, alcoholism, or marital infidelity, such patterns may become more extreme or more damaging to the relationship after the diagnosis.

The task of caring for the ill child may produce such physical and emotional fatigue that parents are unable to be physically intimate. When one spouse desires physical intimacy for reassurance, the partner may resent an invitation to erotic play when their child's condition is so serious. Thus, invitations to sexual intimacy may be judged inconsiderate and uncaring, rather than close and supportive. Obviously, when or how often partners have sexual relations is less critical than the manner of their decision making on this issue.

Research indicates that even with considerable stress the marital system is a source of substantial support. Table 6.2 demonstrates that 65.6% of the married parents in the sample report their spouses as being "very" helpful during the illness, making spouses the most helpful persons in the social environment.[3] In response to questions on how marital attitudes are affected by the illness, an overwhelming majority (72%) of married couples report that the marital relationship presents no problem. In addition, 54.6% indicate that they now feel more positive toward their spouse; 40.6% indicate that there was no change; and only 4.7% indicate that they feel less favorably toward their spouse.

Medical stress is significantly related to parents' assessments of marital quality and perceived spouse support. As the number of hospitalizations increase, parents report that marital quality ($r = -.23$, $p < .05$) and spouse support ($r = -.21$, $p < .05$) decrease. Hospitalization forces mothers and fathers to worry more and to spend more time away from

Table 6.2
Perceptions of Marital Quality and Support from Spouse
Among Parents of Children with Cancer

A. Spouse Support (*N*=64)

Very helpful	Somewhat or quite helpful	Not helpful or a little helpful
65.6% (42)	15.6% (10)	18.7% (12)

B. Marital Quality (*N*=64)

Illness-related changes in attitude toward spouse:

More positive toward spouse	Same	Less positive toward spouse
54.6% (35)	40.6% (26)	4.7% (3)

Marital problems:

No problems	Moderate concern	Major concern
72% (46)	22% (14)	6% (4)

home, attending the child. In both ways it may escalate tensions in their relationships.

Parents who are within three years of their child's diagnosis rate marital quality slightly higher than parents who are three years or more beyond diagnosis (Mean=6.9 *v.* 6.3, $F(1, 63).=2.7. p. <.10$). In the "pile-up" phenomenon discussed by McCubbin and Patterson (1982), parents may overlook marital problems in the initial stages of their child's illness, while they concentrate on the medical crisis facing their child. As issues of the child's survival become settled and life returns to normal, these "piled-up" issues reemerge, resulting in less positive ratings of marital quality (see Chapter 3). The quality of their relationship may or may not have changed, but in time parents may be more aware of and have time to discuss and deal with these problems.

The sibling subsystem. The second major family subgroup is the sibling subsystem, in which children learn to share, compete, and compromise with others close to them in status. By most recent accounts siblings are the *most* left out and unattended to of all family members during the experience of serious childhood illness. A foremost researcher reports that "siblings' emotional needs were met at a level significantly less adequate than that of other family members" (Spinetta, 1981, p. 137). Cairns, Clark, Smith, and Lansky (1979) also indicate that siblings in families of children with cancer are under substantial stress which may result in escalated anxiety, an increased sense of isolation, and fears about their own health problems. When they are treated differently than the ill child, it may lead to resentment.

Sometimes when both Sara and I are goofing around and both of us should get into trouble, I'm the only one that does. They don't like to yell at her much. It bothers me for a while.

Some of the issues siblings face stem from the nature of the sibling subsystem itself. If competition and love are part of the siblings' ongoing relationships, the constraints that the illness places on that interaction are likely to be painful. If, because a former competitor is ill, siblings cannot compete with one another any longer, or even for a while, their prior relationship clearly has been altered. Similarly, if love for one another now can be expressed only occasionally, by means of long-distance telephone or in a hospital room, it may not come as easily. Siblings who feel close to and concerned about the ill child want to be protective and often assume an adult caretaking role.

I try to read stories to him and stuff. Get him what he wants. Like when he had his biopsy he wanted a vanilla malt, so I got it for him. Little things like that, when you're not well, you don't get. When you're sick, they make you feel better. I play with him and get his school work. I go talk to the teachers and the principal.

I worry about what happens to him ... like when he goes to the hospital for checkups.

I worry when he's out playing. He's a normal active kid, he runs, jumps, plays, fights – getting cuts, infections. . . .

Siblings often identify with one another and link their fate with one another's experiences. Some siblings may even think that they caused the illness, perhaps by being too rough with their brother or sister. Moreover, if one sibling gets ill, the other may expect to get ill as well. Newman (1981) argues that parents must attend to this possibility by reducing uncertainty and confusion about the genesis of childhood cancer:

Siblings also need reassurance that they are healthy, especially if the ill child dies. Life after a death is never the same. The parents' loss affects their relationships with the surviving children. Children's reactions to the death of a sibling may be the frightening realization that it could happen to them. "Is something wrong with me?" and "Will I die when I reach my brother's age?" may be thought but never expressed. (p. 5)

Under these circumstances it is no surprise that Hewett and Newson (1970) report that one third of the mothers of cerebral palsied children feel that their physically normal children were jealous of the disabled child to some extent. And Cairns and her colleagues (1979) report that siblings of chronically ill children with cancer see their mothers as overprotective and overindulgent of the ill child. Of course, parents may be overprotective, and reports from mothers bear out the reality of some of these perceptions. There also are numerous examples of siblings who play positive family roles as safety valves or alarm bells, wherein they help draw their parents' attention to these overreactions. However, in some circumstances siblings may have distorted perceptions of their mothers' attention, distortions borne of their own sense of loss, jealousy, and concern. Regardless of the accuracy of siblings' perceptions of mothers' behaviors, they reflect feelings that must be responded to as real and important.

In analyzing families of children with cystic fibrosis, Burton (1975) emphasizes that the age and maturity of siblings significantly influence their reactions. Whereas some children, especially older siblings, display great warmth and participate actively in caretaking the ill child, others, especially younger children, "tended to react less positively. Indeed, they occasionally experienced extreme jealousy" (p. 192). In most families of children with cancer, siblings also have mixed and contradictory reactions.

> *Sometimes I feel bad and sometimes I feel a little jealous. I feel sad when I hear that he had all these needles and stuff stuck in him and I get jealous when he comes home and gets all this attention and doesn't have to clean and make the bed.*

Twenty-five percent of parents in the sample indicate stress from siblings' reactions to the illness (Chapter 3). On the other hand, 56% report that siblings are "very" or "quite" helpful to them during the course of the illness. Siblings can be both a source of stress and a source of support for parents.[4]

Parents are not the only ones concerned about and taking steps to facilitate coping within the sibling subsystem. Reports from the University of Missouri Hospital (Columbia, Missouri) describe a growing trend in efforts to help with these issues — a peer support group for siblings of children with cancer (Lysen, 1982). Providing an opportunity especially for younger siblings to discuss their feelings about the child with cancer and the distribution of parents' attention can be very helpful. In similar but less intensive programs the Children's Hospital of Michigan (Detroit) and the Children's Hospital in Milwaukee hold a yearly clinic open house. On this day the clinic is open to families of children with cancer; and siblings examine, play with, and encounter some of the machines, instruments, waiting rooms, and staff members that ill children deal with on a regular basis. Strong Memorial Hospital, in Rochester, New York, operates a special summer camp program for siblings of children with cancer. These experiences help make the ill child's situation more realistic and understandable for their siblings, and help remove siblings' concept of the ill child's condition and need for extra attention from the realm of mystery and fantasy.

Adapting Flexibly to New Tasks

The experience of childhood cancer brings many practical changes in family life, often disrupting routines that provide continuity and stability. Moreover, other negative changes may occur, such as a decrease in the frequency of social/recreational activities and home upkeep. This stress and related coping task involves finding ways to preserve as much of a sense of normalcy and stability as possible, while at the same time accommodating to new situations. Whereas the task discussed previously relates to family emotional processes, this challenge is concerned with family duties and role assignments. For instance, the jobs of caring for the ill child and of transporting the child for clinic treatment or hospitalization often force parents to reduce or alter their responsibilities as homemakers or wage earners. Some fathers cut back on the amount of time spent at work in order to perform family chores or to spend more time at the hospital, and mothers often cut out or cut back from full-time employment in order to be available to care for the ill child. As they curtail work time or even refuse relocation opportunities, parents sometimes give up career and financial advancement. Maintaining the household and caring for younger children at home also require considerable adaptation, cooperation, and sharing among family members if the family is to adjust well over the course of the illness.

The difficulty of achieving a balance between change and continuity is exacerbated when families lack sufficient resources to handle all the jobs involved. Time and energy are often at a premium and parents, especially, face the problem of whether and how to renegotiate their work roles and their involvement in home management and child care. In 59% of the families, mothers took sole responsibility for caring for the child in the hospital and for monitoring the child's health care; in 6% of the families the fathers alone monitored treatment; and in 34% of the families, both parents shared the task.[5] Mothers often characterize this responsibility as unpleasant, because it involves long waiting periods in which they are confronted with their child's pain from procedures and with isolation from their family and their normal adult world.

Some fathers respond to the illness by maintaining traditional work schedules that limit their accessibility to the ill or hospitalized child. Others try to tailor their work schedules to hospital plans, so they can spend more time during the day with the child and family.[6] Many fathers are poorly prepared for these new activities, or have rarely experienced the unremitting demands of being at home alone with their children.

In some families siblings assume increasingly responsible roles in helping around the house or keeping the ill child's school informed. The family's flexibility in reallocating roles and juggling schedules often determines whether family members are able to overcome traditional role barriers to mutual involvement in the care of the ill child.

Some families redistribute chores or duties around the house, sacrificing individual needs and comforts so that the family will function more smoothly. Some relocate and move to a neighborhood closer to the hospital and medical care facilities, or move closer to extended family members who can contribute to the care of the ill child. Families also may cope with the intrusive nature of the illness and its treatment by altering or rescheduling family vacations and participation in holiday festivities.

The most effective coping strategy may go beyond balancing change and stability and may involve opportunities for emotional growth and social maturity for all family members. Thus, marital partners can examine their experiences and coping patterns to seek pleasure and growth, not just emotional survival; parents can plan physically and intellectually stimulating activities for siblings, and everyone can plan for the ill child's appropriate educational experiences and social relationships.

The ingenuity with which these tasks are handled also influences the relationship in the marital and sibling subsystems. The flexibility that spouses bring to altering their accustomed roles affects how they view their marriage. Wives' favorable perceptions of marital quality relate to their husbands' active participation in the care for the ill child and information seeking about the illness and its treatment. Conversely, the more often wives report assuming sole responsibility for staying with the child in the hospital and managing medical decision making, the less favorably they evaluate marital relations. Husbands' reports of spousal support significantly relate to the extent to which wives spend time at home as opposed to the hospital. Tucker (1982) describes a couple's feelings about these issues:

Sally realized that Brian loved Ellie and had to work to support the family, yet she resented the fact that she was so much more

*involved than he was in Ellie's care. She suspected that he came
to the hospital less often than he could have because he could not
bear the idea that Ellie might not survive. Perhaps by avoiding the
illness, he was trying to make it go away. Brian, on the other hand,
resented Sally's total absorption in Ellie's care. It just wasn't normal for a mother to be with a child all day and all night. As a result,
he was left at home with all the responsibilities and the housework,
deprived of physical contact with his wife, emotional support, and
a normal family life. (p. 76)*

Flexibility in changing parental tasks may not come without emotional costs in the sibling subsystem as well as in the marital subsystem.
As mothers' and fathers' roles shift to accommodate the ill child's regimen, siblings may have to adapt to new-found distance from mother
and interdependence with father. If parents express love for each other
and for their children through a devotion of their time and energy, shifts
in the amount and focus of parental attention may be perceived by the
siblings of an ill child as evidence that their parents no longer love them
or that they love the ill child more. This may intensify or re-create more
primitive feelings of sibling rivalry and result in new forms of competition for parents' attention. Similarly, as parents focus attention upon
the immediate demands of the illness, they may fail to engage in or may
defer long-range planning or activities essential for siblings' development, such as schooling and clothes buying. Even when siblings understand this phenomenon and the rationale for it, they may feel shunted
aside or put on hold.

*I feel sad and left out sometimes. He (ill child) can get away with
anything. He uses his illnesses and mom and dad will let him stay
home from school. They wouldn't let us get away with that.*

*My mom's changed a lot. Sometimes she ignores us and pays more
attention to Dave (ill child), but that don't bother me. But Brent,
my brother, he can't take it.*

Managing External Relationships

Coping with extended family, friends, employers, co-workers, church
groups, and community agencies increases in importance when a family
experiences a crisis such as childhood cancer. In Chapter 9, "Getting
Help from Others," we elaborate on the interpersonal issues of stigmatization, isolation, and awkwardness in social contacts between parents
and their close friends. The family must decide how open or private it
wants to be in its contacts with others, whether it will include others
in responding to family issues, or if it will minimize external contact.

For their part, friends may not know what to say or do or how to be helpful to the family.

Because the demands of caring for a child with a chronic illness such as cancer may exceed the family's resources, outside help is often required. The family must cope with burdensome medical expenses, and insurance rarely covers the wide range of costs that families incur. When inadequate insurance or insufficient resources makes it impossible to ensure competent or complete treatment for the child, or requires submission to a humiliating charity structure, guilt and shame are often experienced.

Assistance may be hard to get, and some persons outside the family may react with indifference or insensitivity. Siblings may be particularly vulnerable to social slights from outsiders who draw back from or express pity toward members of a family with childhood cancer. Under such circumstances Burton (1975) notes that siblings may be torn between loyalty to the family and a desire to avoid stigma. Friends and neighbors who shower the ill child with special attention may increase sibling jealousy. Grandparents who urge siblings "not to make a fuss" or "not to make it any harder on your parents than it already is," and teachers or other representatives of community agencies who do not deal skillfully with the impact of the illness on siblings, may escalate the problems that siblings face inside the family.

When families are so overwhelmed by the burdens of childhood cancer that they are unable to respond to one another in helpful ways, turning to an outsider may be essential to family survival. The COPE *Torch*, a newsletter prepared by a self-help group in Cincinnati for parents of children with cancer, emphasizes the importance of coping by going outside the family for help (Eickhoff & Eickhoff, 1985):

> *You may need to seek help. Perhaps that is not good news, but it may be the best news to hear. If you see these problems, do not be ashamed to admit you need help, because there is no shame attached. A person who never needs help is either a saint or a fool. The hospital staff recognizes childhood cancer as a family problem, and they want to help by helping the family better help the patient. But, and this is important, you must seek help and ask for help. The staff cannot read your mind and cannot be expected to know your needs. The more they know about your problems and the faster you can seek help, the better the chances they have to help you. Talk to other parents and share your fears. You'll soon find out you are not the only one in the world with a particular problem, and, perhaps, that parent can tell you the particular person to contact. COPE can help you in this way, but again COPE does not pry into your life—we act when you ask. (p. 4)*

THE MEANING OF COPING AS A FAMILY

Patterns of family coping can be observed in the ways in which families manage intra- and extrafamilial relations and adapt flexibly while preserving continuity in family life. The coordination of individual coping responses is sometimes represented in turn taking, such that members compromise and give up the satisfaction of their own needs at one point with the conviction that their turn for satisfaction will come at some later point. It also is reflected in negotiation or redefinition of roles, as old tasks may be reassigned and new tasks distributed in more effective or satisfying ways. It also is reflected in the development of a shared perspective on the stressful situation, especially with respect to the meaning attached to stress, interpretation of its causes, and perceptions of responsibility for solving problems (McCubbin & Patterson, 1982).

A prolonged stressful situation, such as childhood cancer, imposes such a wide array of new tasks that no one family member can cope with them all. The advantage of having a family unit available is that while each member can contribute individually the unit can make a coordinated response to stress. Coordination of family members' contributions permits a division of labor, which precludes many persons from doing the same task and leaving other tasks undone. Family coping is distinct from individual coping as members take on different roles and coordinate their activities to enhance the effectiveness of the entire family under stress (G. Nelcamp, 1980).

> *And every member of the family is going to approach the problem a bit differently. That can create a great deal of tension. Though sometimes the husband is the strong one, often the husband will bury himself at work or deny the fact that his child has cancer and put the whole burden on his wife. The patient's brothers and sisters also have to be considered. Some may hide their feelings and suffer in silence; others may be irritable. So parents have to be careful; otherwise they might save the patient and lose the others. (p. 11)*

One way of assessing the degree of family coordination is to examine the extent to which spouses, in particular, are the same (symmetrical) or different (complementary) in their use of specific coping strategies.[7] Table 6.3 indicates that more couples adopt symmetrical than asymmetrical or complementary patterns: The greatest symmetry occurs in help seeking (77%), denial (61%), optimism (61%), emotional balance (58%), and religious beliefs (58%).

The implications of intracouple differences in coping strategies have

Table 6.3
Proportion of Couples with Symmetrical and Complementary
Coping Patterns (*N*=32 Couples)

| Coping Strategy | Symmetrical | | Complementary |
	Used by Both Parents	Used by Neither Parent	Used Only by One Parent
Information seeking	10%	35%	55%
Problem solving	29	26	45
Help seeking	3	74	23
Emotional balance	26	32	42
Religious beliefs	16	42	42
Optimism	29	32	39
Denial	26	35	39
Acceptance	29	24	47

rarely been considered in studies of childhood cancer or other pediatric illnesses. Under certain conditions, symmetrical coping strategies may lead to more favorable outcomes (perceptions of high spouse support and a stable satisfying marital relationship): When partners exhibit reactions such as anger or despair at similarly high or low levels, each may reinforce or validate the other's response to the illness and thus increase cohesion and support within the marital dyad. Moreover, when both share equally in instrumental tasks, such as taking the sick child to the hospital and caring for siblings, feelings of support and reciprocity may be engendered. It may be especially important for parents to adopt symmetrical coping styles in approaches to treatment. In the case of juvenile diabetes, Anderson and Auslander (1980) review research suggesting that "parental consensus regarding treatment requirements fostered adaptation to treatment by other family members" (p. 698). On the other hand, symmetrical use of some coping strategies may lead to less favorable outcomes: When both partners exhibit anger or despair, each may be too depleted to respond to and comfort the other.

Asymmetrical patterns, in which one partner exhibits despair and sadness and the other restraint and optimism, also may lead to favorable outcomes: As one partner expresses the sadness common to both, the other can support his/her distress while also expressing the positive feelings that both may have. Similarly, a useful division of labor may occur when one parent relies on emotion-focused coping strategies (denial, optimism) and the other utilizes action-focused strategies such as information seeking and problem solving (Sabbeth, 1984). However, the salience of different responses also may challenge or invalidate each partner's unique reaction to the illness, cause tensions, erode empathy between spouses, and undermine the marital relationship. An example of the problems caused by asymmetrical coping is provided in Tucker's (1982) report of Ellie's parents:

> *Instead of uniting them, the disease had begun to accentuate their fundamentally different styles of coping and relating. Sally was confronting the crisis head-on and being too hard on herself, whereas Brian was running away from it. Initially the disease had touched him deeply and brought out a variety of emotions, but they had been too painful and threatening and he had quickly pushed them back down again and tried to ignore them. (pp. 75–76)*

OUTCOMES OF FAMILY COPING

In Chapter 5 we discussed how difficult it is to agree upon a standard criterion of effective personal coping. The same problems occur with effective family coping. We asked all parents themselves to assess the impact of the illness on family life.[8] Forty-two of the 84 parents (50%) report that family life has improved as a consequence of the illness; 35 (42%) report that the quality of family life is the same; and only 7 parents (8%) report that family life is worse (see Table 6.4). The 50% who report improvements in the family do not differ from others with regard to the age of the child, the child's diagnosis, parents' age, or parents' education or income.

Parents who report coping better as a family do report less personal stress associated with the medical situation (as measured by responses both to the stress charts and to questionnaire items). It is difficult to separate the relationships of these two factors. It may be that because the ill child is doing well, parents experience less personal stress and, therefore, more positive family coping. On the other hand, positive family coping may result in parents' feeling and reporting less stress. Some hints about the relationship of these factors, and details about the family's success and failure in coping with the impact of the illness, are provided in parents' direct reports. Parents who report that the illness has a positive impact on family life (e.g., is handled well, the family copes well) generally report satisfaction and improvement on one or more of the major family coping tasks. One common result is a change in the quality of the marital relationship.

> *It definitely brought my wife and me closer together. We did a lot of talking we'd never done before. It made us the best of friends*

Table 6.4
Parents' Reports of Stress and the Impact
of the Illness on Family Life

Parents' Ratings of	Impact Positive (N=42)	Impact Neutral or Negative (N=42)	F Value
Medical Stress (from stress chart)	29.8	46.6	4.2*
Medical Stress (from questionnaire)	9.5	10.5	5.1*

*p. <.05

along with being husband and wife. We now spend more time together.

Our marriage was in trouble before. We were going to separate but my husband said he couldn't leave our child, so he stayed. We had to bring our troubles out in the open and work on our problems so we could live together. Now we're closer than we've ever been and have real strength in our marriage.

It made our marriage 100% permanent.

We've learned to be more aware and sensitive to each other's needs. My husband and I had needs in our own lives that we needed to become aware of, and we learned to be more positive with each other.

Of course, the language of "it improved our relationship" is only a manner of speaking. "It" didn't do anything but provide opportunities for growth or decay, for an improved or worsened marital relationship. It is parents' wise and energetic ways of dealing with each other and the illness that lead to improved family relationships.

Parents reporting that the family is coping well also note greater closeness and pulling together by all family members – in both the marital and sibling subgroups – and a willingness to subordinate personal preferences to family needs.

The kids and us stick together more in general, not just with the child with cancer. Before it was easy to say, "Oh, I'm tired," if the kids wanted to go for a bike ride or something. Now I say, "Let's do it." Of course, there are times we don't. But we do have fun and enjoy being together more now because maybe tomorrow we won't be able to.

I think our strength as a family has helped us a great deal, and our family has gotten even stronger. I think the fact that we've gone our own way as an entire family, that we've pulled together and really gotten to know each other and depended on each other has helped a lot. I think we've become terribly strong as a family and that's going to be important for our daughters for the rest of their lives.

Even when a child dies some parents feel that their family has grown closer as a result of the experience (Roach, 1974):

We had become closer through our mutual sharing and concern over Erin's well-being. Although we had friction, misunderstandings and frazzled nerves, there was a strong basis of mutual caring and the realization that we were two fragile human beings facing an enormous problem. In the end we knew that each of us had given all our love and had experienced together the deepest of human emotions. We learned to love unafraid. We had invested immense love and that love, we have learned, was not lost when Erin died. Rather, it became the better part of us. (p. 22)

Some parents who report that the family copes well with the illness also report positive and supportive relationships with their extended family members.

We've always been very loving in our immediate family, but I think it's brought the extended families closer.

I think we've learned to share more with our parents, the grandparents. They are terribly concerned about the children and now share so much of their lives, and that would not have happened if he hadn't gotten ill.

Although many families learn these lessons or make these changes on their own, some families find it helpful to seek professional counseling as a way to maintain or improve the quality of family life.[9] Counseling objectives may focus upon the renegotiation of roles within the family, so all members may be enabled to reallocate tasks and responsibilities. Equally important may be assistance in enhancing mutual communication or empathy, to improve family members' abilities to understand one another's feelings, and to share these feelings. In addition, professional guidance may enable family members to more effectively deal with a variety of external agencies (e.g., school personnel, medical staff, employers). Just as individual parents may need assistance in learning how to cope better with the stresses accompanying chronic childhood illness, so may the family as a unit gain from such assistance. Such counseling may not only improve the current quality of family life; it may help develop patterns of family sharing and problem solving that prevent problems from occurring later.

As a practical guide to the creation of a close and quality family life in the face of childhood cancer, Adams and Deveau (1984) suggest parents do the following:

1. Give their partners sympathy and understanding rather than blame and criticism;
2. Make their sick child a priority; both parents come together to learn about the diagnosis and treatment;
3. Recognize that they must continue to share in caring and loving for their other children;
4. Share their own feelings of anger, sadness, sorrow, and hope with each other;
5. Accept the help of family, friends, and neighbors whom they love and trust;
6. Maintain loyalty to their husband or wife in the face of criticism or blame from relatives or others. (p. 37)

Our own data and experience certainly support these suggestions. However, we also suggest:

7. Alter traditional husband-wife roles so that the work of caring for the child, the home and other family members is done in an efficient and satisfying manner;
8. Talk together about how all family members may experience the illness situation very differently; listen carefully to each person's expression of how he/she feels and what he/she wants to happen;
9. Look for opportunities to do new things together as a family.
10. Don't assume that family members fit any single pattern suggested by research or medical staff, but find your own way;
11. Carefully but positively explore options for professional assistance.

CHAPTER NOTES

1. Studies examining the marital impact of childhood illness in general include Crain, Sussman, and Weil (1966) and Marcus (1977). Evidence of increased marital discord specific to childhood cancer has been reported by Kaplan, Smith, Grobstein, and Fishman (1973).

2. They generally were small sample studies, conducted on a one-time basis, with no substantial control or comparison groups. Moreover, they concentrated on families of chil-

dren who died. They also typically asked parents only to enumerate or respond to questions about problems and deficiencies, rather than asking simultaneously about positive coping behavior or outcomes.

3. This and subsequent analyses of the marital unit are based on the reports of a subsample of the entire sample, involving 32 married couples or parents of living children in which both spouses were interviewed.

4. The combinations of sibling stress and support, discussed further in Chapter 7, can take many forms.

		Sibling Stress	
		Hi	Lo
Sibling	Hi	A	B
Support	Lo	C	D

In A, both support and stress from siblings are high; it is essential that they be dealt with. In D, neither stress nor support from siblings is potent, representing young siblings who are unaware of the illness and its impact on them and others, or older siblings beginning to separate from the family. B and C represent mixed stress creation and support provision. These permutations of roles and reactions might be a useful guide into research on the complex world of sibling dynamics.

5. A similar trend toward primarily maternal involvement in the medical care of the child with cancer is reported by Cook (1984), and in studies of other childhood illnesses (Featherstone, 1981; Burton, 1975; Strong, 1979).

6. Cook (1984) describes fathers' common conflict between maintaining their workload on the job and fulfilling their responsibilities at home.

7. Bateson's (1972), Jackson's (1965), and Burke and Weir's (1976, 1979) research on the ways in which the coping strategies of one spouse related to the coping strategies of the other indicate that couples tend not to adopt similar or symmetrical coping strategies; frequent use of a particular coping strategy by one partner is not related to frequent use by the other. Instead, they observed a predominance of complementary or asymmetrical patterns; when one partner adopts a particularly active style, the other tends to adopt a passive style; when one partner shows a preference for avoidance or withdrawal strategies, the other tends to use direct attack or problem-focused strategies. Most common are asymmetrical patterns in which husbands predominate in instrumental, task-oriented, and problem-solving areas and wives predominate in expressive and emotional areas (Jackson, 1965).

8. Data from all parents in the sample, and not just from married couples, are analyzed here.

9. Discussions of family counseling occasioned by chronic childhood illness once again emphasize the problem of treatment assumptions (Kaplan et al., 1973; Masters, Cerreto, and Mendlowitz, 1983; Tylke, 1980). The traditional psychotherapeutic concern with family pathology may not be well suited for aiding otherwise healthy families trying to cope with the abnormal stress of childhood cancer. Moreover, parents may not wish to utilize services oriented to pathologic processes, partly explaining why some social workers report "difficulty in engagement" and refusal from oncologic families (Tylke, 1980). Supportive counseling that deals concretely with stress, and that helps the family utilize their positive histories to cope with such stress may be more appropriate.

CHAPTER 7

Parenting Children with Cancer

Parents have the awesome responsibility of preparing children for a successful adult life. Basic child-rearing tasks involve the selection of developmentally appropriate standards, and the application of discipline, so that the child acquires approved attitudes and skills. The typical child-rearing process is complicated by illness and treatment, pressures to treat the child in a special way, and reactions of others to the child and family.

BASIC CHILD-REARING TASKS
FOR THE NORMAL BUT SPECIAL CHILD

Preparation for adulthood entails intense parental involvement in providing for the child's physical and psychological well-being. It includes development of social behavior, moral reasoning, self-control, and achievement. As the child approaches adolescence parents must gradually yield control and permit the child greater autonomy and freedom to make choices about his/her personal, educational, and social goals.

Most parents' limited preparation for these tasks is based on observations of the success and failures of others; there are few reliable principles or trustworthy guidelines on how to act in any given situa-

Portions of this chapter first appeared in: Chesler, M., Barbarin, O., & Paris, J. "Telling" the child with cancer: Parental choices to share information with ill children." *Journal of Pediatric Psychology*, 1986, *11*(4). Reprinted by permission.

tion. Most parents use trial and error, developing and testing their own methods and rules as they go along. Even without the complications of a chronic childhood illness there is much doubt and uncertainty about how best to prepare children for adulthood.[1]

Childhood cancer increases the complexity of the child-rearing process. The child's physical and emotional condition and parental uncertainty about the future may produce confusion on how to administer discipline. Moreover, treatment and its side effects may interfere with normal maturation processes. The impact of medication on the child's self-control and emotional stability is captured by one parent:

> *Living with him has been hard. He can be super angry and two seconds later he can break down in tears and then be sound asleep. This can all be in two minutes. The medicine really messes him up.*

The emotional and physical disruption brought on by the illness and treatment may make typical developmental milestones inappropriate for the ill child. For example, language competence is an important signal that a child has moved from infancy to toddlerhood, but young children with cancer may experience developmental delays in language as a result of their surgery or extended hospitalization. Similarly, bladder and bowel control are important accomplishments for children moving from the toddler to the preschool stage; children in treatment may regress or fail to develop normally as a result of drugs that cause constipation or bladder irritation. The development of appropriate eating habits and dietary preferences also may be affected by radiation and chemotherapy, which may destroy a child's appetite and/or create preferences for salty or sugary foods. The rules and practices that parents employ to deal with a child's refusal to eat anything but junk food, or to reinforce toilet training, may be ill-suited for a child being treated with toxic chemicals. The achievement of independence and autonomy, the litmus test of normal adolescence, may also be difficult for children with cancer. They may experience temporary but strong needs for dependence and nurturance as a result of the devastating effects of cancer and its treatment. These physical and psychological factors add to the frustration and mood swings of what is already a volatile period of life. Adolescents' regression to earlier periods of emotional and physical dependence may require new behavioral and emotional rites of passage through which they gradually regain their sense of autonomy and personal responsibility.

The determination of the child's progress as normal and age appropriate may be clouded by questions about whether immature behavior or developmental lags are caused by physical effects of treatment, psychological reactions to stress, or whether the child is not emotionally ready to take on new responsibilities. Emotional immaturity can flow equally from physical effects of the illness experience and from the child's unwillingness or incapacity to behave as parents expect. Parents' attribution of the cause of such failure to meet their expectations is critical (Comaroff & McGuire, 1981). Parents who sense that their child's difficulties are the result of the impact of drugs or anxiety usually alter their standards and expectations. Parents who suspect that their child is willfully taking advantage of the illness situation are more likely to insist upon adherence to prior standards. It is difficult to distinguish the physical impact of drugs and other treatments from their psychological impact, let alone to distinguish youngsters' psychological fears and needs from their willful disobedience.

Underlying all these distinctions is the problem of determining what is normal behavior, and thus what should be normal behavioral standards for the child with cancer. Parents face a dilemma in simultaneously treating their child normally and acknowledging the child's special condition. Children with cancer are special if only because they are seriously sick, often uncomfortable, and often worried about their illness. While seeking to protect their child, and to adjust hopes and expectations for the child's future in terms of the illness, parents must stimulate the child to achieve his or her potential and to live as normal a life as possible – now and in the future. Burton reports that when parents of children with cystic fibrosis were asked about their ideal goals, "the majority stressed the need for normality, and believed that any marked change in attitude would probably be detrimental to the child's overall growth" (1975, p. 140). So, too, parents of children with cancer seek to normalize the life of the child and family. As one parent notes, she was

Trying to avoid overprotection of my child, and coping with life as usual without panic or stress.

Burton further reports a frequent disparity between parents' ideal goals and their actual child-rearing practices. "Parents who seem most secure and happy in their rearing of the sick child . . . claimed that their child was definitely different, and argued that it was therefore ridiculous to treat him as normal" (1975, p. 141).

There are many ways of resolving this tension and many ways of defining normalcy. Whereas parents want to protect their child, not to make unreasonable demands upon a vulnerable youngster, they also wish to avoid a spoiled child, or a child cured of cancer but emotionally crippled or obnoxious (Van Eys, 1977b). Fortunately, most long-term survivors are not emotionally or behaviorally abnormal (Koocher & O'Malley, 1981). But fears of such outcomes often make parents tense and uncertain about their child-rearing competence; and newsletters, social workers' talks, and parents' informal conversations often focus on these concerns.

For some parents, normalization means ensuring that the child with cancer is indeed treated "just like everyone else," "with no special favors." This ideal goal is impossible if lifesaving medical regimens must be followed.

Other parents temporarily jettison or delay normalization, by placing protecting and assuring the life and emotional comfort of the child foremost. These parents argue that when the crisis is over, or if their child lives, they then will return to normal disciplinary and child-rearing measures.

A third approach treats the child like other children, while providing room for the child's unique and special situation and needs. Parents anticipate that their ill child may not conform to all their prior expectations, but try to specify and consider carefully just where and how deviations make sense and can be permitted or encouraged.

As parents of children with cancer consider these alternative approaches to normalcy, they must deal with several important parenting issues, some of which are quite unique: (1) exerting discipline about behavior and responsibility for household chores; (2) communicating in an open or closed manner with the child regarding the illness – the "telling" process; (3) helping the child manage or respond to the illness; and (4) helping the child prepare for death.

PARENTAL APPROACHES TO DISCIPLINE AND CHORES

Deciding when and how to discipline an ill child is a significant problem for many parents, as is the maintenance of family routines and household chores. In an informal study conducted by the Candlelighters Childhood Cancer Foundation (Lawrence, 1978), two thirds of the parents responding to a mail questionnaire report difficulty disciplining their children. A number of these parents note that the real problem of discipline is not their children, but themselves (Lawrence, 1978):

Our greatest problem was trying to discipline ourselves. How do you punish a two-year-old when you know he may never have another chance? Then we observed another child at the hospital who was so lost because of lack of discipline; she was so scared and insecure, this really helped us. Things became easier, and, even at two years, he knew it was the way things were meant to be. We feel this gave his short life a sense of being "normal." (p. 2)

Discipline is not an abstract problem, but relates to other child-rearing issues and ultimately to parents' definitions and goals for a normal life for their child.

A concern for effective discipline often involves parents' fears of spoiling their child or their experience that their child is becoming spoiled. Thirty-two percent of the parents of surviving children who responded to this inquiry (21 out of 66) report that a fear of the ill child becoming spoiled is a moderately strong concern; 12% (8/66) report that this is a very strong concern.

He's a spoiled monster and gets away with a little more than his sisters and brothers. He bends my rules more than anyone else. Sometimes now I'm extremely hard on him because everyone is very easy on him.

Anytime my son gets a cold, cough, sniffles, etc., it sends my husband into a tailspin. He doesn't handle it very well and over-protects him and lets him get away with things.

I don't spoil him anymore. During the first year he was spoiled, that is, he was given many presents and material things, but now he's not.

The potential for spoiling may be created by others outside the immediate family, by relatives or neighbors who, overcome with grief and concern, constantly pamper and overreact to the child's imagined or real discomfort or shortened life span. Parents' inability to ward off or correct neighbors' and relatives' behavior contributes to this problem. When parents do not know enough about their child's medical condition, they are especially unable to know what standards they should establish or encourage. In some cases, conversations with the medical staff can provide such information and direction. However, even the most knowledgeable staff members sometimes cannot determine whether a child's reactions are primarily the result of psychological or physiological factors.

The Association for the Care of Children's Health provides one useful response to parents' concerns about disciplining an ill child (*The Chronically Ill Child and Family in the Community*, 1982):

Should I discipline the child who is ill or has a handicapping condition?

The aim of discipline is to help a child learn to control his or her own behavior.

Setting limits in a firm but loving way offers security and is reassuring to any child. It is no different for a child with a health problem.

Children who do not have limits set for them are frequently frustrated. Too much freedom makes a child feel insecure and frightened.

It is often easy to attribute some behaviors like moodiness, temper tantrums, and avoiding schoolwork to your child's illness. Many of these behaviors are normal for children at certain ages and are not related to the health problem. If you are concerned, you may want to talk to your child's teacher, to health professionals, or to others who know your child.

Brothers and sisters who experience a double standard of discipline or feel favoritism shown a handicapped sibling may have problems relating to their sibling or parents.

Parents frequently feel that by "giving in" to the child and by being permissive, they can lessen their own guilt feelings and make up to the child for some of the things she or he will miss in life. This is usually not helpful for the child.

Let grandparents, teachers, and hospital staff know about the need for consistent discipline so that they will have the same expectations for behavior as you do.

In disciplining a child, help the child verbalize his or her own feelings. . . . "I know you are angry, but I cannot let you hit your brother." Let your child know that feelings are always acceptable but certain behavior may not be. Try to offer an acceptable alternative to the unacceptable behavior.

Many parents are reluctant to set limits for fear that their children may hurt themselves in a temper tantrum. It is best to ask your doctor, but some crying is not usually dangerous for a child, even a child with a heart condition or seizures.

Similar problems and resolutions apply to household chores and family responsibilities. Just as effective discipline normalizes the child's life as a child, effective responsibility-taking normalizes the child's relation to others in the family. Assignment of regular chores to ill children requires a judgment that the child is physically and emotionally ready to take on the responsibility.

Some parents report that ensuring that the ill child shares chores and family responsibilities is not a significant problem:

Definitely she does her chores. Leukemia is not an excuse to get out of chores unless she is really sick.

She still does the dishes and I still holler at her. I don't baby her and I don't let her get away with anything.

Other parents report that the ill child is difficult to handle but that the resistance seems quite normal. Ill children, like other children, sometimes resist doing their chores, and this may be taken as a sign of healthy development.

She does her share of work. You have to argue with her just like any other kid, but she still does it.

He does his share of chores when I get down on him and make him.

He does the dishes, the lawn, whatever I make him do, he does. If I don't sit right down on him and make him, he doesn't. I think this is typical of an 11-year-old boy. Actually, none of my children like to do their chores, they think mother was put here to wait on them all.

Probably most parents of ill or healthy children appreciate the child-rearing dilemma presented by the last mother. For parents of ill children it is a special pleasure to wrestle with problems that are "typical of an 11-year-old boy."

Some parents report that they have substantial difficulty deciding whether or how to assign chores to the ill child. As noted earlier, it is sometimes unclear whether the child *can not* do the assigned chores or *will not.*

I don't push her as much, and am a little quieter towards her. She is still very slow and lazy.

The development of his sense of responsibility has passed. Chores became trivial to me when he was so sick. And now, because he has been sick for such a long time, some of his development of responsibility is lagging behind. So now that he's well, he isn't interested in chores such as cleaning his room, helping in the house and garden, and things like that. Now that he's well, we want him to do these things and he refuses. These skills and attitudes are built into other children a step at a time, but they are missing in

*him, and it's hard for me to be patient and build them in now, little
by little.*

At other times parents are clear that the ill child is not resisting but
is just too ill to perform to normal expectations.

*Last year she really couldn't do the same chores, but this year she
can do more.*

*She used to clear the table and do the dishes, but now she really
doesn't do much of that anymore. When she feels good, she does
things, she cooks or works in the garden or helps with the housework, but it's more dependent upon how well she feels.*

Several different definitions of normal behavior and normal child-
rearing expectations and styles are in operation in these reports. Some
parents are pleased that their child does just what he or she used to do,
like their other children; other parents are pleased that their child resists
chores, just like other children; some are pleased that their child tries,
even though he or she is too sick to really accomplish chores; and other
parents struggle with their child's resistance or delayed development.

"TELLING" THE CHILD WITH CANCER

A unique child-rearing dilemma that parents of ill children face involves the need to decide what and how to tell the child with cancer
about the illness. How this issue is managed depends upon the parents'
views of the normalization process and their child-rearing values. Slavin,
O'Malley, Koocher, and Foster (1982) argue that the real issue is not
necessarily "what to tell," but what kind of emotional trust, communication, and support exists between parents and children.

Adults constantly struggle with their capacity to communicate important and complex issues, such as sex, religion, death, and illness in
ways that make sense to children. In childhood cancer no physician can
predict the impact of general advances in treatment on the health and
life of a particular patient. Since the long-term future cannot be predicted or shared with confidence or accuracy, the problem of what to
tell the child about the disease and treatment occurs within an atmosphere of uncertainty.

There are two quite different approaches to "telling" the child: the
protective approach and the open approach.[2] The protective approach

shields the young patient (and siblings) from full knowledge of the disease. In support of this policy, advocates contend that detailed knowledge of the disease and the possibility of death is likely to be harmful to the young patient because it elevates anxieties and fears, which is counterproductive to effective coping. A second rationale argues that an atmosphere of normalcy should be maintained in the family, and the frightening reality of the diagnosis/prognosis should not be allowed to interfere with a calm and supportive family life.[3] Moreover, open acknowledgment of the illness and its implications may publicize a parent's inadequacy "as a person without meaningful control over his own and his family's destinies" (Futterman & Hoffman, 1973, p. 15). By protecting children from knowledge of their illness, parents may delay their own loss of stature and authority before their children.

It is now more common, although by no means universal, for physicians to counsel open communication of a serious diagnosis/prognosis with the patient and the family, and for parents to tell their children important details of their illness and treatment. Shielding children from awareness of the diagnosis does not necessarily alleviate anxiety or fear, but may in fact heighten these emotions. Waechter argues, "The anxiety of meaningful adults is conveyed to them through an altered emotional climate in their homes and through the false cheerfulness or evasiveness of those around them" (1971, p. 1168). In a study of the long-term psychosocial adjustment of survivors of childhood malignancies, parents who did not initially disclose the diagnosis and prognosis report their "lack of candor" as a source of stress or other difficulty both during and after the treatment period (Slavin et al., 1982).[4] Some children may even conceal their own knowledge and avoid conversation in order to protect adults. As parents or the staff convey their reluctance to talk freely by avoiding or ignoring questions, changing the topic of discussion, or leaving the room, children who note these signals of unwillingness to deal with their condition may begin to practice mutual pretense.[5] Thus, children caught in a conspiracy of silence learn to accommodate to adults' needs for a charade and conceal their own needs for candor and openness.

Whereas the protective approach may be of constructive use for a short while, eventually the pretense fails and awareness generally is inevitable. Glaser and Strauss (1965) discuss how the medical staff often leaks information and Bluebond-Langner (1978) and Vernick (1973) suggest children find out about their illnesses from other children in the hospital. Young patients often talk with one another when adults (parents or nurses) are out of earshot and may compare records, medication labels, and even the specialties of attending physicians.

What Is Told? How Do Parents Deal with This Choice?

We gathered information on what parents told their children through questions such as, "What did you tell your child about his/her illness?" and "Was there anything he/she was not told?" All responses were read several times and a five-category typology was developed of the amount and type of information told to the child.[6]

Fourteen parents (19%) chose to tell their children nothing regarding the illness.

> *She was not told that she was sick or had a chronic illness. I was told by the doctor to treat her like all the other kids.*

> *Nothing. He was too ill to be told anything. If he would have asked, I still wouldn't have told him.*

Twenty-one parents (29%) provided their children with information limited to a discussion of "here and now" or day-to-day procedures and activities.

> *I just told her that she was going into the hospital for an operation to have her lump removed, etc. She was told nothing about having cancer or being ill.*

> *I didn't tell her what she had. I always told her she was going in for a big shot that would hurt a little, but would be over fast.*

> *He knew what he had to know. Whenever there was a major test that I knew was serious, I told him. I explained to him that it had to be. He just knew he was sick but he didn't know what or why.*

Sixteen parents (22%) told their children something about their illness and the reasons for various procedures, hospitalizations, and so on. However, they did not mention cancer or discuss the serious implications of the illness.

> *We told him that he had a blood disease and that he needed to have some treatments. We did not tell him the fact that he had cancer.*

> *When she was in the hospital, we used the words disease and tumor. We used tumor a lot. I mean, we weren't really lying to her, but we just told her she had a tumor.*

> *We just told him that it meant there was something in his blood that shouldn't be there, some kind of blood cell and it was bad. It*

would make him sicker if he didn't take the medication and the IV's. The medicine he got might make him sick, but that hopefully he wouldn't have to be in the hospital too long.

Twelve parents (16%) gave their children information on almost all aspects of the disease and treatment, except that they excluded discussion of death or possible death.

We decided to be truthful about the whole works. We told her everything. But we didn't say that she had a 5% chance to live. She wasn't told exactly what her chances were.

He was two years old, but we told him everything. We didn't tell him that he might die, of course. He doesn't understand that concept probably. We told him what he had was cancer and that we were going to try and make the cancer stop growing.

The doctor told her that she had a bad tumor and let it go at that. She started asking a lot of questions and then they explained to her what had to be done (amputation). They (doctors) didn't tell her that she could possibly die because we felt she couldn't handle it.

In the final category, 10 parents (14%) disclosed everything they knew to their children. Parents' reports illuminate the distinctive nature of this approach quite clearly.

We told her everything, exactly the way it was. Why hold back because she was going to hear it sooner or later. By us telling her, she wouldn't have to get it from someone else. There was nothing she was not told, as far as I know. She knew she had to cope with it and she did. Sure she was scared. I bet if someone told you that you might die, you'd be scared, too.

She heard everything from the doctors right from the beginning. There was nothing she was not told, she was old enough.

Told him the truth . . . that it was cancer and what kind it was. (Anything not told?) No!

The evidence that only 30% (22/73) of the parents responding told their children about all or almost all aspects of the disease (categories 4 and 5) suggests that despite the greater popularity of the open approach in recent professional and scholarly literature, it is not readily adopted by parents and practicing professionals. Some of the reasons or correlates of these parental choices are explored next.

Factors Related to What the Child Is Told

Table 7.1 presents correlations between parents' reports of the amount of information they told their children at the time of the diagnosis and various demographic and social factors. The age of the child at diagnosis is significantly and strongly related to the amount of information parents share with the child about the illness, treatment, and prognosis. Parents of younger children tell significantly less than parents of older children, and their comments indicate why:

We did not get into cancer and this and that because she wouldn't have been able to understand it anyway. Probably a few years later when she got a little older she could understand.

I never really told him about the cancer until he was old enough to understand.

The data further indicate that parents' gender, education, and income are not related significantly to what is told the child, but that parents' age and religion are.[7] Older parents share more information about the disease with their ill children than do younger parents; in all probability parents' ages reflect children's ages, and older parents tell more because their ill children are older. Catholic parents tell children significantly more than do Protestants, other, and nonreligiously affiliated parents.

Table 7.1
Sociodemographic Correlates of "How Much Was Told"

Sociodemographic Factor	Pearson Product-moment Correlation
Child's age[a]	.63**
Parent's age	.46**
Parent's religion (Catholic)	.31**
Number of siblings	.27*
Number of siblings over 6 years	.35**
Extent of sibling problems	.25*
Extent of support from siblings	.32*
Extent of support from social worker	.23*

*$p. < .05$
**$p. < .01$
[a]When the variables in this figure are entered as predictors in a multiple regression analysis, the child's age continues to have the most potent and significant relationship with "telling"

Detailed reading of the interviews indicates that Catholic parents often demonstrate a concrete and tightly organized cosmology or system for explaining the role of God in their experience with childhood cancer. Perhaps a more concrete image of their child's dying and "being with Jesus," or living because "God will take care of my child," helps these parents face the illness with more comfort and security; they can then act on that basis in conveying fuller information to the child.[8]

Parents with more other children tell the ill child significantly more about the disease and treatment than do parents with fewer or no other children. This relationship is especially potent when the ages of siblings are analyzed; parents with more other children over the age of six years tell significantly more to the ill child than do parents with fewer or no children over the age of six years. In addition, parents who report greater stress in their relationship with the ill child's siblings tell the ill child more about the disease, as do parents who report greater amounts of help and support from their other children.[9] Both of these findings lend additional weight to the importance of siblings in family relationships. Prior research does not identify the sibling structure as having potential impact upon the telling process. However, it is reasonable that parents with larger numbers of children would find themselves in a situation in which they must share more information. If the ill child is to be given the special attention a chronically and seriously ill child must have, siblings must be forewarned about how to behave (caution about spleenic injury and infections) and prepared for shifts in family chores and parental attention. If there are older siblings in the family, parents may share more information with these siblings simply because they are responsible family members, perhaps themselves "old enough to know" and to be of assistance in the caregiving process. Once explanations are made to siblings, parents can expect that siblings might tell or leak that information to the ill child. Thus, they may be more willing or forced to share more information about the disease or reasons for treatment with the ill child.

The amount of help and support parents report receiving from social workers also significantly relates to the amount of information they share with their child; the greater the social worker support, the more information that is shared. This relationship does not hold for parents' reports of the support they receive from doctors and nurses, however, suggesting that something unique occurs between parents and social workers. If social workers, as the most psychosocially advanced members of the medical staff, encourage or urge parents to share information more fully (within the bounds of age-related understanding), then parents who are closer to the social worker, who report receiving more support from this professional's role and activities, may be expected to tell their children more.

The "Telling" Process Changes Over Time

Decisions made at one point are remade several times as the child matures or as the disease and treatment progress. As the child's medical situation changes and new procedures are required, it may be important to share more information with the child.

> He wasn't told immediately about the potential of surgery, because at the time we weren't sure of it ourselves. But as soon as it looked like it was the operation coming up, and that we might have to make that decision, we discussed it with him.

> We were given a book that we could read parts of to him. We didn't do it right away. Eventually we talked to him and read to him about the bone marrow aspiration and the spinal tap before they had to do it to him.

Glaser and Strauss (1965) report a similar dynamic in their studies of terminally ill adult patients, noting that the need to justify or explain certain procedures often requires new sharing of information between patient, family, and attending staff. As a child suffers a relapse or enters a terminal phase, it may be necessary to share more information to prepare for forthcoming crises. As the child enters a stage of reliable remission, or is ready to go off treatment, parents may take advantage of these good times by reviewing history and providing a fuller perspective on what the child has been through or may look forward to.

As parents adjust to the crisis of diagnosis and begin to reorder their personal and family lives, they may rethink a decision to withhold information and share more about the disease; this is especially true for families characterized by an open communication pattern in general.

> We told him what he had to know when we fully digested it and understood it. It took us a while.

> At the beginning, we didn't tell him anything. The doctors said not to tell him unless he asked and we went along with this. But it made quite a strain. We would walk into his hospital room, look at each other, and not have much to say that was meaningful. Then he would turn on the TV and tune us out. If we couldn't talk about what was really happening right then and there, what was there to talk about? After a few days, we began to get our feet on the

ground and decided that he needed to be told the whole story, and
by the doctors, and that we would insist on this. We did insist, and
they told him, very nicely. As soon as they told him, our family
was able to talk together like always. He no longer turned on the
TV and we could all talk about being scared or getting ready, or
getting better, or the future, or whatever. Our family was returning
to normal even though we had this terrible new problem to deal with.

In some cases, parents are not able to control what their child is told
about the disease, especially as their child interacts with other ill children or with other social groups. Not only does sibling structure play
a key role in the telling process, information shared with grandparents
or other relatives, or conversations between relatives and the ill child,
may cause the child to raise questions that require more parental disclosure. In like fashion, classmates, neighborhood acquaintances, or
teachers may inadvertently talk about cancer in ways that advance the
child's knowledge of his/her own situation and/or make it necessary for
parents or medical staff members to share more information with the
child.[10] Thus, decisions to tell ill children about their medical condition
cannot be isolated from what is told to or known by their family and
community. "Telling" is not only a child-rearing issue, but a lifestyle
issue for both parents and children.

MANAGING THE CHILD'S RESPONSE TO THE ILLNESS

Parents of living children were asked about their child's response to
the illness. As Table 7.2 indicates, the overwhelming majority of parents
report that their child's response is positive.
A similarly positive outlook emerges in parents' responses to ques-

Table 7.2
Parents' Reports of How the Child Has Responded to the Illness

Response	Number of Parents (N=56)	Percent of Parents (100%)
Strength and courage	27	48%
Denial	6	11%
Acceptance	5	9%
Optimism and hope	3	5%
Self-pity or regression	3	5%
Other negative	6	11%
No response to the illness	6	11%

tions about whether their child is developing like others of the same age. Sixty-two percent (43/69) of the parents responding report age-appropriate psychological or emotional development. Some (13/69 or 19%) feel that the illness and how they handled it has caused their child to mature or develop more rapidly than their peers; another 13 parents (19%) feel that the illness and treatment may have a negative impact on their child's emotional development.

Some particulars of these responses are quite dramatic. As Table 7.2 indicates, the most common positive response parents note is their child's demonstration of emotional strength and courage.

> *I'm pleased with my daughter's strength and courage. She took it real well.*

> *One day my son came home and told me that he had just run "the mile." In a way I was shocked, I asked him if the other children had also run "the mile," and he said, "Oh yeah, they ran it the first week." All I could think about, was how much courage it must have taken to keep trying like that. I was very proud of him.*

> *I was pleased by my son's courage especially when he lost his hair and decided he would go to school without his hat.*

Other parents are pleased with their child's acceptance of the situation and his/her ability to continue with life.

> *I think she has accepted it.*

> *My son accepts his illness. He knows that he has cancer and that he has to live with it. He caught up on the school work he missed and he gets good marks. My son's a very strong and a very brave boy.*

One parent notes that her child struggled with depression and worry but still came through the most difficult parts of the treatment in a positive frame of mind.

> *At first my son was very scared, upset and confused. Now I think he understands his illness, and I think he is accepting it really well.*

Under such circumstances, Cook (1984) reports a central parental function is to help keep up the ill child's morale; it apparently is successful in these cases. Moreover, some of these youngsters' reactions must boost parents' morale!

Not all parents are so positive about their child's reactions. Some feel their children are emotionally quite depressed or otherwise unable to handle the situation well. As one parent noted:

This illness has really taken a toll on my daughter, I think she still gets very angry about it. She is often angry and bitter and never happy. I even feel she might be a bit suicidal.

Parents found their children's reactions especially bothersome when they regressed, were cranky, and acted spoiled. Sometimes parents are quite clear that these problems are a by-product of the child's medication.

When my son was on his medication, he was very sensitive and emotional. If you just looked at him funny, he would cry.

My daughter was very cranky for three to four days after she had her chemotherapy.

In other cases parents are unclear whether the negative behavior is the result of medication or the normal problems of growing up.

Nothing really bothers me except, like any child that has something they can use, my daughter might use her illness as an excuse to get out of something she doesn't want to do, like her homework.

This confusion about the source of problem behavior reflects the more general issue of disciplining an ill child, discussed previously.

Parents who report positive psychosocial development and reactions to the illness were asked what they do to create this response. The most common answers reflect an intense commitment to create a normal situation and to treat the child as normally as possible.

We just treated him normal . . . the same way as the other kids.

We made sure our daughter did as much as she could. She used this form of denial, telling herself that she was just like everybody else, to keep going.

We try to treat him like we always did which isn't always easy. Sometimes we tend to pamper him a little more, but in general, we try to go on like before.

Several parents suggest that open communication within the family, and with the ill child, creates bonds of trust and confidence that gives the child strength.

> *I think the reason my daughter is ahead of her age group is that we told her everything. There was nothing that she didn't know was going to happen; therefore, there was no fear of the unknown. I think that is why she was able to handle it.*

If parents can help children conquer their fear of the unknown, one of the major debilitating aspects of cancer can be brought under control.

Given parents' own fears for their children, and differing definitions of normal behavior for ill children, success in helping children deal with illness is never easy. Parents' successful child-rearing tactics often involve gentle but firm pushes for children to continue with their prior life and work. They support denial at times, but also welcome open communication and discussion. When parents treat their children as if their illness can be managed and their life can continue normally, youngsters often adopt this stance themselves.

PREPARING A CHILD FOR DEATH

For parents of children who die, unique child-rearing issues develop. Foremost among these are the ways in which parents talk about or prepare terminally ill children for death. Parents of deceased children were asked if their children had ever asked them if they were going to die and how they had answered this question.

A number of parents indicate that they were honest and direct with their children; while they encouraged the child to have hope, they were ready to face together the reality that the child was going to die.

> *A week or so before my son's death I told him bluntly, "Son, you're dying." We never held anything back from him. I don't think there's any benefit in lying. My son would have been tremendously disappointed in me if I hadn't told him the truth.*

> *We learned to "open the door" so that whenever my daughter wanted to talk we were there. It always ended dramatically but the door was always open.*

In addition to being honest with their children about impending death, some parents tried to pacify their children's fears by telling them that they would be going to heaven and would no longer be in pain.

I told my son that if he died he would go to heaven and that he would be able to see me but I wouldn't be able to see him. I also read him the book The Smallest Angel.

We always used to go visit our relative in the cemetery. When my daughter found out that she was dying, she wanted to know if we could move next to the cemetery. I think she said this because if we lived close to the cemetery we could visit her often. I told her that it was not bad to die and that she would go to a beautiful place and there would be no more pain. I think just talking about it helped her.

Some parents, on the other hand, denied the seriousness of their child's condition or didn't know that their child's illness was terminal until shortly before the child's death. These parents generally did not prepare their children for what lay ahead.

She would say things like "I'm not afraid to die, but I wish I didn't have to leave you all." My response was to cry. I told her that nobody knows for sure when they are going to die and that she should just proceed with her life. Medically, I knew that she was going to die, but I just kept hoping for a miracle that would save her.

I didn't realize the extent of my son's illness until five months before he died. Most of the time, we didn't know that he was going to die.

Several parents report that they didn't prepare their child for death because their child was just too young to understand the concept of death or because they didn't want to frighten the child.

She was never told that she was going to die because she wasn't old enough to understand death.

We never told our daughter that she was going to die. She loved life so much that if she knew she was going to die she would have died much sooner.

It appears that the age of the child, as well as the degree to which the parents themselves prepare for their child's death, are key variables in determining how parents of children with childhood cancer deal with this issue.[11] Sometimes older siblings, with or without their parents' knowledge, also play critical roles in teaching terminally ill children how to behave and in preparing them for death.[12]

CONCLUSIONS: PROMISES AND MEMORIES

Children represent the future; for parents, children often represent their own unrealized futures, their own promises and hopes. Parents of seriously ill children find that promise threatened. As they rear their children, as they imagine their children's futures, and as they reflect upon their children's pasts, the illness constantly reminds them of the limits of that promise.

Parents of children living with cancer consider the future from a variety of viewpoints. Some parents, because their children are doing well or because they themselves are optimistic, approach the future with positive images of normal lifelines and careers. When asked, for instance, about their images of their child's future, several parents respond in these terms:

> *He's got the right personality and is a pretty all around kid, able to handle his handicap and everything.*

> *I am sure she will lead a normal life. She is a leader, not a follower, and so whatever she wants to do, she will do.*

Other parents feel their child is well ahead of other children and has an especially bright future.

> *I think of him becoming someone who will help others . . . he's a very loving child.*

> *She will grow into being a very beautiful and talented young lady, being very strong from the experiences that we've gone through. There might be some discrimination because of her illness, but I don't have any fears as far as what her strengths are. She's different, she really is, and she's going to be very successful.*

Other parents express worries or fears regarding the future.

> *He's going to have a hard time, that's for sure. His learning capacity is low and he is lacking.*

> *His career choices will be limited because of the problems of getting insurance and possible physical disabilities.*

And some parents think of the child's future with dread.

> *I just want her to get far enough to have a future.*

Death. I see death in the future for him.

I hope she finishes college. She feels she is a freak and her future is limited. It is very sad.

These hopes and fears are all realistic. Just as the first set of parents expresses their hopes for normalcy and the second set their grand hopes, the third set presents their realistic concerns and the fourth set their deep anxieties and fears. All are real. Their juxtaposition reflects the dilemma facing parents of children with cancer – great hope and promise versus great fear and anxiety.

Parents of children who have died of cancer no longer have these promises or these fears. However, they do have memories of their children and of their children's struggles with cancer and with life itself. We asked these parents to describe their deceased child. Some indicate that the child was just like everyone else:

Happy, cheerful, regular young kid.

She was a very quiet child. She liked doing things with her hands and making things to hang on the wall.

But some parents remember their children as quite unusual, outstanding in many ways:

He was very bright and intelligent. He was a marvelous little boy, superb in everything.

She was an unusual child in many ways. She had a winning personality with both adults and children and was an excellent student. She had received many college scholarships, was an accomplished musician, a cheerleader, and tended to help the underdog.

He was the kind of child you wished everyone had. He didn't demand anything and was a very happy boy. Everyone loved him.

One parent states, "God makes them better," and others suggest that God only picks out the strong and the beautiful for this travail.

Why is it that so many parents of children with cancer speak with such respect of their child's coping, of their strength, of the courage of those who are still living, and of the beauty of those who have died? Are parents unrealistic in their hopes and memories? Are the parents of children who have died preserving their memories in a selective fashion, thus memorializing their children? Are the parents of living children looking at their offspring through rose-colored glasses? Or is there something in children that comes out under trying circumstances that is very impressive?

Perhaps it is the sheer enormity of the illness that children with cancer must deal with that so impresses parents and other adults. After all, these children face a threat that adults can only imagine and thus may fantasize. As they continue to live, or even as they die, perhaps their suffering and their struggle draw adults to them. Small victories may loom large, and these children may seem larger than life to those who love and care for them. Involvement in their struggle may require adults to acknowledge and deal with existential dilemmas and deep feelings of hope and tragedy that are generally avoided.

One test of effective child rearing is whether parents feel good about their children and, on reflection, about their own roles as parents. Although these parents of children with cancer are not able to protect their children from this disease, or even in some instances from death, they are able to help them cope with it. And although they are not always happy with their own child-rearing efforts in the midst of the disease and treatment, they are generally quite positive about the ways their children cope with the illness. They "like" their children, often respect them, and sometimes are in awe of their strength and beauty through great travail. What better measure of effective child rearing could there be?

CHAPTER NOTES

1. The great popularity of experts, media presentations, and books on child rearing may be helpful, but they also testify to the fragile confidence many adults have about their parental functions.

2. The relative merits of these two approaches have been debated on both theoretical and practical grounds, with the open approach gaining greater popularity in recent years. The general issues are well advocated and summarized in Bluebond-Langner (1978), Evans (1968), Share (1972), and Slavin, O'Malley, Koocher, and Foster (1982).

3. These rationales for the protective approach can be found in Howell (1966), Morrissey (1965), Plank (1964), Sigler (1970), and Toch (1964).

4. Several authors report that those children who were aware of their diagnosis or prognosis, but whose parents did not want them to know about it, experienced additional loneliness and isolation as a result of this lack of communication. Thus, when trust may be vital, parent-child reluctance to discuss the vital facts of diagnosis may make it difficult to talk about anything else important (Binger et al., 1969; Bluebond-Langner, 1974; Karon & Vernick, 1968; Showalter, 1970; Spinetta, 1974; Spinetta, Rigler, & Karon, 1973; 1974; Vernick & Karon, 1965; Yudkin, 1967).

5. Bluebond-Langner (1978) and Glaser and Strauss (1965) discuss the dynamics of mutual pretense.

6. Three raters read all responses and initially agreed on which of five categories was appropriate in 78% of the cases. Outstanding disagreements were resolved by discussion among the raters.

7. Education and income approach statistical significance but do not achieve it. Other research suggests educational level should be related to telling, because more highly educated parents can be expected to read more of the popular and technical information about medical and psychosocial aspects of the disease. However, the data do not support this speculation.

8. As noted (Chapters 3 and 5), a strong religious or theological orientation may provide parents with a stable explanation for their child's illness, a clear sense of where responsibility for the prognosis lies, and a comforting view of death, should it occur. Other scholars address the positive importance of a theological or existential explanation for parents' own coping and adjustment, although they do not relate this to a particular religious orientation nor to the dynamics of sharing information (Spinetta, Swarner, & Sheposh, 1981).

9. The significance of both sibling problems and sibling support repeats a theme discussed in Chapter 6 (see pp. 126–127 and note 4).

10. These dynamics, especially potent for older children, are why Glaser and Strauss (1965) argue that secrecy, or the protective approach, is an inherently unstable condition.

11. Our sample of parents of deceased children is not large enough to determine statistically age-related influences on the process of preparation. However, it appears that parents who are most open about death are dealing with older children, and that this openness increases as the terminal phase of the illness advances.

12. In one family of a deceased child, the parents both report that they did not discuss death with their young son. The ill boy's older brother and sister, however, report (in separate interviews) that they often discussed death with the terminally ill child. They did not do this within their parents' hearing because they knew such a conversation would be upsetting to their parents. This loving family eventually shared with one another this information about their different approaches to death preparation.

CHAPTER 8

Being a Child with Cancer

Although childhood cancer is a shared stress to which families develop coordinated responses, the illness affects the child differently than it does other family members. In this chapter we focus on ill children, especially adolescents, and the ways they describe and respond to this challenge.[1] Adolescence, in particular, is a trying time of life for most young persons, a time when adjustment to a changing body, relationships with peers of the same or different gender, growing independence from parents, and career futures present paramount struggles (Havighurst, 1951). Having cancer and dealing with the stresses of cancer often make it especially hard to cope with each of these developmental tasks (Kellerman & Katz, 1977).

The most recent literature on children's and adolescents' experiences with cancer has put to rest earlier concerns about psychological abnormality. Studies indicate that most children with cancer are as psychologically normal as physically healthy children. Of course, some ill children have emotional and psychological problems, but so do some physically healthy children. Tavormina, Kastner, Slater, and Watt (1976) reach a conclusion, based on research with youngsters with a wide range of illnesses, that is shared by many contemporary scholars and practitioners:[2]

The normalcy rather than the deviance of these children (was demonstrated). Although exceptions were noted, the children's functional strengths and coping abilities noticeably outweighed their weaknesses. (p. 99)

Moreover, Koocher and O'Malley (1981) indicate that long-term survivors of childhood cancer are generally well adjusted to their adult
roles, with only a small percentage experiencing serious psychological
distress or needing professional treatment for emotional problems. Recent work (Teta et al., 1984) also indicates that the frequency of a major
depressive syndrome is no greater for children with cancer than for their
siblings, and that values for both groups are quite similar to values for
a nonill population.[3] How does this come about? How do youngsters
with this terrible illness manage to be relatively well adjusted?

COPING WITH THE STRESSES OF
CHILDHOOD CANCER ... YOUNGSTERS' VIEWS

Figure 8.1 presents the composite of 17 adolescents' stress charts,
(filled out in accordance with instructions noted in Chapter 2 and parallel
to parents' charts, Figures 2.3 through 2.8). Whereas adolescents' charts
often indicate the same strong stresses as their parents' charts (i.e.,
diagnosis, surgery, relapse), they also specify hair loss and school reentry as powerful psychosocial events. Whereas these events certainly
matter for parents, they are much more potent for youngsters.

As with parents (Chapters 2 and 3), two categories of stress appear
in our own and others' research with children and adolescents with
cancer: those with an immediate medical focus and those with a psycho-

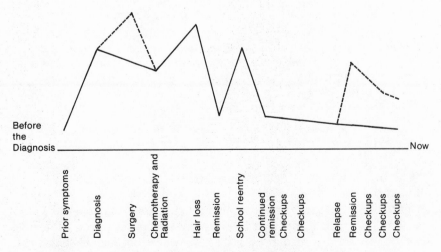

Figure 8.1. Composite stress chart for adolescents with cancer

social focus. In the following list of stresses that youngsters identify, the first two relate primarily to the medical situation and its threats and necessary adjustments, and the latter three relate to relations with the external social world:

1. Understanding the diagnosis, prognosis, and treatment;
2. Adapting to treatment and side effects, including pain and fears of death;
3. Relating to the medical staff;
4. Relating with one's family and peers;
5. Dealing with two worlds – illness and health, specialness and normalcy.

Understanding the Diagnosis, Prognosis, and Treatment

At the diagnostic stage and immediately thereafter children may experience stress in understanding the seriousness of the situation and in dealing with uncertainty. How do children become aware that they are in a serious situation, that they have a condition they ought to worry about? Sometimes parents or staff members tell them directly (Chapter 7). But information may be incomplete or delayed. Then the child draws a conclusion using many cues (such as parental distress) and reading between the lines of what is said directly and what is whispered out of earshot. Many children note the rapidity and drama with which they are hospitalized; siblings are allowed to stay home from school in order to be at the hospital, grandparents travel long distances to come to the bedside, and friends and relatives visit in large numbers.

> *I had been sitting in my doctor's waiting room for about 30 minutes when my mother came out, her eyes red and watery, looking slightly swollen. I knew that she and my pediatrician had been talking about me and the symptoms I'd been having. I knew from her look that something serious was up.*

> *I knew it was serious when my dad, who is divorced from my mom, started to come around a lot more than he used to.*

Children's initial anxiety often is exacerbated when they are not allowed to be active participants in discussions of their illness. In the absence of adequate information, children may fantasize an even worse scenario. As Orr, Hoffmans, and Bennetts (1984, p. 50) note, adolescents report that "they immediately feared the worst because they did not know what was wrong with them." These researchers and the adolescents with whom they talked recommend early and full disclosure of the diagnosis in clear and supportive ways.

Zeltzer (1978) and Koocher and O'Malley (1981) suggest that of all the coping strategies used by adolescents with cancer, information seeking and denial seem to be the most common. Information seeking, which is closely related to the psychological defense mechanism of intellectualization, is an attempt to manage stress by cognitive mastery, by learning enough about it to establish a sense of intellectual control and by being able to convey the nature of the illness to others. Denial as a coping strategy involves the avoidance of information or experience that may unnecessarily increase one's anxiety about the illness. Both strategies represent efforts to deal with information and its emotional meaning. Although each has the potential to help the child respond positively to the stress of the illness and treatment, overuse or extreme forms of each strategy have negative potential. Information seeking may lead to understanding, but information overload may lead to a lack of attention to feelings that accompany facts. Denial may prevent great anxiety and permit the youngster to continue to live normally, but its overuse may lead to a premature cessation of caution and medical compliance (Katz & Jay, 1984).

Marten (1980) and Geist (1979) write that intellectualization, as a common coping strategy for older adolescents, leads many to become interested in studying biology and psychology. One youngster reports his attempt to cope with Hodgkin's disease by studying it.

Oh, yes, I've read a lot. Last year I did a research project on what it was and how long it would last. It'll stay with you for about twenty years. I also learned how dangerous it was and the risk involved. It was quite eye opening.

The pages of the Candlelighter's Childhood Cancer Foundation's Youth Newsletter are often filled with youngsters' efforts to write about and to make intellectual sense out of their disease and struggle.[4]

In contrast, other youngsters use denial to cope with the same kinds of issues. Lazarus (1981a) notes the prevalence of this strategy and argues that under some conditions it is a very successful way of coping with great uncertainty and fear.[5]

Actually I never really think about it and I don't care to read about it.

A relapse is not going to happen! So I am not going to worry about it.

Younger children, especially, are more successful in using denial than are their parents. Some youngsters even ask their parents to stop asking questions or to stop talking to them about their cancer.

As noted, denial can be carried too far.

Unfortunately, I dealt with it the wrong way, wanting to be like everyone else. I made the mistake of trying to pretend there was nothing wrong with me.

Most youngsters who utilize denial do not carry it to such extremes.

Adapting to Treatment-Induced Side Effects and Fears

As treatment progresses, the seriousness of the situation may be brought home to the child by drastic medical procedures. Surgery, chemotherapy, radiation, repeated hospitalization, tests, and injections all debilitate the child physically and emotionally. In addition to pain, the illness and the side effects of treatment disrupt family life, school attendance, and friendships. Zeltzer et al. (1980) indicate that youngsters with cancer feel that their illness has a greater impact on their lives than do youngsters with other chronic or serious illnesses (e.g., diabetes, cystic fibrosis, cardiac problems). In particular, they emphasize disruption because of treatments that are "worse than the disease" (p. 134).[6]

Radiation and chemotherapy produce a number of painful side effects (Seltzer, 1983):

A feeling of nausea starts churning in my stomach. Not an uncommon feeling. I lie there just feeling numb. A medical student comes in to examine me. I feel like his homework, not a person, and I cannot even gather the strength to tell him. He pokes, looks, listens, and finally leaves. Now the nausea has increased. I feel it down in my toes and up to my ears. I reach for the familiar pan and begin my routine. It doesn't even upset me anymore. I've grown too used to it. My mother takes away the pan filled with clear bile. I don't even have that bad taste in my mouth. I just lie back and shut my eyes. Do I feel relieved? No, I never do, the feeling comes back too quickly. I know it will. (p. 3)

Young children, especially, describe the illness and treatment in terms of the needles, chemotherapy, infusion pumps, cat scans, bone marrow aspirations, and complex machinery.

Many children cope by using self-control procedures that minimize anxiety, pain, and discomfort. Some report the use of progressive relaxation techniques, in which they imagine pleasant scenes and do deep-breathing exercises to remain calm during spinal taps, bone marrow tests, or chemotherapy. Many articles describe the use of hypnosis and other behavioral techniques as part of regular program for youngsters undergoing aversive procedures.[7] Establishing an active and self-controlling posture over medical or hospital routines also aids adolescents' needs to feel independent and autonomous in the face of medically forced helplessness and passivity.

Chemotherapeutic and radiologic treatments sometimes make children feel as if their bodies are not their own. Their well-remembered physical responses often are thrown out of kilter by the mood-changing and physique-altering effects of drugs. Changes in body image stem from both the physical effects of treatment and the wrenching feeling that there is an internal battle going on between good cells and bad cells.[8] Orr et al. (1984) note that, for some adolescents, changes in their appearance are even more troublesome than the pain of treatments. One youngster's comment upon the impact of hair loss emphasizes this embarrassment (Pendleton, 1980):

> *I hated being bald. I hated wearing my wig. I hated talking to anyone about it. I wore my wig, outwardly pretending it was my hair, but hating it. I only let a few select people see me without my wig on. A year later I quit college after one quarter because my hair had started falling out again and I was afraid it would all go — I chose to quit rather than wear a wig. (p. 127)*

Other youngsters facing this issue adapt differently (Pendleton, 1980):

> *For a while there, losing my hair really got to me. Nobody wants to lose his hair. But I got to thinking that there are so many people who lose an arm or a leg or maybe even their eyesight. Your hair can always come back. Eyesight can't. That's the way I looked at it, and I was able to say, Okay, I'm thankful I've got my arms and my legs. And I don't have to lose them.*

> *My hair fell out about two weeks after chemotherapy. It was real thin anyway, so it didn't really take much to fall out. But my parents didn't let me have the mirror, and when I finally got them to, it was not really that bad. It was just the first shock of it. (p. 126)*

Loss of hair and consequent baldness generally are more traumatic for girls than for boys, and for older children than for younger children.

An adolescent describes in some detail how he began to cope with the amputation of his leg because of osteogenic sarcoma:

The doctor came in and knelt down and talked to my parents, who were sitting next to me, real quietly for about a half hour. Then he rose up and told me that they had to amputate my leg. I asked him what amputate meant. He explained it, and then it hit me. I cried for about five minutes and then calmed down. That night my parents stayed with me. That night I started making fun of my leg and doing certain things to it because I thought it was coming off anyway. My mom and dad told me to stop it. When they put me back into my bed after recovery, they put me on my right side. I reached for my leg and couldn't feel it and I started to scream. It still seems like a dream or a real long nightmare that I haven't woke up from, but you have to face facts and deal with it. It's weird having it happen so fast.

Of all the treatment-related issues that children with cancer find difficult, the unremitting, continuous, prolonged course of treatment, having to "deal with it from week to week," is most debilitating. There is no respite, no escape from the inevitable series of events.

You think, wow, twenty-four of these to go, and I'm on number one, and I have twenty-three to go. It was just tough. Once over the hill, it doesn't get any easier, every week, at least not for me. It's something I had to get all psyched up for and I had a lot of trouble. I was getting sick beforehand, before I get it, so Godawful sick. I knew I was going to get sick, but there was nothing I could do about it. So my subconscious, with sympathetic nerves, took over. They couldn't give me anything. I was getting sick before they even gave the medicine to me.

The thing that people don't take into consideration or don't realize is that you have to live with it every single day, twenty-four hours a day of your life. There is nothing you can do about it. This is part of you, now, and there are times when you'll be down, and people just don't realize why.

In addition to prolonged discomfort, frequent hospitalizations or confinement at home often lead to social isolation. Although most children with cancer experience a great deal of attention at first, some feel forgotten and eventually isolated.

I got flowers all the time, just hundreds of cards, and visitors all the time. It brightens every day a little bit. Then it slowly diminishes off and off and off and soon nobody comes.

Over time, the cumulative discomfort of prolonged treatment, and the gradual isolation from friends, may lead to hopelessness and despair. About 10 months into treatment, continued illness and the miseries of monthly hospitalization caused Val's spirits and will to live to ebb dramatically. She became depressed, rebellious, angry, and bitter – all common reactions among childhood cancer patients. As she reported in a series of interviews (V. Nelcamp, 1980):

"As my veins 'ran out,' so did my patience," Val admitted. "I began to get irritable and hyper a couple of days before I had to go back to the hospital. At any comment about going back, I'd burst into tears and say, 'I won't go and you can't make me.' On the way to the hospital I'd get nauseous. I was angry at my parents for making me go through all that without giving me a choice. I thought no one cared about how much I suffered – not my parents, not the doctor, no one.

"That was my darkest time," Val said. "I felt I couldn't go on. What was the use of living, if it was all pain and suffering? Much later I realized that my vision had been narrowed by the pain. The doctors didn't exactly discourage me, but they didn't encourage me either. The interns were often insensitive and insisted on trying veins I knew were 'no good.' I began to panic whenever one approached to draw blood or start an IV. I know now that the doctors do care about their patients, but I still wish they could be a little more empathetic with them.

"I was also upset that after being away from school for a year it was time to go back," Val continued. "I was petrified of returning. I had left high school as a sophomore with two legs and would return as a junior with one leg. That in itself is 'mind-blowing' for a teen. Dad had told the principal why I wouldn't be coming to school, so everyone knew that I'd had cancer and had had a leg amputated. I worried that I would be a spectacle – stared at and whispered about. I secretly worried about whether the boys and girls would still like me. I desperately hoped the kids would realize that amputation of my leg didn't mean I'd changed inside. I remember thinking bitterly, 'If I can accept myself as an amputee, others certainly have no right to do less. I'm the one who has to face the reality of amputation everyday, not them.'" (p. 16)

Youngsters who respond well to initial treatment, and who surmount the side effects of treatment, often feel quite well. When they are in remission they generally are able to resume a full schedule of activities. Although over 90% of children with cancer enter this state of remission, almost half suffer a relapse, a reemergence of their disease at some time. Some youngsters deny the possibility of a relapse, whereas others openly discuss their feelings about it:

I've thought about that a couple of times. It would be tough. I don't know how I'd react. Right now I can forget about it. It would probably upset me more than the first time, because I'd start to figure maybe I'd never get rid of it.

Yes, I've worried about a relapse but I put it off. I go to the hospital every three months now. I really do worry about it now because I would hate to have to go through all the treatment again.

As the amount of time spent in treatment increases, children inevitably experience the death of other children whom they have befriended. These deaths bring home very clearly the life-threatening nature of their own illness. One young girl was devastated when another young girl with whom she shared a hospital room died. She had hoped and believed earnestly that they would survive the illness together. The fragility of her own life became apparent when she realized that death could affect her as well. Several youngsters discuss their concerns about death (Pendleton, 1980):

It's terrifying. I think about how it could just start spreading faster and faster and just take me like that. The best part about having it is that you have a half-and-half chance of living. You can be treated, and hopefully, it could go away. I can't just give up, though. I haven't seen everything I want to see, and I thought this cancer was going to keep me from doing things. But it hasn't. Everywhere I go, I want to keep a smile on everybody's face for me. I want them to know me. I wouldn't want to die and have them say, "Who was he?" At night I lay there thinking about where I'm going to go when I die. I'm like some kind of walking time bomb. I make my peace with Him everyday.

Anybody who has a terminal illness will tell you that dying is something that goes through your mind a hundred times a day. You're always thinking that maybe they'll do something about it. Maybe they won't. It makes you more aware of things like the Jerry Lewis Telethon to help people out who are pretty much in the same boat. You feel more charitable toward people.

It makes you realize that you haven't got much time left and what you do now they're going to remember you by. That helps out. You want to make each day nice. The way I see it, you just live for today. (pp. 156–157)

We do not know how these children dealt with the imminence of approaching death, but their clarity and straightforward approach, in these conversations, represent a powerful coping strategy.

Relating to the Medical Staff

In addition to adapting to the disease and its treatments, children with cancer also experience stress arising from relationships with staff members and medical personnel. In general, youngsters desire the same relational qualities with their doctors and nurses as those reported by their parents (Chapter 4). Orr and his colleagues report (1984, p. 53): "Physicians were expected (by adolescents) to be open, honest, non-judgmental, and respectful, and to include the patient in the formulation of treatment plans." In contrast, Zeltzer (1978) reports what ill adolescents *do not want* from their physicians, what they indicate are characteristics of the least trusted and most disliked physician:

1. *One who is dishonest ("He lies to you or doesn't tell you the whole truth").*
2. *One who talks only to parents and excludes the adolescent ("as if you were a kid and didn't matter! After all, it's my body!")*
3. *One who seems uncaring or distant ("I don't think my doctor likes me; he never talks to me; he only looks at my chart").*
4. *One who acts in an authoritarian manner ("My doctor is so bossy; he's always telling me what to do; he should join the army!").*
5. *One who uses scare-tactics to insure patient compliance ("Doctors are so dumb! They think that if they tell you you'll lose your leg if you don't take good care of your diabetes, that that'll make you test your urine! That just makes me so scared that I try to forget I even have diabetes!"). (p. 249)*

When physicians are distant from and lack communication with young patients, ill children may feel like nonpersons. Adolescents' reflections reinforce this interpretation (Pendleton, 1980):

I really don't like it when the interns stand outside the door talking. They don't stand outside my door and talk about me, but they stand there talking about somebody, and I know that at one of those doors they're talking about me.

In the hospital they really take away your personality. They take away your clothes, your privacy, they decide your schedule, when you take a bath, when you eat. All the bars are down. And if they don't explain anything, it can be really traumatic. You feel like an object that's out of order the doctors are trying to figure out. (p. 112)

Young men and women do not lose their personal or sexual identity when they enter a hospital. The protection of privacy and modesty, no matter how hard to come by, is especially essential for young people whose bodies are being assaulted by a disease and its treatments.

Youngsters' critical comments about their doctors and/or nurses do not mean they are generally disappointed or dissatisfied with the medical staff. Formal and informal reports are filled with young patients' expressions of respect, gratitude, and even love for their caregivers. However, they also want a full relationship and often seek ways to personalize medical transactions. When staff members respond with personal overtures, or obvious demonstrations of caring, they are appreciated.

Young patients' attempts to influence or actively manage their relationships with the medical staff take many forms. One adolescent woman reports that she deliberately prepares for her clinic appointment as if she were preparing for a school test, an athletic event, or a date.

> *One thing that I like to do when I go in is to make myself look good and talk good and feel good and stuff. I think I want the doctors and nurses to also think I look good, and that at least I'm here for something and something good is happening.*

This young woman does not intend to fool the medical staff but to have an impact upon the relationship. Her strategy is to behave as a good patient—as obedient, as "up" for treatment, and as a success.[9]

Another way to have impact on the staff members is to treat them with humor. Indeed, on occasion the staff is the target of biting humor (Pendleton, 1980).

> *This new nurse came on the floor one night. I wanted to kind of break her in. So I poured apple cider in the urinal, and when she came in to take it, I pulled it out from under the sheet and held it up to the light. Then I said, "Gee, looks kinda cloudy. Better send it through the filter again," and drank it. That wiped her out.* (p. 112)

One young man and his father drew pictures or mazes on his pelvis when it came time for a bone marrow aspiration. These drawings were designed to lead the staff to the right spot for needle entry, but often contained humorous messages that the staff began to look forward to reading. Such efforts to cope with the anxiety of medical procedures and relationships place the patient-jokester in the posture of an active and assertive person, rather than that of a passive victim.

For adolescents, the desire for a more personal and interactive relationship with the medical staff often has a special importance. As teenagers draw away from dependence upon their parents they often wish to relate directly with medical staff members – to make their own appointments, to monitor their own drug dosages, to receive information directly and to select their own physicians and treatment sites (Chesler & Anderson, 1985). As older adolescents, or young adults, struggle to achieve independence from their families, the medical system should adopt approaches that support this growth, that treat them as young adults, and that avoid keeping them in a dependent or passive relationship.

Relating with Family Members and Peers

The research literature suggests that seriously ill youngsters tend to become more dependent upon their parents, at least temporarily.[10] For young children this may be an extension of preexisting dependency. For adolescents, however, it may involve regression from a new-found independence into a prior dependent relationship. Several adolescents discuss their feelings about this change in their relations with their parents (Deasy-Spinetta, 1981):

When I was first diagnosed my mom came every single time I went to the clinic. When I turned 19, I told her, "That's it, right here; I'm going alone and you can't come." She accepted it. I still have a problem. She is overprotective. She's always telling me to take my medicine, to come home early. The other day I came to the clinic on a Wednesday instead of Friday because the doctors wanted to check me. I called her from campus and told her where I was going. She panicked. She called the clinic; she called the main hospital searching for me. "Was I ok? Did I arrive at the clinic safely?" So there is really no way I can tell my mom to let me handle things myself. No matter what I do, she will always be on top of me to try to protect me.

I lived away from home for two-and-a-half years before I was diagnosed. I was used to taking care of myself. I did my own wash; I cooked; I handled my finances. Then I came home and had to be taken care of. It was a real drag. I wanted to do things for myself but couldn't. It really had me down. I talked it over a few times with my parents because I thought I was being a drag on them, but we worked it out just by talking it through. I had to accept the fact that I had to be taken care of for a while. (p. 193).

As youngsters and their parents try to deal with or to discuss the illness with one another, they sometimes discover that they have quite different coping strategies. Just as symmetry in coping strategies is an important factor in spousal interaction, it affects child-parent interaction as well. Parents may want to discuss issues with their children that the children do not wish to discuss, or vice-versa. Parents also may express emotional distress quite differently than their children. One young person reports this conflict:

> *My parents wanted to talk more, and they were not as calm as I was. I still find it hard to talk to them about certain things.*

Other youngsters report that when they and their parents both are ready to talk they do so easily and at the same emotional level.

Some young people with cancer also desire to protect their parents. Perhaps out of guilt for what their parents are going through, or perhaps just because they can see how upset their parents are, youngsters may try to shield them from some of the things they themselves worry about.

> *I try not to show my parents when I'm uneasy about going for checkups. When I start to worry they start to worry.*

> *My mother gets upset easily, and I was worried about her driving home from the doctor's office.*

> *You hate to tell them some things because you know it's going to get them upset. You even put on a front for your folks sometimes.*

In addition to dealing in new ways with ones' parents, youngsters with cancer recognize that their illness has an effect on their younger brothers and sisters. Comments from ill youngsters often confirm many parents' reports (Chapter 7) that their brothers and sisters feel left out, get less attention, and feel jealous:

> *Jealousy was a big thing. My little sister said, "You never give me as much attention when I'm sick as you do when Harriet's sick"; and "She got all the attention and I should get it now." I remember there were so many fights over that. It's not my fault I have leukemia.*

> *I think she felt that I was getting a lot of attention. She also thinks that I'm lazy and that I expect everybody to give me attention.*

Other youngsters report their siblings' deep caring and concern, and ways in which they are comforted by their brothers' or sisters' reactions.

This is especially characteristic of relationships with older siblings, who sometimes adopt a parental role toward the child with cancer.

They all know it's very serious. I can talk to them all about it. They were worried that I wouldn't come home from the hospital.

They're glad that I'm better. They're not upset about special treatment or anything because it would have happened to them if they were sick.

These heartfelt concerns and reactions are as much a part of the ill child's family experience as both the jealousy they create and the special responsibilities they bear for informing and reducing their sibling's fears.[11]

Among the coping strategies youngsters use that help them deal with their illness is open communication with family members and friends. Those who do not engage in open communication often feel that their problems are exacerbated.

At first I did not talk about having cancer with anyone, and I mean anyone, my closest friends, my brother and sister, even my parents. Unfortunately, although I was glad at the time, most people sensed my attitude and did not bring up the subject in my presence. But not talking about it was some mistake because everyone knew I was sick. I wore a wig, I was absent from school, I was pale and skinny and there was no hiding from it. Yet, not talking made things worse. People did not know how to deal with me and so they spread rumors and whispered behind my back, and all the while I tried to pretend nothing was happening. But, I hurt inside — more than I can ever describe, and more than I would ever let myself feel.

Relationships outside the family, particularly with friends, often are a source of stress. Frustration and pain from social isolation and stigmatization by peers are captured in youngsters' comments:

I don't mind sitting home and watching TV all day. Sometimes I just want to do something with somebody. When I get done with chemo I want to move into a dorm so bad so that I can just be with people. I think that my last year in high school was really bad. I didn't like it. . . . Hearing my friends talk about going to the show and them not asking me, just stuff like that. That you are standing right there and they're all talking about it but it's too hard for them to turn and say, "Hey, do you want to go too?"

I think a lot of them were afraid of me. I know a lot of them were because that's what a couple of the guys said. The girls were just scared to death of me. I think they were scared that I was going to give it to them or something.

Zeltzer et al. (1980) report that youngsters with cancer are most likely, compared to adolescents with other illnesses, to report that the illness decreases their popularity with peers. This may be in part the result of chronic and repeated hospitalizations that decrease access to their peers. However, it may also relate to the stigma of cancer and to ill youngsters' experiences (or fears) of rejection.

Issues in peer relations arise early, often at the point of diagnosis. Just as parents must decide what to tell their children about the diagnosis, youngsters with cancer must decide if, when, and how to share this information with their friends. An even more delicate issue is what and how much to say about their illness to new acquaintances. Two young women discuss sharing information about their diagnosis with their friends:

I try to keep it quiet. I don't tell people unless they ask or inquire about it. It changes a relationship because people shy away and don't want to talk about it or don't know how to.

This one friend of mine was worried and didn't know what to do. She didn't come to see me much and that bothered me and that bothered her. Now I don't say anything about it unless I'm explaining something. Like the other day I told someone I had leukemia. She said, "I didn't know that." And I said, "I know you didn't know." I don't walk around with a label on my head saying I AM A LEUKEMIC.

How do friends react? According to adolescents' reports some friends are scared, run away, and back off. The loneliness and hurt created by friends who are scared and pull back is described clearly by a teenage girl:

When I went back to school last year for my senior year I was closer to my teachers. I couldn't get close to any of my old friends. I got close to one new girl who was a junior. She had never been my friend but she started asking me questions and talking to me. But the girls who were my closest friends from when I was in seventh grade were scared. I always felt they were scared of me so they wouldn't talk with me. If I tried to talk with them they would back away. Last year was the worst year of my life in school because I've always had friends and then for all those friends to just back away . . . it's hard.

One young man with cancer wrote a paper for school in which he returned to his elementary school friends of three years earlier and asked them how they had reacted to his illness.

> *Friend A said: "I was out of touch with it because you weren't in school. It didn't seem real, and I didn't know much about leukemia so I didn't really understand. I was worried about you but was also worried about myself. If something like that could happen to you then it could also happen to me."*
>
> *Friend B said: "When I found out you were sick, I was shocked and confused. I didn't know much about leukemia, just that it was a type of cancer. Again I asked myself, 'Why?' Cancer had taken my mother and was now threatening my best friend. The thought of not seeing you never crossed my mind. Not only did I try to offer my support to you, but to your parents and younger sister."*
>
> *Friend C said: "I was very surprised and didn't know much about the disease except that it was serious. I was worried because I didn't know about the cures that they had discovered. I couldn't understand why this guy was given this serious disease, and I thought that if he could get it, then why couldn't everyone else? I had never come in contact with someone so young getting a serious disease without any warning, but knew of people who were born with diseases, or old people getting them, but not someone whose life had already started, whose life was just like mine. I was then told more about it, and found out that you were doing very well, and that you felt better."*
>
> *Friend D said: "I was very scared when I found out you had leukemia. I thought you would die and didn't know how to talk to you about it. I asked my parents about it, and they said leukemia was hard to control. The thought of not seeing you again was very scary to me and when I would come over to visit you, you seemed very depressed. It was hard to talk to you and I was afraid of saying the wrong thing."*

Faced with such varied reactions, youngsters with cancer may lose confidence because of their uncertainty about whether and how they will be accepted. When loss of opportunities for social interaction with peers is severe, it is experienced as a major deprivation that multiplies other stresses of the illness. When positive interaction with peers occurs, it helps ease the stress of coping with the illness and renews youngsters' adaptive capacities.

Some young people become emotionally very close to one other person on whom they rely heavily. A teenager reports how she received great support from her boyfriend who remained with her throughout the ordeal. In fact, because the boyfriend lived closer to the treatment setting, her parents permitted her to stay with his family.

I was only going with Henry for two months when I got sick, but he stayed with me through the whole thing. I don't know why he stayed, we've talked about it. He says, "I know what's inside you and I didn't want the scars from what happened to you to change how I felt." He's really different. He is mature, he took care of his parents' business since he was 14. He's been like a rock throughout this. When I first started going home I had a lot of trouble with my mom because she wanted to be there, she wanted to be that rock instead of Henry. With my mom being sick, I felt that I couldn't do that to her. I was afraid if I told her something serious about me that something would happen to her. I didn't want that to happen because she had more kids to take care of. So I went and stayed at Henry's house.

Orr et al. (1984) report several approaches that adolescents with cancer find useful in coping with peer relationships:

1. Having people around who understand ("One good friend on your side who will fight for you if need be");
2. Having parents who are strong;
3. Thinking that you can get better and refusing to feel sorry for yourself and having everyone around you do the same;
4. Realizing that your appearance is less important than who you are ("You're the same inside with or without your wig");
5. Learning new skills; and
6. Being willing to take responsibility for maintaining a conversation with peers ("Make up for what they can't do; make them talk to you. Understand that they may be scared—that they may not know what to say to you. Use the word cancer"). (p. 52)

Orr's findings, and youngsters' comments, suggest that not only is it helpful to have friends who will reach out, but that it is part of the ill child's responsibility (and therefore the parents' responsibility as well) to reach out to friends and to create opportunities for positive peer interaction. If youngsters with cancer are awkward about relating to former peers and unsure how much to share about their illness, so are their peers. Whereas some are lucky enough to have assertive and sensitive friends, others are wise or skillful enough to send the right cues to their former friends, cues that indicate a desire to talk, to share, to play, and otherwise to continue a friendship.

Dealing with Two Worlds

As a consequence of dealing simultaneously with normal social situations and with a unique medical situation, children with cancer sometimes feel they are living in two social worlds. One is a world of health, and children in remission and doing well spend most of their time in this world. The other is a world of medicine and illness, and even children doing well continually enter this world for checkups and treatments. There are different rules in these different worlds. At home and school, ill children try to be normal and to live according to the same rules as everyone else, trying to grow up and master the many challenges of everyday existence. In the hospital and medical center, they are special people – patients, struggling with life and death, seeing sickness and pain on every side. Here they relate to doctors and nurses, not solely to parents, teachers, and friends. Here, too, they often see friends die and may have to confront their own mortality.

Young people with cancer overwhelmingly report that their primary goal in relation to these two worlds is to resume a normal path through a normal life as soon as possible. At the root of this quest is a concern about being different or being treated differently than other young people. Most resist this, avoid an identity as a person with cancer, and try to remain physically and socially active. Since it is impossible to do everything in quite the same way as before, some youngsters report unique attempts to be normal:

> *If anything I try harder. Maybe some of my friends feel sorry for me, so it makes me work harder.*

> *I realize that I can't meet up to the other people's standards. My favorite sport before all this happened was football. I can't run now, so I was made team statistician. If I played I would have been a hazard to the other team members, because they would have been watching out for me. So I'm going on to other things.*

Children who have been in lengthy remissions and who are ready to come off treatment make more permanent transitions between these two worlds, from the medical world to the normal social world. For many, getting better brings its own stresses and strains. Koocher and O'Malley (1981) titled their book about long-term survivors *The Damocles Syndrome* to dramatize the fragile thread by which even recovered or cured youngsters live. Koocher (1984b) also discusses crises that youngsters who are off all treatments and who are long-term survivors can expect to face. Continuing attention to lumps or symptoms that might indicate a return of the illness and heightened reactions on the anniversaries of diagnosis or treatment-cessation are reminders of the ill world, even in the midst of health and recovery.

We asked youngsters with cancer what advice they would give others who are coping with these two worlds – with the need to deal with their illness and with the need to get on with their lives. Children under the age of 11 provide the following advice:

I'd tell them to fight hard and you'll make it through.

Make sure you drink milk. It gives you strong bones and it's better for you than pop.

Don't be too sad.

Be nice to the doctors.

Be sure not to wiggle when they try to give you a shot, because they'll miss the vein and have to poke you some more.

Older youngsters, adolescents, provide the following suggestions:

Don't give up and don't take advantage. When you're not doing anything you feel more helpless, that's why I have a garden.

Don't think bad thoughts alone. When I was alone I'd think about it and cry. The worst thing I ever did was to keep it all to myself.

The only way you are going to make it is if you fight. If you fight it back it's going to back up and slowly go away. Take your chemo as it comes and realize that there's things you can do to stop yourself from getting sick. You can wear a wig, you know, and most of the people you meet will be nice. It's going to be hard to handle what's going to happen to you, but you can handle it. Your mom and dad and other people also have to come in.

You've got to be considerate of other people and not take advantage of the situation. When people do what you want them to do it's hard not to enjoy it, but it's really bad if you don't stop.

First, I would tell them to keep up their hope and that all isn't lost. You have a long way to go, but keep fighting and you're going to win. I was told that and so far I feel I'm doing a pretty good job of winning. I'd tell them to do what the doctor says to do. If you don't want to do it, do it anyway. It's all to help you.

You have to say to yourself, "I have it and I'm going to live with it." You have to take the treatments and medicines as well as the pain of the treatments. You will soon overcome the pain, and when the pain dies, so do many of the possible feelings of death and dying. In its place come stronger feelings of hope, courage, and feeling for others who are struggling.

Several themes are clear from these excerpts: don't get depressed or sad, especially do not cry alone; have hope; don't give up—fight for your life; work with the staff and treatments; don't take advantage of others' kindness and generosity. Not a bad set of prescriptions from one group of young people to others.

PSYCHOSOCIAL OUTCOMES

Parents and professionals often express concern regarding the long-term effects of childhood cancer on psychosocial development. The degree of disruption cancer has on youngsters' lives can be gauged not only by their physical survival, but also by the extent to which they can resume pre-illness activities. Many independent reports suggest that adolescents who are living with cancer do continue their involvement in most prior activities, although some who experience extended hospitalization or amputation may find this a greater challenge. Beyond the resumption of their normal social lives, many children with cancer report that their lives have changed for the better. Orr et al. (1984) indicate that the adolescents they interviewed "believed that there are some positive aspects of having cancer or of having recovered from it" (p. 55). This is not to say that anyone would deliberately seek such a learning activity, but that making the best of it does produce positive outcomes.[12]

Adolescents with cancer often suggest that they have become more serious or intense about life, cherishing each minute in its own right.

All this has helped me to realize that there are a lot of things out there that we take for granted that we ought to stop and look at. The other night I was going home; it was cold out but there were so many stars out I had to stop and look at them. I think that before I would have just jumped in the car. I enjoy each simple moment.

Among the positive outcomes reported by Orr et al.'s (1984) informants are a sense of mastery or confidence, a feeling that now one can handle anything, and a greater sensitivity to other people. Our own interviews with children and adolescents reveal similar reflections on how they feel they are different from their peers now.

> *I feel I've experienced something that most kids haven't and probably never will and I feel that I know a lot more about what I got.*

> *I've become more daring and take more chances. I go to a farther point than I probably would have if this had not happened to me. Persons with a handicap try to prove themselves and I feel I've tried to do that. Sometimes it works and sometimes it doesn't.*

> *I can handle more — I'm more courageous than my peers. I'm probably stronger than my friends mentally.*

> *I think I'm more realistic about life — thinking more about what can really happen.*

All of the adolescents we interviewed report that they receive encouragement concerning their future and do not feel that their ambitions are curtailed by their illness. Some change their goals as a result; many more now are interested in using their talents in a medically related field. Although such interests may be a natural outcome of direct experience and expertise in the medical field, it also may represent an attempt to contribute to the welfare of others, to deal with the feelings of being a survivor. According to Koocher and O'Malley (1981):

> *Many interviewees (survivors of childhood cancer) believed strongly that the illness had brought about a change in their conduct of living and reported feeling driven to repay that "debt." Those who believe that they are "special" as a result of surviving seem to do so to find a personal explanation of why they were spared while other cancer patients they knew were not. Their feeling of specialness did not correlate with increased risk-taking activities, as one might predict. Nor did they define their specialness in specific religious terms. Rather, they felt that whatever "life force was controlling life and death," they were spared. (p. 84)*

These conclusions are especially valid for adolescents who are doing well, whose cancer is under control. For many, there is good reason for optimism. However, there are also many unknowns, both of a physical and social nature.[13] Deasy-Spinetta asked a group of adolescents with cancer about their long-term social outlook (1981):

> *Since I am newly diagnosed, I have suddenly learned a lot about insurance: my parents' insurance, group school insurance, and med-*

ical insurance. I was forced to learn a lot quickly. My parents worry about it somewhat, but I worry a lot.

I just got a job, but I was very concerned about the initial job interview. What would I say on the health report? Would I be honest about my medical history and risk losing the job, or would I not tell the truth and hope that nothing would happen. (p. 191)

Children with cancer who grow up to be adults often have to pay exorbitant rates in order to obtain life or health insurance. In addition, those who desire to enter the military may find themselves rejected by virtue of their prior illness (Teta et al., 1984). Other subtle prejudices and job discrimination exist for adults who once were children with cancer. It may be a long time before these impediments to full social participation will be eliminated. In the meantime, children with cancer go on with their lives.

SUPPORT SERVICES FOR CHILDREN WITH CANCER

These reports from young people illuminate the threat and poignancy of childhood cancer as well as youngsters' coping strategies. Obviously, children's strategies and even their ability to meet the challenge of childhood cancer vary with their intellectual, emotional, and social development. Maccoby (1980) proposes a set of principles that relates stress and coping to the developmental process. First, she argues that even very young children experience considerable stress and anxiety. However, younger children are more likely than older youngsters to be reassured by their parents' authority and by the expertise of the medical staff. The trust and dependence that underlie this reassurance act as a buffer against stress. Older youngsters are more likely to generate and use a wide repertoire of coping behaviors and to engage in social comparison; thus they are more vulnerable to their peers' reactions. With increasing age, responses to stressful situations are better planned and more likely to fit into an overall value system or philosophy of life. There is little research on age-related or developmental differences in coping strategies of children with cancer, but even these potential differences merit serious attention in the provision of familial and medical support services.

One response to these developmental issues has been the creation of special (and separate) hospital units for young children and for adolescents with cancer. Lang and Mitrowski (1981) describe the advantages of such units, including the development of peer relationships among youngsters experiencing many of the same crises and stresses in their lives. Concentration of youngsters with cancer in an age-appropriate grouping also makes it easier for the hospital to focus appropriate psychosocial services.

A growing number of hospitals and/or community groups have also sponsored special camps for youngsters with cancer (Buttino, 1983; Camps for Children with Cancer and Their Siblings, 1983). With medical supervision and specially designed activities, youngsters' recreational needs are accommodated in supportive and age-appropriate settings. Being together in a relaxed setting with other children with cancer permits youngsters to escape from overprotective parents and peer stigma. There is a certain comfort in being bald, or in taking IVs, in the presence of other young people in the same situation. One teenager with Ewing's sarcoma reports (Vaughn, 1985):

> *It's different than other camps because you don't feel like an out-sider, there you are just another camper having a great time at camp. No one looks at you differently or wonders what's wrong because everyone has been through it at one time or another. It's nice to be able to talk to so many other teens who have or have had cancer. You don't have to explain yourself or worry about what your peers might think. (p. 6)*

The camp environment also may provide each camper with a vision of how other ill children overcome their problems. Enthusiasm for these special camps should be tempered, however, by the realization that they may not suit the needs of all children with cancer. Just as the negotiation between normal and special worlds proceeds differently for each youngster, not all may prefer being in a special camp.

Another important support service for children with cancer is described by Karon and Vernick (1968). At a time when secrecy was still in vogue, their central intervention was openness and honesty with the young patient about the illness. Social workers and medical staffs used a life-space interview technique to encourage children to discuss their illness and relate fears and experiences. Weekly group sessions also were held, with topics for discussion based on material that had arisen in social workers' interviews the previous week. Tape recordings of these meetings were provided for children who were unable or unwilling to attend group sessions.[14]

Several recent reports also describe discussion sessions and mutual support groups for youngsters with cancer.[15] Such groups (inpatient or outpatient) generally deal with a range of issues, including both normal developmental needs of adolescents and particular medical or psychosocial issues relevant to youngsters with cancer. In the latter category, themes include reintegration into the peer social group, conflicts concerning health maintenance, death and dying, sexuality, and self-image. The peer process that occurs in such groups helps counter the fear and loneliness so common among ill youngsters who are removed by hospitalization and illness from their regular family and social networks. One adolescent discusses her interest in a peer support group (Young Board Member Plans for Youth Groups, 1983):

> *I am not a member of a hospital youth group for teenagers, but I would very much like to be. I definitely feel that such a group would be helpful. Young cancer patients need others like themselves to whom they can relate and who can honestly say, "We understand." With something so deeply personal in common, I believe that members of a youth group could provide genuine support, encouragement, and acceptance for one another. They also could help each teenager to gain insight into his or her own emotions and problems by serving as points of comparison. (p. 1)*

Although such groups generally are organized by social workers and psychologists, they don't always proceed according to these professionals' inclinations, as noted in an insightful and sensitive report by Lewis (1984).

> *By the second group meeting, it was clear that the teenagers' agenda was different from mine. There was less talk of problems and more socializing. . . . This avoidance could also have been related to anxiety generated by topics raised in our previous session, particularly the brief discussion of death. However, their preference for recreational group meetings is consistent with teenagers' expressed interest in being "normal," like their well peers. (p. 302)*

Beyond talking and sharing feelings, some groups organize large peer support networks, phone chains, public presentations, and movies or videotapes of their experiences with childhood cancer (Panke, 1985). As they embark upon an outreach program to provide resources to other chronically ill youngsters, or to the public at large, group members expand their own lives by making positive contributions to others.

Individual psychological counseling is another service that should be available for children with cancer. As with camps and support groups, not all youngsters need or will utilize such opportunities, but some will. In the provision of counseling services it is important to retain the distinction between psychological normality and abnormality discussed earlier in this chapter. Most youngsters with cancer are and will be psychologically normal. When the stresses of their illness and treatment, or the reactions of others around them, make it difficult to master developmental tasks, they may profit from preventive and supportive counseling. Some youngsters may be overwhelmed by these stresses, or by preexisting personal and family problems, and need more intensive forms of psychological counseling or psychotherapy.[16]

Hospital staffs and parents will have to engage in vigorous outreach efforts if they are to support and improve the psychosocial adjustment of children living with cancer. Collaboration among the medical staff, the family, and a variety of other people, such as school personnel, religious youth leaders, and so on, is essential for positive outcomes. It is obvious that many youngsters are ready to adapt well to their illness and its ramifications; whether the social communities and organizations of which they are a part will help or hinder them remains an important issue.

CHAPTER NOTES

1. The data base for this chapter is somewhat different than that utilized in other chapters. Because our original interviews were limited to a sample of 26 youngsters with cancer, we have expanded the data base with more recent interviews with other youngsters and with excerpts from other important works that present adolescents' experiences in their own words (Deasy-Spinetta, 1981; Pendleton, 1980; and several issues of the Candlelighters Foundation Youth Newsletter).

2. Kellerman and Zeltzer and their colleagues (Kellerman et al., 1980; Zeltzer et al., 1980) support this finding in their research on adolescents with cancer.

3. Any study that utilizes siblings (alone) as a comparison group for ill children is somewhat suspect, as considerable research suggests that if ill children are negatively affected by their illness, so are their siblings and other family members. Thus, ill child-sibling comparisons may underestimate the degree to which ill children experience more psychosocial problems than does a healthy population. Fortunately, Teta et al. (1984) partially avoid this trap by using as an external comparison group general population data. Of course, buried within this methodological debate is a larger question of the use of control or comparative groups in such research. A number of researchers have argued that the experience of ill children is so different from that of physically healthy (nonill) children that they need to be understood on their own terms, not in comparison to others who have not had the illness experience. "Norming" ill children on the basis of nonill children may emphasize negative comparisons or deficiencies and fail to draw attention to the unique strengths or "factors that contribute to successful coping . . ." (Pless, 1984, p. 34).

4. One particularly useful book, written especially for youngsters, is *You and Leukemia* (Baker, 1978). Kjosness and Rudolph (1980) have created a potent little booklet composed completely of children's comments and advice about their illness, treatment, relations with the staff, and family issues.

5. Lewis (1984) and Marten (1980) support the Koocher and O'Malley (1981) finding that denial is the most common coping strategy used by ill adolescents.

6. See Koocher and O'Malley (1981) and Katz (1980) for similar reports.

7. See, for example, Katz, Varni and Jay (1984), Ellenberg et al. (1980), Hilgard and Le-Baron (1982), and Jay and Elliot (1983).

8. Several authors comment on the impact of cancer treatments on youngsters' body images (Farrell & Hutter, 1980; Manchester, 1981; Zeltzer, 1978).

9. Orr, Hoffmans, and Bennetts (1984), Kellerman et al. (1980), and Zeltzer et al. (1980) also report that adolescents indicate a desire to deemphasize their illness and to be "up." Chapters 4 and 5 discuss a similar stance on the part of parents as they relate to friends and to the medical staff.

10. See, for example, Blum and Chang (1981), Kellerman and Katz (1977), and Zeltzer (1978).

11. In Chapters 6 and 7 we report parents' simultaneous experience of stress and support from their other children; a similar duality is evident in ill children's comments about their siblings.

12. To be sure, it is not the cancer that has changed their lives for the better, it is their response to the cancer.

13. See the discussion of potential late effects of treatment and insurance and job discrimination in Chapters 1 and 2.

14. This program was an early effort to counter the protective approach to telling, described in Chapter 7.

15. See, for instance, Blum and Chang (1981), Lewis (1984), Spinetta et al. (1982), Thomas (1980), Worchel and Copeland (1984).

16. A good discussion of the need for psychological support services, and of the distinction between services directed toward pathology or toward normality under crisis, is provided by Spinetta et al. (1982).

CHAPTER 9

Getting Help from Others

Regardless of the different stresses and specific coping strategies that people use to deal with childhood cancer, almost everyone reaches out for some kind of social support. In a conceptualization of this process, in Table 9.1 the first column lists the five major categories of stress faced by parents of children with cancer, and the second and third columns identify the forms and agents of social support that are most relevant to each stress category.

The form and source of help that are most useful to parents often depend on the nature of the stress experienced. In some instances informal helping systems, such as family members and friends, are most useful; in other circumstances, formal service agencies, such as health care providers, are particularly helpful. In the face of the intellectual stress of the diagnosis, the medical or social service staff is likely to be the most appropriate and helpful source of support. For practical or instrumental stresses, the hospital staff, family members, or friends and neighbors all may be helpful. Support for dealing with interpersonal stresses or emotional problems is most likely to come from people with whom parents have frequent contact (intimate friends and family), although social workers or psychologists also may help parents deal with

Portions of this chapter first appeared in: Chesler, M., & Barbarin, O. Difficulties of providing help in a crisis: Relations between parents of children with cancer and their friends. *Journal of Social Issues*, 1984, 40(4), 113–134; and Chesler, M., & Yoak, M. Self-help groups for families of children with cancer: Patterns of stress and social support. From H. Roback (Ed.), *Helping Patients and Their Families Cope with Medical Problems*. San Francisco: Jossey-Bass, 1984. Reprinted by permission.

Table 9.1
Stress and Related Social Support

Category of Stress	Forms of Social Support	Source of Social Support
Intellectual Confusion Ignorance of medical system Ignorance about who the physicians are Ignorance about where things are in the hospital Lack of clarity about how to explain the illness to others	Information Ideas Books, newsletters	Medical staff Social service staff Scientists and researchers Other parents of ill children
Instrumental Disorder and chaos at home Financial pressures Lack of time and transportation Need to monitor treatments	Problem-solving activities Practical assistance at home or work Financial aid Transportation to the hospital	Social service staff Family members Friends Neighbors and co-workers Self-help groups Community agencies (e.g., school)
Interpersonal Needs of other family members Friends' needs and reactions Relations with the medical staff Behaving in public as the parent of an ill child . . . and stigma	Affection Listening Caring Being there	Family members Close friends Medical and social service staff Other parents of ill children Church congregations
Emotional Shock Lack of sleep and nutrition Feelings of defeat, anger, fear, powerlessness Physical or psychosomatic reactions	Affirmation Counseling Clarifying	Close friends Spouse Social service staff Other parents of ill children
Existential Confusion about "Why this happened to me" Uncertainty about future Uncertainty about God and fate and a "just world"	Reflection on God and fate Creating a community	Clergy Church congregations

a psychological crisis.[1] Clergy may be the most useful form of assistance for parents struggling with existential stresses. These are not rigid distinctions, and people may find just the right assistance from unexpected quarters. However, part of the skill involved in asking for and receiving support involves identifying which persons or agencies may be helpful in which situation or for which tasks.

A number of scholars argue that social support buffers or reduces the stresses of life crises,[2] and this general theory has been applied to discussions of parents of chronically and seriously ill children, including those who have children with cancer.[3] However, as noted in Chapter 3, the same significant others who are sources of positive help and support also may be sources of added stress. As researchers report in other contexts, not all potential helpers actually deliver helpful assistance, and some may even add to patients' or parents' pain, isolation, or sense of inadequacy.[4] Thus, the process of seeking and receiving help is neither automatic nor easy.

To assess the overall use that parents make of various support agents, we provided them with a list of 14 common "sources of support and help" (spouse, close friends, physicians, and the like), and asked them to indicate, on a five-point scale (5= very helpful, 1= not helpful) "how helpful each of those sources has been."[5] Table 9.2 indicates that parents report receiving a substantial amount of help from many sources.[6]

Sixty-eight percent of the parents report that their spouse is "very" or "quite" helpful. Close friends and nurses are rated as next most helpful, whereas psychologists/psychiatrists and social workers generally are rated least often as "very" or "quite" helpful. To deal with the possibility that some parents did not have a spouse or close friend available or did not have contact with a social worker or psychologist, a second set of calculations control for whether there has been any contact with these sources. Under this system, 83% of the parents with spouses available report that their spouse is "very" or "quite" helpful and close friends are reported as "very" or "quite" helpful by 73% of the parents who have contact with them; social workers and psychologists/psychiatrists are reported as "very" or "quite" helpful by only 54% and 44% of the parents who have contact with them.[7] A similar pattern of responses is reported in a survey of parents actively involved in self-help groups for families of children with cancer (Morrow, Hoagland, & Morse, 1982).

Table 9.3 presents the correlations among parents' reports of the amount of help they receive from various sources outside the family. The many significant correlations among these sources indicate that parents who make use of one source typically make use of many. For

Table 9.2

Sources of Help/Support Reported by Parents of Children
with Cancer, Rating Source as Very or Quite Helpful*

Source	Percentage of Parents	
	Not Controlled for Contact or Availability (%=100)	Controlled for Contact or Availability (%=100)
Spouse	68	83
Close friends	59	73
Nurses	58	64
Physicians	53	62
Other parents of ill children	47	64
My parents	45	70
School staff	44	68
My other children	42	62
Other relations	41	52
Neighbors	40	55
Church people	39	66
Other friends	37	45
Social workers	26	54
Psychologists/psychiatrists	9	44

*The total N for the sample is 85, but the particular Ns for different sources vary slightly, because of variations in response rate.

instance, the highest correlation in this table (+.78) occurs between parents' reports of help from close friends and from neighbors; it indicates that parents who get help from one of these sources generally get it from the other, and that parents who do not get help from one do not get it from the other. The low correlation between help from neighbors and from physicians (+.07) indicates no relationship between these sources. Interestingly, support from close friends is most often and most highly correlated with all other sources.

Because close friends are ranked highly as a source of parent support, and because help from close friends relates so highly with support from all other sources, the chapter focuses on this particular source. We asked parents of children with cancer how they share their experiences with their close friends and what kinds of help and support they ask for and receive. We also asked them to describe the nature of that helping process. In addition, we interviewed a number of close friends whom families identified as being particularly helpful, and asked them about their roles and reactions.[8]

Table 9.3

Correlations Among Parents' Reports of Support from Extrafamilial Sources (Total *N*=85)

	Close Friends	Neighbors	Other Friends	Physicians	Nurses	Social Workers	School People	Church Leaders
Friends								
Close friends								
Neighbors	.66**							
Other friends	.78**	.68**						
Medical Staff								
Physicians	.38**	.07	.33*					
Nurses	.50**	.33*	.29*	.61**				
Social workers	.27*	.19	.25*	.22	.34*			
Community Institutions								
School people	.46**	.49**	.44**	.08	.32*	.37*		
Church leaders	.36*	.46**	.25*	.29*	.40**	.13	.30*	
Self-help								
Other parents of ill children	.40**	.29*	.27*	.33*	.34*	.38**	.18	.44**

*p. < .05
**p. < .001

WHO GETS HELP FROM FRIENDS?

Analyses of the relationship between parents' demographic status and their reports of help and support from close friends reveal few significant distinctions; parental age, gender, and income do not relate significantly to reports of the amount of help received. However, parents who are college graduates do report slightly more support from close friends than do parents with some or no college (mean=4.3 v. 3.7 and 3.6: Anova F [2,82]=2.6, p. <.10). This finding is substantiated in a good deal of literature on life stress and support systems.[9]

Several characteristics of the child and the disease also relate to parents' reports of help from close friends. Parents of deceased children and living children who have relapsed report receiving more help than do parents of living children who are in first remission (mean =4.2 v. 3.9, F[1,81]=3.5, p. <.06). The obvious tragedy of death or relapse, and public knowledge of a great need, may make it easier for these parents to ask for and receive help, and for their friends to provide it.

Parents of living children between 6 and 11 years of age (at the time of the interview) report slightly less support from close friends than do parents of children under 6 years of age or over 11 years (mean=3.5 v. 4.2 and 4.0). However, the age of the child at diagnosis and the length of time elapsed since diagnosis do not relate to parents' reports of support and help from their close friends.

Parents of living children with different diagnoses also report significantly different amounts of support and help from their close friends (F[4,59]=3.5, p. <.01); parents of children diagnosed with Wilms' tumor report receiving less help from close friends than do parents of children with other diagnoses, and parents of children with lymphoma and osteogenic sarcoma report substantially more help. Wilms' tumor generally is diagnosed at a very early age (under two years), and these youngsters have the shortest treatment duration (six months to a year) and one of the highest long-term survival and cure rates of any of the childhood cancers. Youngsters diagnosed with osteogenic sarcoma and lymphoma generally are the oldest age group at diagnosis, their treatment generally extends over a longer time period, and recovery rates, at least for osteogenic sarcoma, are not as high as for Wilms' tumor. Although age at diagnosis and elapsed time since diagnosis do not by themselves relate significantly to parental reports of social support from friends, these factors may interact with the prognostic and treatment characteristics of each particular type of childhood cancer to influence parental support systems. For instance, it may be easier for parents of older children, with an illness with a poorer prognosis, longer treatment period, and visible disfigurement (e.g., osteogenic sarcoma) to ask for and receive help from close friends. Parents of preschool children, who also have an illness that is less severe or noticeable and treatment of a shorter duration (e.g., Wilms' tumor) may be seen as deserving or needing less help or may require or ask for less help.[10]

KINDS OF HELP

Several scholars emphasize the complexities of social support and informal help, noting a great many variations in form and substance.[11] Sometimes the most important help is a nonspecific response to a generalized emotional need for contact and connection with others. Many parents report that they are grateful that someone "was there" or "listened" or "cared." Parents provide examples of this form of help:

> *They helped me as far as feelings. I could talk easily with them about "What am I going to do when she dies?"*

> *One friend would go out for coffee with me and just talk. Mostly this guy just listened. Knowing he was there was great.*

Friends of parents also discuss the ways in which they provide such emotional support.

> *We talked about the quality versus the quantity of living. If you can talk about it, consider it, share some of your feelings about it, then it doesn't loom out there as a catastrophe.*

> *What I did in those situations was to listen, support, advise, help with problem solving, let them express anger and do a lot of anticipating of grief.*

Caplan (1979) calls this "psychological support" and Gottlieb (1981) refers to it as "emotionally sustaining behavior."

A second form of help that parents report is a quite specific response to practical tasks or needs. Many mothers and fathers report receiving help with key household or caretaking chores, such as cleaning, cooking, ironing, mowing the lawn, changing light bulbs, shoveling snow, and fixing bicycles. In addition, some tasks related to the care of the ill child (visiting at home or in the hospital, checking doctor's appointments) and to the care of siblings (babysitting, transporting, entertaining) were picked up by others. Caplan (1979) labels these "tangible supports" and Gottlieb (1981) refers to them as "problem-solving behaviors." Some of these specific forms of help require friends to know the family well enough to know what is needed, and some require just common sense. Parents' examples of practical help include:

> *Our friends took turns coming in and staying with the kids when my daughter was in the hospital. If I was at the hospital all day and one of the other kids got sick one of our friends would go and get them from school.*

> *Our friends and neighbors would come over and spend the night with our sick child so we could get some sleep.*

In turn, friends also report examples of such practical assistance to the family.

> *I cooked several meals and sent them. We took her to one of her medical appointments. When the child was released we took her up North with us for the weekend.*

> *Unfortunately we cannot take their pain away. But we can and did make their life less complicated so they can deal with it.*

Several helpers indicate indirect help they provide to parents of ill children. Rather than, or perhaps in addition to, engaging in intimate interpersonal assistance, they organize the larger neighborhood or community to generate extra resources.

> *It is important to find someone in the neighborhood to organize help. I was like a cog in a large organization. When one couple called and said today is our day to take food to the family up at the hospital, I went and did it.*

> *I was one of the principal people who helped organize a raffle drive to get some extra money for them. They got the money when the child was in his last stages and they didn't have enough money for the trips to the hospital and for the funeral. So what we raised from the raffle came in handy.*

Although parents indicate that they receive this form of help, they do not necessarily know how it is organized.

Whether the form of help is direct or indirect, instrumental or emotional, the process of giving and receiving help is not always easy. It is sometimes characterized by awkwardness and tentativeness on the part of both givers and recipients.

DIFFICULTIES OF HELPING AND BEING HELPED

The parent/friend interaction of seeking and providing help is initiated when parents announce or share the diagnosis. Sometimes this is a deliberate attempt to seek specific assistance, and sometimes it is part of a larger pattern of information exchange among friends. Parents' willingness and ability to share the diagnosis can be the initial, and perhaps the critical, step in gaining help from friends. When parents fail to share this intimate information with friends, support and help are less likely to materialize. Because of the trauma, fear, and stigma attached to the diagnosis of cancer, parents often experience difficulty in telling even the child, siblings, and extended family.[12] Telling friends is no exception. Forty-one percent of the parents indicate that they had considerable difficulty in sharing their child's diagnosis with their close friends. As might be expected, there is a statistically significant relationship between parents' reports of difficulty in such sharing and their reports of receiving support from their close friends (chi square$=4.5$, $df=1$, $p<.05$): the more difficulty in telling, the less support received.

Some parents obviously are not comfortable telling their close friends of their child's illness, or at least not at first. Why not? Clearly, "going public," even with close friends, is stressful. Moreover, parents' new concerns and friends' responses represent the beginnings of a potential helping relationship, a new phase in a friendship. How this new phase is managed and the ways a well-established relationship responds to challenge depend upon resolution of several issues: (1) concerns about emotional impact; (2) maintenance of privacy and prior boundaries of a relationship; (3) concern about stigma; (4) usefulness or effectiveness of help; (5) attempts to deal with traditional sex role behaviors and stereotypes; and (6) chronic and long-term needs.

Emotional Impact of Childhood Cancer

One difficulty that both parents and their friends report relates directly to the emotional shock and stress of the diagnosis of childhood cancer. The psychological trauma and turmoil that parents and child experience at diagnosis have a parallel in others closely related to the child and family. Wortman and Dunkel-Schetter's (1979, p. 131) discussion of adult cancer patients' interpersonal relations suggests that for others in the social environment, cancer " . . . arouses fear and feelings of vulnerability." Several scholars also report pain, stress, and even burnout of medical practitioners dealing with pediatric oncology patients.[13] Close friends of the parents of children with cancer, more closely identified with the family than these professionals, may be profoundly affected by their concerns for both the ill child and the parents. Reasonably sensitive parents may anticipate such reactions from their friends, especially when they have observed them in themselves and other family members. As DiMatteo and Hays (1981, p. 141) indicate, "patients often are distressed by the 'burden' that they place on their loved ones. . . " when they seek psychological support.

Parents in this study report their concern about their own feelings and those of their friends. Some parents note that the prospect of talking about the situation with close friends makes their pain even more unbearable:

I denied what was going to happen and therefore didn't want to deal with people who would tell me differently.

I didn't want to talk about it because it was something I wanted to shut in the back of my mind and have go away. It doesn't go away but I want it to. I didn't want to talk about it because that brought up my unconscious fears.

And many parents indicate that they knew talking would bring shock and similar pain to their friends.

It was harder for my friends. They would be on the phone with me and would just choke up and just couldn't take it.

It was difficult talking about it with them because our real close friends were really shocked. They were shocked and cried and didn't want to believe it. It was just like us at first.

The remarks of friends support parents' perceptions that sharing the diagnosis has a major impact on them and on their lives.

I felt absolutely like someone had hit me. I was just very shocked.

Amazed. Shocked. Incredulous. How could this be happening to anyone we know?

The compassion that friends feel for the parents of ill children is complicated by their own emotional distress. Several friends report the combination of these concerns in the following terms:

We had a lot of our own grief and anger about what was going on but there wasn't any place to dump it. To some extent we could share it with the parents, but we didn't want to add to their overload.

*I remember trying to figure out what they needed, on the one hand,
and trying to deal with how I felt on the other hand.*

Other friends indicate that one initial response was a concern about their
own children and an increased awareness of the fragility of life.

*The impact has been that I really took a good close look again at
my own children and how much time I spend with them. I just
thank God that they are healthy.*

*It's almost snobbish, but thank God it didn't happen to me and I
hope it never does. I wish it had happened to someone I didn't
know, yet I don't want it to happen to anybody.*

This last friend echoes many people's desires to push the illness further
away from their own experiences and lives. Some parents notice the
ambivalent behavior of friends that arises from the emotional impact
of the illness.

*Understandably, many people were afraid to call or meet us, either
from fear of disturbing us or from fear of their own emotions.*

Invasions of Privacy

A second difficulty reported by both parents and their friends is the
potential for the mutual invasion of privacy or for dramatic alterations
in the prior relationship. Close friends are embedded in an ongoing
relationship that is guided by norms and rules derived from prior experience (Froland, Pancoast, Chapman, & Kimboko, 1981). As parents
and friends deal with issues triggered by childhood cancer, they may
need greater flexibility in the boundaries and rules regarding mutual
disclosure and intimacy. Several parents comment on their own privacy
and emotional openness.

*My husband's friends weren't able to be real helpful because he
didn't want to see or talk with them while our daughter was sick
because he was afraid he'd break down.*

*It was hard to tell my friends because it was a long time before I
could talk about it without crying. In a way I wanted to talk with
them and in a way I didn't.*

Some parents report that it is hard for their friends to be really helpful
to them because they aren't really sure they want to talk with anyone
else about their private worries.

The way I am, when it first came out and everyone wanted to help, I just wanted to be left alone. If everyone stayed away it was the best thing they could do to help me.

In addition to their own concerns, parents note that their friends often have difficulty redefining these boundaries or overcoming barriers to communication.

Some friends who came to visit didn't want to hurt our feelings by discussing it (the illness), so they would sit in silence, which made us feel very uncomfortable.

Some friends we didn't hear from. They didn't want to say the wrong thing so they didn't say anything. That's the wrong decision.

Although many friends see these parents in need of help, they often express ambivalence and discomfort about being intrusive and "invading parents' space." Concerns about intrusion form an invisible barrier to being helpful.

There were a limited number of things asked of me and I felt it was hard to invade their space and say what I would do.

I didn't want to be intrusive, in terms of where they were at, but I wanted to be supportive.

Not all friends experience the issue of privacy or of a changing relationship as a difficulty; some feel they know parents' expressions and needs well enough to have cues about what will be helpful (DiMatteo & Hays, 1981). Even when good cues are not available, some friends feel that the preexisting relationship is strong enough and/or the boundaries certain enough that potential intrusion is not a problem.

When it first occurred I didn't know what to do. I wasn't sure whether to approach them or not, but decided I would call and offer to help and let them make the decision.

As far as intruding was concerned, I don't think that was a problem. We're close enough that they know I wouldn't be hurt if they said, "That's enough."

Even when friends decide to be assertive in offering help, caution and ambivalence often characterize their efforts. General assurance from parents or specific feedback about boundaries and limits of privacy are very helpful.

Stigma and Denormalization

A third difficulty for parents and friends is rooted in the social label attached to the parent of a child with cancer. Parents who are prepared to "go public" are aware that in this society cancer is a frightening disease, often associated with mystery.[14] The illness sometimes alters the status of the child and the family in their social environment, and some friends and neighbors may avoid social contact with both parents and child.

> *I found out that people are scared of the word cancer.*
>
> *They asked how he was doing but never came to see him. They acted like, "Keep him away from me, it's catching."*

In addition, parents often worry whether they are acting normally or will be perceived and treated normally by their friends. They fear that if they express their grief and despair they may be viewed as weak and pitiable, and be treated as needy or abnormal.[15]

> *I didn't like that kind of pity or sympathy.*
>
> *It was hard not to break down when I talked about it. But I didn't want my friends to feel sorry for me everytime we got together, so I covered it up.*

Goffman (1968) and others note that people close to a person with a stigmatizing condition often treat themselves and are treated by others as stigmatized. One report of a family's experience in a small town identifies how routine interactions with acquaintances may be altered by public awareness of the diagnosis (Roach, 1974).

> *It became uncomfortable for us even to shop in the local market. Fellow shoppers and clerks we had known for years suddenly became very occupied when they saw us coming. They avoided eye contact and we soon realized that communication was up to us. (p. 26)*

In the face of such social stigma, some parents are hesitant to share much information and eventually limit their disclosures.

Friends seldom report a concern about the cancer label in quite the same manner as parents, but several identify their attempts to avoid treating the parents in inappropriate or condescending ways.

We'd tried not to pity them. We knew they didn't need pity, just companionship.

I wanted to help them feel normal, that everyone in their situation experiences strong feelings, and that they're not strange or sick or crazy because they feel sad or want to cry.

The last report comes from a close friend and helper who herself is the parent of a child with cancer. She understands the concern about normalcy quite well!

Usefulness or Effectiveness of Help

A fourth difficulty reported by parents and friends centers around the utility or potency of the help provided. Several observers suggest that parents of children with cancer feel powerlessness and a loss of control in the face of this diagnosis (e.g., Futterman & Hoffman, 1973), and the same may be true of close friends. Researchers suggest that such powerlessness, and concerns about whether or not they have the energy and ability to utilize help, may affect the likelihood that parents will seek help and that friends will provide it.[16]

Parents indicate that some friends respond in ways they experience as ineffective, or worse. Perhaps some friends are not sure what help is needed or how to offer it; it is hard to avoid the twin pitfalls of not raising issues and of pushing too hard. In these excerpts, parents illustrate their feelings about help that is intended to comfort them but which is too pushy.

It wasn't helpful when one said, "Maybe you'll get pregnant again and replace her." They didn't understand that you don't replace a person.

Some friends kept trying to push help on me that I didn't want.

A lot of parents we talked with said they wouldn't have put their child through chemotherapy, but they didn't know what they were talking about.

Although parents are hard pressed to anticipate all the things their friends might do that would be distressing, they clearly object to empty gestures and platitudes.

Friends offered help by saying, "If there's anything that we can do just call." That was the most difficult type of offer because we knew we would never call for help and perhaps they did too.

The most beneficial support was totally unsolicited. The friends who provided the greatest relief were those who treated us natural-ly and spontaneously, offering casseroles instead of platitudes. Sympathetic bystanders were definitely a liability rather than an asset. In fact sympathy, even from family and friends, was often just what we didn't need. It was empathy and understanding that were always welcome. (Roach, 1974, p. 27)

Parents who are uncertain about asking for or receiving help un-doubtedly communicate this ambivalence to their friends. When such mixed cues interact with friends' own caution or confusion, the helping process flounders. Some friends agree that it is hard to help some parents.

I gave the same kind of support to her as to him, only it was less intense and more distant. She had less impulse to use me as a re-source.

I tried to indicate to him that he mattered and wasn't expected to be quiet, strong and long suffering.

Several friends indicated that cues given by parents regarding the type of help they desire are useful:

Sometimes they would say, "People are afraid to ask us because they don't want to bring up the negative topics, so they rely on us to do it." So they gave us clues to know what they did want people to notice and talk about.

It was clear we were useful and helpful. They've been very direct and open about their appreciation of our support.

Good cues make it easier for friends to distinguish between the different kinds of help parents want — psychological/emotional or tangible/prac-tical. Perhaps more importantly, specific and direct feedback does more than provide corrections or directions to friends; it also rewards them and makes them feel effective and appreciated.

The sheer magnitude of the medical and emotional traumas faced by the family sometimes overwhelms helpers. Some friends note their frus-tration in feeling helpful at all, or as helpful as they want to be.

A lot of it was easy to know what to do. But the hard part was that I always felt that I wasn't doing enough, or that I wished I could do more.

You never feel as though you're quite as useful as you think you should be. You think, "I should be doing more."

Some close friends report that the most important kind of help simply is not within their power to provide.

The best help that anyone could give them would be to find a cure.

No matter what you wanted to do, no matter what you did for them, you could never take away the pain from them or their child of this sickness.

These friends reflect an important aspect of this tragic illness and a realistic constraint on the helping process. They also mirror parents' own occasional feelings of powerlessness and loss of control.

Sex Role Differences

Although parents' gender does not relate to the amount of help they receive from close friends, their comments do suggest the relevance of sex role issues in the helping process. One father of a child with cancer presents the issue of sex-role differentiation openly, as he discusses his pain in not getting the help he needs. He indicates how he may contribute to the situation by withdrawing from dealing openly with his feelings.

I think if I knew someone in my position one of the things I'd like to ask him is how are you coping. I did not experience that much, only a couple of people asked me how are you doing. I think my wife experienced that a lot with her friends, but I only had a couple of friends who asked me. If I could wish for anything it would have been more of that. Probably there are things I could have done to make that happen though.

Some friends also comment on the gender-related issues they encounter in their attempts to provide help to mothers as compared to fathers.

He was in a position of having to be the rock. I felt bad for him because he couldn't draw that much support from anyone, because everyone was drawing support from him. We were there for him, too, but I'm not sure I helped him emotionally that much, even though I tried to. We didn't talk like she and I did.

Both reports suggest that some fathers avoid dealing with their own feelings and withdraw from their friends' potential help.

Other research on sex roles and life stresses indicates that women seek and use help more often than do men.[17] Knapp and Hansen (1973) report that fathers of children with cancer tend to be less open and emotionally accessible than mothers; a similar phenomenon has been reported in studies of fathers of children with other serious and chronic diseases, such as cystic fibrosis (Boyle et al., 1976) and hemophilia (Mattsson & Gross, 1966). Male images of strength, of denying or dealing covertly with feelings, of competence and independence, and of family leadership may stand in the way of expressing emotional needs and receiving certain kinds of help from friends. It also is easier for friends to assume some of the tasks generally performed by women (e.g., household chores, cooking, shopping, and sibling care) than men's typical tasks, such as working outside the home.

These gender differences are complicated further because male helpers may be as reluctant or cautious as the fathers of children with cancer. Several male helpers indicate that their role is limited, partly because of available time and partly because they, too, are uncomfortable dealing with intense feelings.

> *My wife was running back and forth a lot and I was babysitting at home. I was sort of a backup person and didn't see as much of them as my wife did.*

> *I would have liked to talk with him more about what was going on with him in terms of his thoughts and feelings. I didn't feel comfortable that he would have felt comfortable talking with me about those sorts of things. I felt a little helpless in that regard.*

Thus male friends, who might be in a particularly good position to help fathers, often are unavailable or feel awkward about inquiring into or responding to their needs for help. This may be especially true when help takes the emotionally oriented form of sympathetic listening, advice, and self-disclosure. Male friends may be more able to help with chores and practical assistance and less able to raise painful issues, discuss personal feelings, and provide emotional comfort to fathers—especially to fathers who are themselves emotionally cautious. Friends may have to deal with their own well-socialized barriers to expressing feelings as well as with fathers' caution. These barriers may require male friends to use different tactics. One male friend, who overcame these barriers for himself and the man he related to, reports a particularly energetic and creative process of helping the father of a dying adolescent.

> *I would bake bread, bring it to the home, and just shoot the breeze with the father. As our relationship grew, I invited him to go*

*fishing and then take a weekend trip in the woods. Later he told
me that these vacations and our closeness helped him deal with
his feelings and cope.*

Although these data, and other research, emphasize gender differences
regarding the helping process, it is important not to draw a rigid stereo-
type. Some mothers are closed and withdrawn and refuse to reach out
for and accept help from their close friends, and some fathers are very
open with their feelings and responsive to emotional help. Likewise,
some male friends express themselves in loving and caring ways, whereas some female friends cannot deal with parents' emotional concerns.

The issue of sex-role differentiation also may emerge primarily from
the context of the marital couple or family as a social unit. Within each
family there may be a well-established pattern of coping, a division of
labor for these emotional and practical tasks and for relating with close
friends. Several friends indicate their attention to the complementary
roles of the couple as a unit in seeking or using help.

*There were times when he (the father) would break down and cry,
but this was hard on his wife.*

I helped him by helping her.

Friends who understand these marital dynamics are able to focus their
efforts on the appropriate individual parent in the context of the marital
subsystem, and thus find indirect ways to help previously inaccessible
men or women.

Long-Term Reciprocity

All of these particular difficulties are exacerbated by the long-term
or chronic nature of childhood cancer's treatment and accompanying
stress, and the long-term demands on the helping relationship.

*This wasn't just a one-month crisis. We're talking about a couple
of years as an intense period of crisis in which the thing was really
impacting on their family and anyone they were relating to — including us.*

The damn thing didn't go away.

The issues in helping relations might have been clearer two decades ago,
when children with cancer routinely died within a few months of diagnosis. Now, with a longer period of life and even potential for cure, the

need for friends' help and support for the child and family is more extended and complicated.

Over time, the chronic nature of the disease and treatment, and thus of the helping process, can be debilitating. As several friends comment:

> *There would be times when my husband and I would be exhausted from talking with them or each other — we'd be zero. We'd go to bed and barely have enough energy to say goodnight to each other, we were so emotionally played out.*

> *I felt drained. You can only bear so much. I love them dearly but I can't deal with the child's illness for seven days a week for a long time, because we have a life too.*

Whereas the duration of this struggle may make it more difficult to help, we indicate earlier that parents of children who die or relapse, or whose treatment extends over a longer time, report receiving more help from close friends. A longer-lasting illness may provide more opportunities to experience both help and difficulty in helping. These difficulties do not necessarily raise insurmountable barriers or lower the quality of help, but they do present challenges to be resolved in an ongoing relationship.

Helping is not only ongoing; it is a reciprocal process, an interaction between helpers and helpees. Most of the difficulties that parents and friends experience reflect the interactive or reciprocal character of their relationships, as portrayed in Table 9.4. As parents ask for or receive help, they are concerned that sharing information may increase their own emotional distress, depress them even more, and recall their initial shock and pain. At the same time, they are concerned that this information will sadden and worry their friends. Friends, in turn, are shocked and depressed by information about the child's illness. They hesitate to raise painful topics with parents and do not want to add to parents' distress. Parents' and long-term friends' mutual concerns about each other's emotional status create reciprocal difficulties in the helping process. Similar reciprocal expectations and interactions occur around the other core difficulties reported by parents and their close friends.

In its most self-conscious and articulated form both helpers and recipients of help see the mutual benefits of giving and receiving help, and both are aware of their vulnerability to risks or costs. In Mead's terms, this is an example of empathy, of taking the role of the other, in which, "The taking or feeling of the attitude of the other toward yourself is what constitutes self-consciousness" (1934, p. 171). Such consciousness of self and others' feelings is critical in creating a relationship that is capable of being sustained over time and under stress.[18]

Table 9.4

Reciprocal Difficulties in the Helping Process for Parents
of Children with Cancer and Their Friends

Source of Concern	Difficulty	Target for Concern	
		for Parents	for Friends
By parents	1. Emotional impact	Become more depressed Relive pain	Make them sad Create more worry
	2. Privacy invasion	Give up privacy Expose feelings	Ask too much of them Alter the relationship
	3. Stigma	Appear weak Mystique of the cancer label	Fear of scaring them off
	4. Effectiveness	Will get no help Will be hurt by unhelpful help	Will be unable to help Will feel useless
	5. Gender role	Father cannot easily ask for help Kind of help available is inappropriate	Men cannot provide help very well
By friends	1. Emotional impact	Make them more depressed Hesitate to bring up painful topics	Feel exhausted and distraught Become depressed and anxious
	2. Privacy invasion	Invade their privacy Not know what they are ready for	Be consumed by parents' needs (and resent it)
	3. Stigma	Not treat them as special	
	4. Effectiveness	Desire not to hurt Not know what help they need	Feel powerless and inadequate Desire to be assertive, to do more
	5. Gender role	Fathers may not be open Comfort in concentrating on mother	Males' discomfort with feelings

ACTION STEPS

The importance of friends' roles in providing the help and support needed by families of children with cancer, as well as the difficulties of giving and receiving help, have clear implications for effective personal behavior and professional practice. *Parents* of children with cancer, as seekers and recipients of help, might specify clearly and as early as possible their needs and the conditions under which help from friends will be most effective. Parents can use the vitally important tactics of feedback and cues to extend their repertoire of effective help-seeking behaviors. *The immediate family* of the child with cancer may help parents by including friends in information sessions or family events and by sharing cues about family members' needs.

Friends or helpers who recognize the importance of sensitivity and assertiveness may realize that the most effective help is empathic, unsolicited, and often quite concrete. Helpful friends can try to anticipate parents' needs rather than wait to be asked, although barging in with help that is not attuned to parents' needs may be counterproductive. In addition, friends may have to keep on trying, maintaining their commitment and energy over the long haul of this chronic disease, and perhaps despite occasional withdrawal by parents. Above all, it appears clear that friends have to prepare themselves for their own potent and chronic stress.

Health care professionals, those persons invested with the social responsibility of providing services to children with cancer and their parents, also can learn from these findings. Whereas substantial prior literature focuses on the importance of the spouse and family system as sources of help for parents of children with cancer, our data also emphasize the value of close friends of the family. Several scholars critique the ways in which professionals and professional service agencies ignore or overlook friends of ill adults,[19] and Sourkes (1982) argues that "relationships which do not fit a clear family category are often overlooked by the caregiving staff . . . (friends are) rarely accorded comparable recognition and support" (p. 39).

New practice built on these findings may include medical and social service staffs suggesting to parents that they quickly involve their close friends in learning about the diagnosis and in establishing a system of social support, that the family "go public" and immediately share information and needs with close friends. Staffs also can routinely inquire about parents' relationships with close friends. Just as some medical staffs are beginning to develop outreach programs to community institutions such as schools and workplaces, professionals also may (with parental approval) work directly with friendship networks and informal support systems. Information about the child's diagnosis and prognosis, as well as potential personal and social stresses, may be shared with individual friends or in public meetings designed for many friends of many families. These sessions should also attend to the stresses that friends face, and not assume that only parents are in pain and in need of help.

Actions that minimize the difficulties of helping may assist parents, informal helpers, and professionals improve the delivery of social support to parents of children with cancer. Current psychosocial research discusses childhood cancer as a family disease, emphasizing how all family members are affected by the stresses of the illness and treatment. Our findings draw attention to childhood cancer as a community disease, emphasizing the ways in which others in the social network of the family of an ill child may be affected by and may affect this crisis.

CHAPTER NOTES

1. As other scholars have observed (Froland, Pancoast, Chapman, & Kimboko, 1981; Gourash, 1978; Kulka, Veroff, & Douvan, 1979), "Typically people do not seek professional help in dealing with personal problems. They use their social networks and individual resources . . . " (Taylor, 1983, p. 1161). Current research emphasizes the importance of informal networks, such as family members and friends, in the process of psychosocial help.

2. See, for example, Antonovsky (1974, 1980), Bloom, Ross, and Burnell (1978), Caplan (1974), Gottlieb (1981), Hirsch (1980), House (1981), Pilisuk and Froland (1978).

3. See, for example, Adams (1979) and Futterman and Hoffman (1973).

4. Cassileth and Hamilton (1979), Coates, Renzaglia, and Embree (1983), Dunkel-Schetter (1984), Hymovich (1976), Katz (1980), Rook and Dooley (1985).

5. In the interviews, parents generally use "support" synonymously with "help." The working definitions, terms, and examples in this chapter are drawn from parents' own responses to what does or might make things easier for them.

6. Everyone is enmeshed in a network of social relationships. As a result, parents often get help and support from others in unknown and unnoted ways. The ubiquitous and subtle character of social support may explain why, in Table 9.2, parents report receiving substantial support from many sources, whereas in Chapters 5 and 6 it was noted that not many parents report consciously utilizing help seeking as an active coping strategy.

7. The relatively minimal change in percent of parents reporting the helpfulness of physicians and nurses, when controlled for contact (9% change for physicians and 6% for nurses), reflects the fact that most parents do have contact with these health care professionals; controlling for contact minimally affects their reports. The more dramatic increases that occur with respect to help from churchpeople (27%), social workers (28%), and psychologists (35%) indicate that much of the low helpfulness of these sources reported in column 1 is not because of their lack of helpfulness, per se, but to lack of contact. The relative ranking of helpfulness of all these sources remains fairly constant, regardless of contact and/or availability.

8. The sample of close friends was created by asking six families of children with cancer (four families with a living child and two families with a deceased child) each to nominate two other families who had been helpful to them. At least one adult from each nominated family agreed to participate in interviews and follow-up questionnaires, for a total of 20 adult helpers in 12 families. The interviews with helpers covered some of the same questions as the interviews with parents of children with cancer but also included specific questions on the helping process: kinds of help provided and by whom, ways decisions were made about what help was appropriate, and issues or problems involved in being helpful.

9. Gourash (1978), Greeley and Mechanic (1976).

10. The interpretation that an invisible or less severe disfigurement makes it more difficult to receive help is supported by an adolescent who notes why his friends had difficulty relating to his illness: "Especially for me it was hard, because I didn't show a leg amputation or hair loss." However, while a highly visible illness or disfigurement may make it easier to ask for and receive help, it also increases the probability of stigma and rejection.

11. Caplan (1979), DiMatteo and Hays (1981), Gottlieb (1978), Hirsch (1980), Wortman (1984).

12. See the discussion in Chapters 3 and 7.

13. Rothenberg (1967), Stuetzer (1980), and Vaux (1977).

14. Sontag (1979), Wortman and Dunkel-Schetter (1979).

15. Some scholars suggest that just asking for help creates feelings of inequality in a relationship and generates a secondary stigma of weakness and neediness (Fisher, Nadler, & Whitcher-Alagna, 1983; Brickman et al., 1983).

16. Brickman et al. (1982), Voysey (1972).

17. Gourash (1978), Greeley and Mechanic (1976), Pearlin (1975), Vaux (1985).

18. Some scholars examining helping interactions apply principles of exchange relationships developed by Homans (1961) and Gouldner (1960). The experiences and difficulties reported here do not conform to such exchange principles, at least helpers do not indicate any expectations of being repaid for their efforts. These interactions more closely follow the principles of a reciprocal or altruistic relationship (Hatfield & Sprecher, 1983; Schwartz, 1977), one embedded in communal rather than exchange norms (Clark, 1983). The sincere desire to help, born of a mutuality of caring among close friends in a crisis, is the dominant theme. It is possible that parents of children with cancer feel indebtedness as a function of receiving help (Gouldner, 1960); one could interpret some parents' reluctance to ask for help and fear of alteration of their prior relationships with friends as concern about becoming indebted or entering an exchange form of relationship. However, there is no direct discussion by parents of exchange norms and no clear support for such an interpretation in parents' reports.

19. Froland, Pancoast, Chapman, and Kimboko (1981) and Wortman and Dunkel-Schetter (1979).

CHAPTER 10

Help from Other Parents of Ill Children

In addition to reaching out to old friends, parents sometimes gain support from new friends they meet in clinics and on hospital wards – other parents of ill children. Connections with other parents often arise spontaneously and are maintained on a one-to-one basis. Parents talk with one another in hospital rooms, hallways, and cafeterias, call each other on the telephone, and visit each other at home. Sometimes, however, parent-to-parent connections are fostered by formally organized parent groups. Such groups provide an arena for bringing together a larger number of parents in programs that continue over time. On an individual or group basis, the process of self-help aids parents to cope with the prolonged and unusual stresses of serious and chronic illness on themselves or on other family members.[1]

Self-help essentially involves people with an identifiable and chronic problem, in a similar situation or with common needs, coming together voluntarily to help each other cope with or solve the problem. This focus on people "doing for themselves" distinguishes self-help from support activities run or guided by professionals. As Smith and Pillemer (1983) note, many support and counseling services "involve people not suffering from an alterable, pressing personal problem attempting to help those who do suffer from such a problem" (p. 206). This describes the professional help generally available from the medical, psychological,

Portions of this chapter first appeared in: Chesler, M., Barbarin, O., & Lebo-Stein, J. Patterns of participation in a self-help group for parents of children with cancer. *Journal of Psychosocial Oncology*, 1984, 2(3/4), 41–64. Reprinted by permission.

or social work staff. In the case of self-help, especially pure forms of self-help, the people with the problem are the ones helping people who have the problem. When professional help and self-help are combined, people can benefit from the mix of these different forms of expertise and assistance.[2]

Self-help is an especially important resource for parents of children with serious and chronic illnesses such as cancer. It can provide parents with medical information, interpersonal contact and identification with others in a like situation, social and emotional support, and quite often practical and material assistance. It may also help bring about improvements in the medical care system and in community services. Although parents utilize a broad range of coping strategies and seek support and help from a variety of sources, some find discussions with other parents uniquely valuable. Parents comment on what experienced parents offer that the staff cannot:

> *Sometimes it's easier to talk to an ordinary person than to a doctor. The doctor doesn't have a heck of a lot of time to sit and hold your hand.*

> *Other parents can answer all the questions that you have as you are going through it, even if their experiences are different. The doctors helped, but I still had a lot of questions, and talking with the parents of another amputee helped.*

Thousands of people participate in hundreds of different kinds of medical self-help groups. In the case of childhood cancer, more or less organized groups exist in at least 300 communities and medical centers across the United States. The work of many of these groups is sponsored and publicized through the efforts of the Candlelighters Childhood Cancer Foundation. Candlelighters is an international network organization of parents that maintains contact with many local groups, publishes materials and a newsletter for parents of children with cancer and professional medical and social service staffs, maintains a hotline for parents with questions about diagnosis or treatment, and often represents parents to other organizations, such as the American Cancer Society, the Association for Care of Children's Health, the Association of Pediatric Oncology Social Workers, and the Association of Pediatric Oncology Nurses. The Candlelighters Childhood Cancer Foundation also helps establish and link local groups in communities and medical centers across the nation.

WHAT SELF-HELP GROUPS DO FOR PARENTS

Several different focuses and activities are common in self-help groups; each of these forms of social support responds to different categories of stress (see Table 10.1).

One focus of group activity responds to intellectual, educational, or informational stress, developing programs to inform parents about the disease and its side effects, potential child-rearing and discipline issues, and the nature of the hospital and hospital staff.[3] Several parents note the importance of such activities:

Other people are going to be experiencing processes that us "advanced parents" have gone through. The whole concept is to prepare them to ask questions and learn more about the disease and treatment and understand it better.

It's a good idea for families to get together and to answer questions.

Information and education are the most common group focus, and such programs are operated by almost all groups at some time during their history. Inviting local physicians to address the group often has the additional benefit of linking the medical staff more strongly with parents. Some self-help groups publish regular newsletters with medical information, and others have developed handbooks for parents of newly diagnosed or newly hospitalized children.[4]

A second major focus of some groups responds to the instrumental stress that parents experience. By helping to solve problems of transportation and child care, for instance, self-help groups provide some of the same material assistance offered by friends, family members, churches, and community agencies. Person power is the most readily available resource for such services, but many groups also have become involved in raising funds. Some groups raise small amounts of money in casual ways, mostly to support a newsletter and informal social events. Other groups raise more substantial funds to underwrite the cost of drug purchases, transportation or parking, childcare, prostheses for children not adequately covered by insurance, wig banks, or in-room televisions for hospitalized patients. Still other groups undertake major fund-raising efforts to help transport children to specialty treatment centers, subsidize or construct low-cost lodging near the treatment center, pay for additional psychosocial services, or support research at the local medical center.

Table 10.1

Stress and Self-help Activities for Parents of Children with Cancer

Category of Stress	Self-help Group Activities
Intellectual	
Confusion	
Ignorance of medical terms	Organize staff presentations
Ignorance about where things are in the hospital	Write handbooks
	Establish library of articles
Ignorance about who the physicians are	Print newsletters
	Share information between parents
Lack of clarity about how to explain the illness to others	Educate the general public
Instrumental	
Disorder and chaos at home	Collect and distribute funds for wigs, prostheses, parking
Financial pressure	
Lack of time and transportation	Provide transportation
Need to monitor treatments	Arrange parent lodging
	Improve local medical care
	Raise funds for research or added services
Interpersonal	
Needs of other family members	Identify with others in the same situation
Friends' needs and reactions	
Relations with the staff	Meet new people
Being the parent of an ill child . . . stigma	Have someone to talk with
Emotional	
Shock	Find professional counseling
Lack of sleep and nutrition	Provide peer counseling
Feelings of defeat, anger, fear, powerlessness	Share intimate feelings with people in the same situation
Physical or psychosomatic reactions	
Existential	
Confusion about "why this happened to me"	Talk about religious beliefs
	Share the struggle
Uncertainty about the future	
Uncertainty about God, fate, a "just world"	

Groups also provide instrumental assistance as they advocate changes in the ways the medical system responds to the problems of parents and children. For example, in a Rhode Island hospital the parent self-help group arranged a dialogue between concerned parents and the health care staff; this meeting "cleared the air" and helped parents and staff work together to change hospital procedures. Another group was able to change the way children moved through the medical system, effecting a greater coordination between the Oncology Department and surgical and radiologic services. The Portland (Oregon) Candlelighters provides an excellent example of one way parent groups can help improve local medical services. In their monthly newsletter the organization announces an award for the health care professional providing an outstanding service to their families and children. It also announces a "Bogie" award, to an unnamed person or institution, for the least outstanding service of the month. Through these awards, described in Table 10.2, the organization provides feedback intended to improve the delivery of services.[5]

A third major focus of group activity deals with interpersonal stress by developing networks of new friends and social relationships. The primary activity of some groups is simply to provide an arena within which people with similar experience can gather and talk with one another. People may ask for help if they wish, but they also concentrate on keeping in touch and having a good time with one another. Groups of this sort may provide a subtler kind of support as well – parents may serve as a reference for one another, as points of comparison for defining or understanding appropriate behavior in a new situation (Powell, 1975; Silverman, 1976). One parent reports:

It helps to talk to people. Knowing that other people have gone through it helps. Sometimes I think I felt isolated, like this was only happening to me.

A fourth major focus of many groups is the emotional stress of childhood cancer. Groups provide opportunities for parents to share feelings of joy and pain, hope and despair, and validate their emotional responses to prolonged and uncertain illness. The problems discussed may cover quite a range: dealing with spouses' and family members' feelings, preparing for death, fighting depression, coping with relapse, dealing with fears or anger toward the medical staff, getting ready to come off treatment, being afraid, bringing up an ill child, dealing with the ill child's siblings, and so on.[6] The topics of these sharing sessions may be quite similar to those covered in information and education

Table 10.2

Guidelines for the Portland Candlelighters Compassionate Care Award

1. The award is to be made to an individual involved with the care of children who have cancer.
2. The individual who receives the award works in a medical setting or has a medically related job.
3. The majority of parents at Candlelighter regular meeting(s) vote to award this individual the Candlelighter Compassionate Care Award for exceptional qualities of skill, compassion, and empathy.
4. The local Candlelighter parents can provide three reasons specifically why this individual is deserving of the award and submit them to the Newsletter editor by deadline.
5. Local groups will take turns presenting this award in their area so that only one group is presenting the award in any one month.

Guidelines for the Candlelighters Bogie Situation Award

1. The *Candlelighters Bogie Award* will be made in reference to a *situation* and not a specific individual.
2. Every attempt should be made to eliminate any identifying information with regards to a specific individual or facility.
3. Agreement by Parent-Members on the appropriateness of this selection should be evidenced by a vote taken at a regular meeting.
4. Suggestion(s) for improving the situation should be included. If possible, consult appropriate professionals for their advice.
5. The Bogie award, with its suggested remedy, should be written up and submitted to the President or other individual appointed by the Board or President for that purpose. This should be done in plenty of time—for example two weeks before the Newsletter deadline of the month that it is to appear.

meetings, but the purpose and style are quite different: Here the goal is for parents to share their experiences and feelings with one another.

I went to the meeting and shared my experiences with them. When I see someone else who is going through the same thing I am and they can handle it, then I can conquer it too.

It would be helpful to have someone who has been through this at the very beginning. No one else knows what you're going through until they've been there. You can tell someone who's been through it how you feel and ask should you or do you have the right to feel that way?

The two-way street of giving and receiving help is a vital therapeutic element in self-help groups for parents of children with cancer. Leiken and Hassakis (1973) emphasize this aspect of self-help groups in their report that "The most frequently used helpful coping mechanism was the 'doing defense'" (p. 55). As parents help other parents with similar problems they may benefit from the helper-therapy principle.[7] Helping others may enable people to work through some of their own difficulties, on the basis that they are doing well enough to have extra energy and resources to share with others. In some groups, parents provide such active emotional support to one another directly; in others, a social worker, nurse, or other staff member facilitates discussions and promotes openness and sharing among group members.

A fifth focus of some groups is the existential challenge of childhood cancer. Although seldom the major focus of any group, it is an issue that often arises as parents share their understanding of the role that their struggle with illness plays in their lives. For some, especially for parents of terminally ill or deceased children, group exploration centers on the meaning of life after death and testaments to their own spiritual faith and commitment. For others, discussion focuses on their secular philosophy and how it has changed as a result of their experiences. As parents see how others have incorporated the meaning of these events in their own lives, they may discover more effective answers for themselves.

Parents may find each of these focuses to be appropriate, depending on how they are coping with their situation and the stage of their child's illness or treatment. Parents coping primarily with intellectual stress may find information sessions and activities most appropriate. Others who have difficulty managing the many practical and instrumental tasks associated with the treatment of childhood cancer may want help or advice on how others have dealt with these matters. For parents in dire financial straits, the benefits provided by fund-raising activities may be most important. Parents who wish to share, express, and reflect on their feelings may be best served by activities that promote emotional sharing and intimate engagement. Parents who wish to know and meet others socially may be most interested in talking comfortably with one another without stigma, or in playing and having fun together without being judged as unfeeling or unconcerned about their child.

The appropriateness of each focus for a self-help group also may depend on the services provided by the treatment center or the community. Parents may start up a group or participate in an existing one to make up for specific deficiencies in available care. By the same token, the availability of certain community services (American Cancer Society support, Ronald McDonald Houses, and meetings of the Society of Compassionate Friends) makes some focuses less important if parents already have access to such resources.

Although many groups address several focuses, most emphasize only one or two. As a result, different groups appeal to parents with different desires or needs. Clearly, parents are not likely to remain active in groups that do not meet their needs. In addition to this process of self-selection, a subtler form of socialization may occur; parents who enter a group for one purpose may become bonded to other members and alter their needs or coping styles to fit with the group's main focus. Thus, parents who enter seeking information may become comfortable and active in a group emphasizing feelings, and parents originally not committed to fund-raising may engage in such activities when a group in which they have close friends moves in this direction. In addition, parents who want to participate in a group not oriented to their needs and styles may exert influence on other members to change the group's focus.

Some groups attain balance among these focuses by forming subgroups: one may meet (perhaps once a month) to receive and share information; one may meet (every two weeks or so) to share feelings or emotional problems; one may meet (once or twice a year) to socialize and have a holiday party, summer picnic, or children's activity. At a more formal level, some groups develop parallel structures, separating formally incorporated fund-raising activities from educational and sharing subgroups. Leadership struggles or subgroups committed to different activity priorities may result in some people and activities dominating and other members leaving or becoming inactive.

PATTERNS OF PARTICIPATION

Participation in a self-help group is influenced jointly by the particular needs of parents and by the operations and activities of a specific group. The following is a description of one local group involving some of the parents in this study. This local self-help group was formed in 1977 by several parents, a social worker, and a clinical nurse practitioner.[8] The group developed out of needs expressed by parents attending a once-a-year educational session planned and run by the pediatric hematology/oncology unit of the hospital. Parents expressed a desire to meet more often to explore and discuss a series of informational and educational issues, to provide an arena for sharing ideas and feelings with one another, and to encourage mutual emotional support, especially for families of newly diagnosed children. A conscious decision was made not to engage in fund-raising activities, and the group did not originally plan to have many social events.

The doctors were not active in the group, nor were they publicly visible supporters, although there was no indication of resistance or antagonism. The group remained largely dependent upon the medical and social work staff for referrals of new families, but this referral system worked only sporadically. The names of newly diagnosed families were passed on to the group by the staff only if parents gave their permission; self-help group members seldom contacted new families without permission from a medical intermediary.

A cadre of 10 to 12 parents and two professionals planned most meetings and managed the group. The group elected to organize outside of the medical system; it had a mailing address outside the hospital and was incorporated as a separate nonprofit entity. In its first years of operation the group held monthly meetings in the hospital schoolroom. Most meetings utilized experts or panels to address topics such as:

The nature of childhood cancer;
New treatments;
Chemotherapy;
Research on long-term outcomes of treatment;
Dealing with siblings;
Death and dying.

Other meetings did not have formal speakers or agendas, but provided opportunities for parents to speak with one another, in an unfocused manner, regarding their experiences or feelings on issues such as:

Relations between mothers and fathers;
Helping the child with cancer in school;
Disciplining the ill child;
Feelings of anger, despair, and hope.

Participation at monthly meetings varied, but most were attended by 20 to 30 people. Twice a year, at Christmas and during the summer, a party or picnic was held with food, drinks, clowns, and even dancing dogs and puppets. These social events drew 75 to 100 people.

The group's participants and its internal leadership cadre included parents of deceased children as well as parents of surviving children with cancer. On some occasions parents of deceased children and parents of living children met together; at other times they had separate caucuses but came together for refreshments and casual conversation after meetings.[9]

Who Participates in This Self-help Group?

Most parents we interviewed (80%) know of the local self-help group and receive copies of the newsletter. Thirty-eight percent attended at least a few group meetings. Even parents who were unable to attend meetings are pleased that the group exists and that they are informed of its activities.

Mothers and fathers typically attend meetings together or not at all. Thus, there is a statistically significant difference in the marital status of group participants and nonparticipants (see Table 10.3); group participants are all married. Why? Perhaps single parents do not attend meetings because of greater difficulties arranging child care, because they feel that the self-help group does not address their special needs, or because they feel out of place or estranged in a group of only married persons. Some single parents report that they do not want to talk about their divorce in the parents' group and do not come because they want to avoid exposure of family squabbles in public. The salience of a married person's culture in this group is not typical of other self-help groups of parents of children with cancer, nor of self-help groups more generally. In many groups single parents attend and are quite active; it also is common for only one parent in a couple to attend.

Self-help group participants and nonparticipants do not differ significantly in gender, education, or income. However, a slightly larger proportion of active participants than nonparticipants completed college (44% vs. 26%), and participants cluster in the middle-income range, with proportionately fewer with less than $15,000 or greater than $40,000 annual income. In contrast to these data, findings from several studies of other kinds of groups show that people who are most likely to participate or become leaders are women, upper middle class, and well educated.[10]

Distance between home and the meeting location in the medical center also has an influence on parent participation – at least for parents of living children. Table 10.3 indicates that parents of living children residing less than 25 miles from the medical center are significantly more likely to attend group meetings than are parents who live further away. Many parents dealing with the time and energy problems created by their child's life-threatening illness find another long drive to the hospital simply too taxing. They also may be reluctant to leave their ill child at home.

We don't go because of the distance. If we lived closer we'd probably participate.

Table 10.3
Parental Participation in Self-help Group, by Demographic and Medical Factors

Demographic Factors	Participation in Self-help Group	
A. Marital Status	Participants (N=35)	Nonparticipants (N=53)
Married (N=80)	100%	85%
Not married (N=8)	0%	15%
χ^2=5.9, df=1, $p.$ < .05		
B. Distance from the Medical Center		
Parents of living children	Participants (N=27)	Nonparticipants (N=47)
Less than 25 miles (N=38)	70%	40%
More than 26 miles (N=36)	30%	60%
χ^2=6.1, df=1, $p.$ < .05		
Parents of deceased children	Participants (N=9)	Nonparticipants (N=11)
Less than 25 miles (N=10)	33%	54%
More than 26 miles (N=10)	67%	46%
χ^2=1.8, df=1, NS		
C. Length of Time Since Diagnosis		
Parents of living children	Participants (N=26)	Nonparticipants (N=45)
Less than 1 year (N=11)	12%	18%
1-4 years (N=34)	69%	36%
More than 4 years (N=26)	19%	47%
χ^2=7.2, df=1, $p.$ < .05		
Parents of deceased children	Participants (N=9)	Nonparticipants (N=9)
1-4 years (N=13)	89%	56%
More than 4 years (N=5)	11%	44%
χ^2=2.6, df=1, NS		

I know about the meetings but we don't go to very many because it's a long drive.

Some groups in rural areas deal with this issue by having a spoke design of a central coordinating group with several outlying subgroups. The outlying groups are arenas for personal contact and sharing, whereas the central body publishes a newsletter, maintains liaison with the hospital, raises funds, and so on.

Table 10.3 also indicates that the distance relationship does not exist for parents of deceased children; if anything, the pattern is reversed, with these active parents tending to come from further distances. The sample of parents of deceased children is too small to draw a definite conclusion, but their need for the reciprocal support of other parents may be greater than that of parents of living children, and they may be willing to travel further to get that support.

Length of time since diagnosis also has a significant relationship with parents' participation in the self-help group. The period of one to four years after diagnosis is the most likely time for parents of living children to become active, and the passage of a similar time period after death appears to influence participation of parents of deceased children. Data presented here and in Chapter 2 affirm reports of health care professionals that the first six months to a year after diagnosis or death is a period of great distress. Most parents need time to adjust privately to the reality of their child's illness before they can deal with it in public. Moreover, for many parents the first few months (after either diagnosis or death) may be too filled with trauma and the need to learn many things quickly to devote the time and energy to group activities.

For many people, becoming active in a self-help group signals the adoption of a new identity as a member of a victimized and socially stigmatized population.[11] When parents are ready and willing to deal with these issues, and to meet other parents of ill children, they may become emotionally attached to and identified with others with whom they may share intimate details of their personal and family lives. On the other hand, parents who have passed beyond these issues, whose children have been well or dead for several years, may no longer need to connect with other parents of ill children or with the medical care organization. They may wish to put the past behind them and to normalize their lives. They may wish to define themselves as other than parents of a child with cancer and may no longer need to participate in a group committed to dealing with childhood cancer-related issues.

Parents of deceased children report significantly more medical stress than parents of living children (Chapters 2 and 3). For that reason, we analyze these subgroups separately when looking at the relationship between stress and self-help group participation. Among parents of living children, participants in the self-help group report significantly more stressful events (chi square=6.8, $df=1$, $p. < .01$) and higher levels of stress (chi square=8.9, $df=1$, $p. < .01$) than do nonparticipants. Since the data are associational, we cannot determine whether parents (of living children) who experience greater stress are attracted to the self-help group as a way of coping with this stress, or whether participation in a self-help group legitimizes greater awareness and discussion of stress, which, in turn, prompts more reporting. However, this relationship does not appear for parents of deceased children; their stress levels do not relate to self-help group participation.

The majority of parents in this sample report receiving substantial support from a variety of sources (Chapter 9). Table 10.4 indicates that such support generally occurs regardless of parents' participation in the self-help group; participants and nonparticipants report similar amounts of support from most sources. On this basis we can conclude that active members of self-help groups have quite normal social relationships; they are neither isolated from other sources of social support nor inundated with them.

The two exceptions to this pattern of similarity involve support from social workers and from other parents of ill children, in which participants report significantly more support from these sources than do nonparticipants. Participants' increased support from other parents of ill children is easily understood, since attendance at group sessions necessarily places people into contact with other parents in a mutually supportive context.[12] Parents who report receiving more support from social workers are also more likely to participate in the self-help group, although this relationship is relatively weak. The pediatric oncology social worker is a key link between the medical staff and the parent group. She not only advertises and attends many of the self-help group activities but also makes most of the referrals, often actively encouraging new parents to contact veterans in the self-help group.[13]

In some communities or medical centers, parents do not participate in self-helps groups, and groups do not survive, because the medical staff discourages them. Professionals who are wary of support groups, especially groups not supervised by professionals, may caution parents not to "waste your time talking with other parents" or not to "go to that group and get even more upset." Lack of public information and positive medical referrals also may prevent parents from becoming involved.

Table 10.4
Parental Participation in Self-help Group, by Mean Rating
of Support from Family, Friends, and Medical Staff
(5=very helpful, 1=not helpful)

Support from Various Sources	Participation in Self-help Group		T-value of Differences Between Means
	Participants	Nonparticipants	
Family as source of support			
Spouse (N=85)	4.06	4.00	.18
Parents' parents (N=84)	3.40	3.57	.50
Other relatives (N=84)	3.11	3.09	.11
Friends as source of support			
Close friends (N=85)	4.06	3.62	1.63
Other friends (N=83)	3.09	2.98	.39
Neighbors (N=84)	3.03	2.96	.22
Medical staff as source of support			
Physicians (N=85)	3.51	3.48	.11
Nurses (N=83)	3.85	3.71	.48
Social Workers (N=78)	2.63	2.04	1.73*
Other sources			
Other parents of ill children (N=81)	3.82	2.60	3.94**

*T-test significant at $p.=<.10$
**T-test significant at $p.=<.01$

BENEFITS OF PARTICIPATION

The range of activities provided by self-help groups benefits parents
in several different ways. Some parents suggest that support from other
parents in the form of reassurance and empathy is a central benefit of
participation.

*I felt the need to talk and be with people who had gone through
it. Your friends sympathize, but at times you need "someone who's
been there." I found it helpful at group meetings. The people were
beautiful, and I didn't feel uncomfortable if I wanted to cry.*

The group meeting let you know that there are a whole lot of other people in the same boat as you.

For parents of living children, participation in the self-help group relates significantly to reports of more positive changes in their lives (chi square=7.1, $df=2$, $p. <.05$). Participants identify more ways in which they have grown or created positive value out of their experience with childhood cancer. Parents with positive views, and/or with the disposition to help others, may be more likely to seek the opportunity to meet and share with others. Or perhaps the experience of being with others in a self-help group, in a setting focusing on thinking and adapting realistically but positively, leads to a more positive and outgoing orientation. It may even help some people reinterpret their feelings and experiences in a more positive light, through a process of social comparison or cognitive reappraisal. These more positive reports also may be a result of social pressures placed on group members to "be happy," or to appear positive regardless of their real feelings. We noted in Chapter 9 that friends often place such pressures or expectations on people with cancer, and it is possible that self-help group members do the same. On the basis of these data it is impossible to distinguish the influence of self-selection from direct effects of group participation.

Other parents report that a substantial benefit comes from giving support to others, as in the helper-therapy principle discussed earlier.

The group which I am working with gives me something positive to do. I feel I am helping someone down the road and changing things in a positive constructive manner.

I talked a lot and hope I helped other people by being there.

Perhaps by offering assistance to others, parents test and affirm their own ability to deal with these issues.

Not everyone benefits from self-help groups, or feels he/she would. Some parents who do not attend group meetings indicate they neither need nor desire the particular kind of support offered there.

I've never been a "go to meeting person," so I never went. I might go strictly to listen, even though I do like to run my mouth, but not in groups, especially with people I don't know.

Personally I don't feel the need to get together with other people in the same boat and get reassurance. I'm a loner.

My wife goes, and she reads the newsletter. I can't take the stuff. It's one sad story after another. I don't want to if I don't have to.

One parent expresses quite clearly the ambivalence created by both positive identification or support and reminders of pain or threat.

I thank God for the group. I hate them because I don't want to identify, and I love them because I can. I have a desk full of books, every drawer is full of them and I have to throw things away constantly, but I have every copy of the group Newsletter. I read every article, I experience a catharsis every time I cry, and I cry every time.

PROFESSIONALS' ROLES IN SELF-HELP GROUPS

A key issue for all self-help groups is their relationship with the medical system and with health care professionals, a relationship that is fertile ground for both cooperation and conflict.[14] Some medical professionals, distressed by the proliferation of self-help groups, warn about their potential for encouraging negative attitudes toward treatment and staff and intruding on the carefully controlled physician-patient relationship (Tracy & Gussow, 1976). However, data on parents' attitudes toward the staff do not substantiate concerns about groups encouraging negative feelings toward the staff. Although participants report slightly more problems with the medical staff than do nonparticipants, this difference is not significant. Nor do participants report greater or lesser changes in their attitude toward the staff (e.g., good feelings, anger, or respect). In fact, parents of deceased children who are active participants in the self-help group are more often positive toward the medical staff than are parents of deceased children who are not active (chi square=11.4, $df=2$, $p. < .01$). Considering the extra effort that these parents must make to stay active and in touch with each other and the hospital, this is an intriguing finding. Despite their tragic experience, some parents of deceased children may have good memories and appreciation of the staff and institution, and therefore a desire to stay in touch and be helpful. Perhaps their judgments that their child had good care permit them to adapt more comfortably to the death of their child and to continue active participation.

These findings challenge the simplistic judgments regarding the negative orientation of self-help groups toward medical staffs. Although groups often focus attention on problems with medical care, such activity is not synonymous with personal antipathy nor with an antiprofessional mood. Participation seems less motivated and maintained by animosity toward the staff than by the group's ability to give parents the support and information that are unavailable elsewhere.

Even if this issue is settled, professionals express other concerns about parent support groups, especially ones that meet without professional supervision, guidance, or control. Belle-Isle and Conradt (1979), for example, warn that,

> *The danger of parents inappropriately sharing their concerns and unwittingly increasing each other's emotional burdens is a constant threat. With professional guidance this danger should be significantly less as staff participants are present to correct misinformation and control inappropriate exchanges. (p. 49)*

Almost the same statement is made by Binger et al. (1969) and by Kartha and Ertel (1976). Although many professionals we interviewed express similar concerns, few of them (and very few parents) actually have observed or experienced such dangers in organized groups.[15]

Professionals' attitudes and actions can make a difference in the operation and survival of local self-help groups. Professionals can provide, or fail to provide, important resources to self-help groups, such as access to members, meeting rooms, and credibility. Although staff members cannot prevent parents from getting together, they can make it either easier or more difficult for parents to find and rely upon one another. When parents are fearful or cautious about joining a group of nonexperts, professionals can allay their fears and assure them that the self-help group is a credible and valuable source of support. An effective and vigorous referral system through which parents of newly diagnosed children are placed into contact with members of self-help groups is especially useful (Levy, 1978).

One resource that parents need, to which medical staff members have special access, is information. To provide this information in ways that lay people can understand easily, some professionals write articles for group newsletters and present lectures, discussions, and panels at group meetings. Professionals often have special expertise in family coping strategies and share information personally or through written materials about the way families can cope with various stresses. Social workers also have special knowledge about the staff, the operations of the local treatment facility, and the financial and social services that may be available in the community or school system. Groups trying to help members get services or improve service availability need such information.

The staff's resources for aiding parents to deal with their emotional stress also can be provided in a self-help group context, through group counseling sessions, at scheduled meetings of the self-help group, or at special meetings. Some professionals encourage self-help group members to provide emotional support to one another, and have trained group members in how to counsel and respond to others' emotional needs. Some groups, especially those led by parents who do not have skills in organizational leadership, have found social workers' skills very helpful in developing sound procedures for electing officers, managing meetings, and so on. In a number of treatment centers, medical staff members have collaborated with self-help groups to conduct inservice training sessions and conferences for school staffs or for medical students.

Groups that raise large amounts of money often collaborate with the medical staff to help tap major local sources of funds and to identify needs for new revenue. In cases in which self-help groups have raised funds to support wigs, prostheses, and incidental expenses for families, the professional staff can identify needy families and help distribute these funds. The staff's links to other hospitals and the broader community can make additional resources available to local groups.

Role Dilemmas of Staff Members

Staff social workers and nurses are the health care professionals most likely to work with a parent self-help group, but this role is fraught with tension and difficulty. Reports from these professionals highlight a series of dilemmas summarized in Table 10.5.[16] Some of the problems that professionals face are rooted in their personal attitudes and feelings, others in nature of their professional role, and still others in the operation of the medical institution.

Lenrow and Burch (1981) argue that collaboration can be fostered when both professional helpers and their clients understand that they have "equally important resources to contribute to their common task" (p. 234). Central to the difficulties between parents and staff may be differences about the relative importance each gives to professional expertise and parental wisdom (Reinharz, 1981). Staff members who are not parents of children with cancer are often locked into the role of giving help, while parents are fixed in the role of receiving help. Moreover, staff members' knowledge is based on academic training and technical experience that are quite different from the experiential, but no less valuable, base of parental knowledge.

Institutional conflicts may arise when the social workers' or clinical nurses' function is not clear—not to themselves, not to their employers, and not to parents. Physicians may expect them primarily to control misbehaving patients and to process insurance forms. Any other acti-

Table 10.5
Problems Social Workers Face in Working with
Organized Parent Groups

Personal Issues of Involvement with Patients/Parents
Feeling close with some and distance (or dislike) with others
Time and energy demands
Need to feel appreciated (get strokes) and supported
Lack of clarity about how open to be personally
Specific questions about going to funerals, parties, socials
Feelings of not doing enough
High emotional stress

Professional Role Responsibility
Concern about not having the right skills (or enough of them)
Avoiding telling (or being seduced into telling) parents what's right
Feeling responsible for parents' emotional safety
Dealing with rumors or fads about treatment
Dealing with intrusive or manipulative parents (who may hurt others)
Watching out for parents who get overlooked
Making sure the group stays on track (does good work)
Feeling like the expert in psychosocial care
Feeling responsible for what group does

Institutional Conflicts
Lack of clarity about own role
Conflict between parents' needs and the medical staff's desires,
    especially intense if part of salary raised by parents
Turf conflicts with other staff members
Feelings about the character (quality) of medical or psychosocial care
Low status on staff
Lack of staff information about parents' needs and experiences
Staff hesitancy to share with each other

---

vities they engage in may be performed on their own initiative and not as part of their formal obligations. Members of the medical team also may be unclear how they can link parents with one another without violating professional norms of confidentiality.

As staff members, professionals are primarily accountable to other staff members, perhaps to an institutional hierarchy; parents are accountable only to themselves and to their children. If social workers or clinical nurses do elect to work with a self-help group, they may be held responsible by the rest of the staff for the group's decisions or actions. If the group does things the staff feels good about, all well and good. But if the self-help group starts to do things the staff does not condone, professional participants may be called on to account for such behavior and to control it. In addition, professionals may feel compelled to defend or express loyalty to the medical staff to parents. In those circumstances in which groups challenge the health care organization, close relations between professionals and group members may blunt the challenge, for better or worse.

Several observers have indicated circumstances under which professionals working with parents and parent groups communicate parents' needs to other staff members, just as they educate parent groups to the workings of the medical staff.[17] Some professionals even may find themselves defending parent activism before the medical staff. However, little attention is given to how professionals may mediate actual conflicts between parent groups and staff members. Any of these roles as advocate, mutual educator, or mediator may strain the dual identification of the professional as a servant of parents' needs and as an agent of the medical facility. Since the professionals working most directly with parent self-help groups generally occupy the lowest status roles within the medical staff, they often have little influence at staff meetings and are buffeted by the medical staff's own concerns and crises.

Sometimes professionals find that their traditional skills and roles are not well-suited for work with parent self-help groups. For instance, social workers trained in individual casework skills may not know how to develop an organization, mobilize a constituency, assist in fund raising, alter institutional policy, and the like. Nurses comfortable with medical and intrapersonal dynamics may have little understanding of the interpersonal issues at work in an organized group. Moreover, their senses of professional responsibility for psychosocial treatment may make them uneasy being part of a "lay treatment" system, a peer support and co-counseling network. Discovering and developing the right mix of skills and roles for effective work with self-help groups may require nurses and social workers to do a lot of "on the job" learning.

Little attention also has been given to the support that professionals themselves may need from their patients or parents, especially when they have been active together in a long-term support group. In the midst of a caring group, staff members occasionally feel uncared for. As they care for others and reach out to share skills with others, staff members may feel left out if parents do not express affection and appreciation in return (such as observing birthdays, weddings, and other events). Of course, staff members are trained to be cautious, a bit distant, and to avoid such emotional interdependence with their clients. But caring is a human feeling, and not to acknowledge and deal with mutual caring ignores the human side of professional work. The natural reciprocity of caring in human relations is made most difficult by strict adherence to roles that rigidly distinguish the givers and receivers of help. For instance, in their work with self-help groups, are professionals supposed to consider themselves part of the group or not? Are they insiders or outsiders? When self-help group members share their deep feelings, should social workers and nurses share the feelings as well? Should they ever criticize the staff? When and how can professionals ask parents for reciprocity in caring? If this is difficult or impossible to do, how do these staff members avoid emotional isolation and burn-out?[18]

Many parents recognize the dilemmas facing the professionals with whom they work closely, partly because they care about them and partly because staff members share or deliberately educate parents about these issues. Under these circumstances, parents and professionals may develop a pattern in which they support and care for each other, thus improving the quality of work and life for everyone involved in providing health care to children.

CHAPTER NOTES

1. The emergence of self-help as a national phenomenon is by no means limited to childhood cancer. Many people struggling with chronic health problems have organized mutual support or self-help groups. Good reviews of this phenomenon can be found in Collins and Pancoast (1976), Gartner and Riessman (1977), Katz (1981), Katz and Bender (1976), Killilea (1976), Lieberman and Borman (1979), Powell (1975), and Tracy and Gussow (1976).

2. Some scholars argue that dissatisfaction with the practice of modern medicine alienates patients and prompts the self-help process (Back & Taylor, 1976). The active and reciprocal support generated in typical self-help may be an antidote to the nonreciprocal and passive roles forced on patients by most medical and social service professionals (Gartner & Riessman, 1977). Other scholars find no link between such dissatisfaction and self-help, suggesting instead that some people seek self-help as an alternate form of social connection and mutual aid, not necessarily as a compensation for negative feelings about current professional practice (Banhoff, 1979; Lieberman, 1979; Tracy & Gussow, 1976).

3. Examples are reported by Adams (1978), Belle-Isle and Conradt (1979), Gilder, Buschman, Sitarz, and Wolff (1976), Heffron (1975), Kartha and Ertel (1976), Martinson, (1976).

4. Such parent-developed handbooks usually provide basic information about childhood cancer and its treatment, common childhood fears and child-rearing issues, and a list (or even a map) of local resources (*Oncology Handbook for Parents*, 1976, 1977, 1978; Schweers, Farnes & Foreman, 1977).

5. Some self-help groups that advocate for change take on the character of small social movement organizations or local voluntary action groups (Katz, 1981; Steinman & Traunstein, 1976).

6. Examples are reported by Adams (1979), Belle-Isle and Conradt (1979), Gilder, Buschman, Sitarz, and Wolff (1976), Heffron (1975), Kartha and Ertel (1976), Martinson (1976).

7. Dory and Riessman (1982), Gartner and Riessman (1977), Riessman (1965), Silverman (1976).

8. This combination of initiators appears quite common: Borman (1982, p. 26) notes that, "A recent review of some major self-help networks that focus around particular afflictions of conditions . . . indicates that distinguished professionals have often played important roles in initiating, advising, legitimizing and guiding a group's development."

9. This is a significant issue for many groups and a focus of scholarly and professional debate. Arguments in favor of parents of living and deceased children being part of the same self-help group include (1) parents of deceased children still have ties to the hospital and to other parents, and they might be sadder and lonelier if these ties were cut; and (2) parents of deceased children can help prepare others for the possibility of death and show that life continues even after the death of a child. Major arguments against such integrated groups include: (1) new parents may be frightened by meeting parents of children who died; (2) parents of deceased children may be at different stages of their lives and not interested in talking about the same things as parents of living children; (3) parents of deceased children may find it too painful to meet with and see parents of living children; and (4) it may be too guilt provoking for parents of living children to take heart in their situation in front of parents of deceased children. Different groups have solved this problem in different ways. Some mirror the dual membership pattern of the group described here, whereas others emphasize the distinct issues or needs of each category of parents and organize separate groups, or generate a culture that makes one or another category dominant. Many groups become concerned that they not avoid the topic of death, but also that they not be perceived as a group of "parents of dead children."

10. See, for example, Borman (1982), Durman (1976), Edwards (1966), Levy (1976), Lieberman and Borman (1976), Wheat and Lieber (1976), Videka-Sherman (1982). These results also reflect the finding that women and people of higher social status are more likely to seek, find, and use support of all kinds, from many sources, than are men and people of lower financial and educational status (Gourash, 1978; Greeley & Mechanic, 1976; Pearlin, 1975).

11. Clearly it is not a simple matter, nor is it comfortable, to accept/adopt such a public identity (Goffman, 1968; Lieberman & Borman, 1979; Powell, 1975; Voysey, 1972; Wortman & Dunkel-Schetter, 1979).

12. Rather than a true finding, this relationship primarily represents a positive test of the reliability of the support question.

13. Reports from other treatment centers indicate that a pattern of physician distance and clinical nurse/social worker closeness to self-help groups is quite common. Nurses and social workers often manage the referral process by which parents of newly diagnosed children learn about the group.

14. See note 2. The evidence for mutual interest and cooperation is presented by Lenrow and Burch (1981), Levy (1978), and Lieberman and Borman (1979); the evidence for conflict of interest is provided by Katz (1981) and Kleiman, Mantell, and Alexander (1976).

15. In a study of over 50 self-help groups throughout the nation, Chesler and Yoak interviewed a large number of active parents and over 50 health care professionals (physicians, nurses, and social workers) who work with these groups in various roles (Chesler & Yoak, 1984; Yoak & Chesler, 1985).

16. The data presented in Table 10.5 are from interviews described in note 15.

17. See the discussion of social workers' roles at the conclusion of Chapter 4, and Chesler and Barbarin (1984), McCollum and Schwartz (1972), Ross (1980), and Stuetzer (1980).

18. The phenomenon of professional burn-out, especially in the context of caring relationships, is explored in Freudenberger (1974), Klagsbrun (1970), Maslach (1976), Rothenberg (1967), and Vachon, Lyall, and Freeman (1978).

CHAPTER 11

Schooling for Children with Cancer

As children with cancer undergo treatment, they also continue with their lives. For children between the ages of 6 and 18, school attendance is an important part of life, and a vital social and developmental activity. Indeed, because school attendance is natural for children, it is one way in which children with cancer maintain normalcy despite their struggle with their illness. For this reason, children with cancer are encouraged to participate in school activities as fully as possible.

One student who had been a cheerleader and a member of the gymnastic team prior to her diagnosis with osteogenic sarcoma continued as a cheerleader soon after the amputation of her leg. She felt this step was important for her own well-being as well as for its salutary effect on her peers:

Students with cancer should stay involved in school activities such as band or other clubs. Then other students would see that they (children with cancer) are fine and that they don't have to be worried about or fussed over.

A 13-year-old male with osteogenic sarcoma, also an amputee, learned to ski and ride a bike with one leg. His accomplishments evidently

Portions of this chapter first appeared in: Barbarin, O., & Chesler, M. *Children with Cancer: School Experiences and Views of Parents, Educators, Adolescents, and Physicians.* Maywood, Ill.: Eterna Press, 1983; and Chesler, M., & Barbarin, O. Parents' perspectives on the school experiences of children with cancer. *Topics in Early Childhood Special Education,* 1986, 5(4), 36–48. Reprinted by permission.

inspired other amputees with whom he had contact. One child whose amputation created difficulty also reports adapting, with a little help:

> *I have trouble getting places, but the only time I leave early from class is before lunchtime, because everyone runs down the steps and I have to get down before them. At the end of school, I usually wait a while and a teacher takes me down and helps me get my books and stuff.*

Such examples of continued activity, with or without help, are legion. The experience of cancer, even when it involves physical impairment such as the loss of a limb, need not necessarily diminish students' interest in academic pursuits nor prevent their participation in extracurricular activities.

Of course, not all children with cancer resume regular school attendance. Some die without ever returning to school. Some are so ravaged by the disease and its treatment (vigorous chemotherapy, intensive radiation therapy, and radical surgery) that they cannot resume their normal activities or attend school for a long period or, when they can return, require a specialized school environment and program. Although the vast majority of children with cancer can and do attend school during and after their treatment, there are some problems that, when they occur, pose significant threats to successful school adaptation and to the student's and family's well-being. These problems include physical discomfort, frequent absence, falling behind academically, peer teasing and avoidance, and difficulties in relating to the school staff. This chapter reviews reports from youngsters, parents, and educators on the nature and extent of these problems and discusses the potential for creating collaborative relationships between the school and family to prevent or solve them.[1]

PROBLEMS IN SCHOOL REENTRY

Both the discussion in Chapter 2 and medical reports indicate some of the physical limitations or compromises that may be imposed upon children by their disease and treatment. For instance, hair loss, weight gain and loss, physical discomfort, and fatigue are quite common in children undergoing treatment. Surgery may be disfiguring and potentially disabling. Drugs and/or radiation may cause short- and long-term neurological deficits. Extended hospitalization may require children to miss substantial amounts of schooling. But in addition to these physical stresses, there also are psychological and psychosocial by-products of the disease and treatment that may affect students' school attitudes and achievements.

Several early research reports and clinical case studies suggest that children with cancer exhibit signs of school phobia upon return to school.[2] Our research, however, suggests that the frequency of school phobia or serious anxiety is quite low. Very few parents and only 5% of the educators we interviewed observed school phobia, persistent uneasiness, or fear of returning to school among children with cancer. Moreover, all of the 17 adolescents with cancer who were interviewed describe themselves as eager to return to school.

Among the most serious obstacles to a smooth reentry are the reactions (real and imagined) of peers and educators.[3] Adolescents with cancer report that the major problems they experience involve considerable teasing, especially because of hair loss, and completing some assignments. Thirty of the 59 parents (51%) with school-age children with cancer report that their children experience problems in returning to school; the most common issues involve missing much school, teasing, or rejection by peers and relating to teachers. And when the school staff was asked about these issues they most often mention teasing, the child's physical discomfort, low academic achievement, and difficulties in peer relationships.[4]

Absence from School and Falling Behind

Less than one third of the parents (18/59) report (in Table 11.1) that their children missed "much" schooling,[5] and less than one tenth of the

Table 11.1
School Problems Reported by Parents
of Children with Cancer

Problems	Number and Percent of Parents Reporting School Problems	
	N=59	Percent*
Mention any problem	30	51
Teasing (rejection) by peers	22	37
Missed much school	18	31
Relationships with teachers	7	12

*Since some parents mentioned more than one problem, the total percentage equals more than 100%.

teachers of children with cancer indicate (in Table 11.2) that absences create serious problems.[6] Approximately one third of the teachers feel that low academic achievement is a serious problem.

Attendance and achievement are most likely to become serious problems in the event of a relapse, as one teacher reports.

He was not absent much initially, but at the end of the school year he was absent a great deal because he had another relapse. But he was an outstanding student. He loved to read and the homebound teacher would come to the school and pick up library books for him and she worked pretty closely with him. I always tried to let the homebound teacher know that he was in great shape but I knew that he always wanted to get his work done and that the absences bothered him a great deal. He had this great concern that when he came back to school, the other kids would know more than he did.

Parents' reports that the child missed "much" school relate to relapse and to hospitalizations. As we might expect, children who relapse miss much school more than children who stay in remission (64% versus 26%; chi square=5.6, $df=1$, $p. <.05$), and children who had more extended hospitalizations are more likely to miss much school than those children with fewer hospitalizations (58% versus 13%; chi square=12.2, $df=1$, $p. <.01$). On the other hand, parents who report that their children missed much school are no more likely than other parents to report that their children are not caught up with school or that they experience other problems, including teasing. Whereas missing some school may be a common experience for children with cancer, they do not all miss

Table 11.2
School Problems of Children with Cancer Reported
by the School Staff (N=23)

Child's Problems	Somewhat Serious Problem	Slight Problem	No Problem
Teasing from classmates	44%	11%	44%
Discomfort from medication/surgery	43	13	43
Low academic achievement	32	18	50
Difficulty in relationships with peers	28	32	40
Frequent absences from school	9	56	35
Taking physical risks	5	36	59
Emotional adjustment	4	39	57
School phobia	5	0	95

a lot of school; moreover, absences do not necessarily translate into poor academic performance.

The majority of adolescent students feel that their overall academic performance does not suffer as a result of the illness. Although two ill youngsters failed to achieve promotion, most describe themselves as caught up with schoolwork, even though it may take a while to achieve this status. Several even note that good grades now seem more achievable than before their diagnosis because of the increased concentration, seriousness, and commitment with which they approach school tasks.

However, children who were not doing well in school prior to their diagnosis sometimes have an especially difficult time catching up afterwards. One mother feels her son's problems were compounded by a lack of help from the school.

My son was different from some others because he was a "C" and "D" student before he got cancer. When he came home from the hospital no one called the house. All the initiative had to be ours, and we had enough to deal with already. I guess they figured that since he was not a good student to begin with, they should not bother. Besides, in their minds he was dying already. I think the school gave up on him, and as a result he gave up on school.

Teasing and Rejection by Peers

Over one third (22/59) of the parents with school-age children indicate that teasing by peers is a concern; 44% of the teachers report teasing as a somewhat serious problem and 28% note the child's difficulties in relationships with peers as an important issue (see Tables 11.1 and 11.2). Parents comment:

There was some teasing. But he didn't want me to talk with the teacher or do anything about it. That would make it worse, he thought.

There was one turkey who really teased him a lot. He hit him and knocked out one of his teeth and that stopped it.

Some parents report that peers' reactions go beyond teasing, to rejection of the child with cancer.

She was treated like a leper.

The kids would make fun of him when he had no hair and when he was on medication and blew up like a balloon. There were remarks made to him that he was going to die.

Parents were particularly troubled by and angry at the reactions of some other parents.

The children were told about it in school, and they weren't too upset. But some parents were upset because their kids came home and they were concerned that their friend was really, really sick. Anyone would be upset. But the parents got mad that the school had said anything about it; they felt that the school shouldn't have told the kids and upset them.

I did have some parents call me and tell me that they did not want my child in school, because they did not want their children to come down with cancer.

These comments identify two different fears that the general public has with regard to children with cancer: that the cancer itself is contagious, and that it is always very sad or frightening to come close to this situation. There is no evidence that cancer is contagious, although this myth does persist in some quarters. In Chapter 9 we reported the emotional shock and sadness that close friends of the family of a child with cancer sometimes experience, and it is not surprising that some parents of friends of the child anticipate a similar reaction. When parents of classmates permit these fears to govern their behavior and encourage their children to withdraw from the child with cancer, peer discomfort, teasing or rejection are bound to occur. In the interest of avoiding potential "upset," these parents also are counseling their children to jettison important friendships and to withdraw from some important realities of life. The experience of being close to a child with cancer may bring occasional sadness, and even fear, but it also can generate many important learnings about friendship and about life itself.

Teachers usually deal preventively with teasing in their own class, but teasing often comes from students in other classes. In one case, the problem got so bad that the mother went to the teacher because the child complained that he was being teased about his hair loss. The teacher reports:

We (principal, teacher, and parents) made arrangements for him to leave a little early one day and I talked to the rest of the class about it. Of course some of the children knew that he had been sick because some of them had been in class with him the previous year, but a lot didn't know. I just said that he was sick and that he had a blood disease. They were very concerned about things like whether they could catch it, why does the medicine make his hair fall out. Some of them became very indignant that anyone would tease him about it. A couple of the boys said if they heard anyone poking fun at him, they were going to belt them. I said that if they heard anyone teasing (him) they should just stand up for him and tell the other kids to lay off and explain that it was the medicine that made his hair fall out. They were very quiet. Later in the year I got up at a staff meeting and talked about it to make the other teachers aware that there was a student in the school who had hair loss and the reasons for it, and that gave them an opportunity to talk to their own students about it.

Teasing is a typical school-age behavior. However, children with cancer are inappropriate targets for such teasing because of their physical disability and their psychological vulnerability. Parents wrestle with what they and the school staff might or should do to intervene in or to prevent these situations. The staff's direct and sensitive handling of problems such as teasing can very effectively defuse a volatile situation, and can help other children grow in their ability to empathize with and care for their peers.

In addition to teasing, older youngsters often report that peers' withdrawal, misplaced pity, and fear may transform previously free-flowing and intimate relationships to distant and awkward ones.

When I went back to school, I felt that students were shying away from me. I thought they were ignoring me at first, but now I realize they just didn't know what to say.

Well, I suppose that some people avoided me because they were embarrassed and didn't know what to say, and others went out of their way to talk to me, and some people treated me the same way.

Other adolescents report that their peers shied away from them at first, not knowing how to react, but eventually returned to normal when they realized that the teens with cancer were still "the same people."

Sometimes peers do not know how to behave or what to expect from the adolescent with cancer. Often they do not know whether or not to talk about the illness (or the hair loss or amputation) and wait for signals from the ill child about how they should behave. Once older peers know what to expect they begin to act more normally. However, it generally is up to the ill youngster to establish the terms of normalcy, and to invite continuity in peer relationships.[7] In relationships with close friends, then, it is often the adolescent with cancer who assumes the role of comforter and supporter. One very perceptive adolescent describes the burden of his concern about the psychological well-being of his friends, especially in the early stages of the illness.

*It was hard enough trying to keep myself together... I felt like
I had to keep my friends together too. Whenever we got together,
they were so worried about me that I had to spend time calming
them down, telling them that I'd be okay.*

Physical Discomfort of the Ill Child

Physical discomfort is a problem about which the school staff can
do little except exhibit patience and understanding. Forty-three percent
of the school staff indicate that the child's pain or physical discomfort
is a somewhat serious problem. One teacher talks about a first-grader
with leukemia:

*She lost some hair and some weight. She was a little pale and tired
a little more easily. She is an average child with lots of grit and
guts and I'm sure she was in school some days when she didn't feel
great.*

Similar experiences are shared by other educators:

*She was sometimes very, very pale — almost white. She was often
very immature after treatment — almost babylike. I think she hurt
and that's when her mother let her bring stuffed animals into class
a lot as a sort of security. I noticed this sort of clinging to something she loved. I think that was very necessary to her at the time.*

*The gym teacher noticed his inability to keep up — he could barely
run. That in turn affected recess times. When everyone would go
out and play, he would just walk around by himself.*

Parents do not spontaneously mention pain and discomfort as a problem, although they include such concerns as part of the reason their
child misses school.

Relationships with the School Staff

Twelve percent of the parents with school-age children with cancer
(7/59) report that their child's relationships with teachers is a problem
for the child. Obviously, not all students are blessed with active and
sensitive teachers. Table 11.3 indicates parents' reports of helpful and
nonhelpful, or even negative, school staff behaviors. Parents detail some
examples of insensitivity and apparent lack of caring by the school staff
(for the child *and* the parent):

Table 11.3
Parents' Reports of What the Teacher Did That
Was Helpful or Not Helpful

Teachers' Actions	Percent of Parents Reporting* Teachers' Actions
Actions That Were Helpful	
Was caring	39%
Treated child as normal	28
Gave special academic help	20
Kept parents informed	14
Actions That Were Not Helpful	
Was insensitive	13
Was overprotective	10
Other	23

*Multiple responses cause the total percent to exceed 100%.

During his therapy, one of the teachers told me he'd have to have a letter from a doctor at the hospital because he did not believe that he had leukemia. It must be all in my mind, he said!

One teacher didn't know she was on chemotherapy and that her memory was impaired. The teacher marked her down because she forgot to hand in some homework.

A lack of staff involvement and concern is discouraging, as one parent's report summarizes her son's encounters with the school system:

He found out the teachers didn't care, so he lost interest.

Even when teachers do care, the ways in which they express their concern for the ill child affect how well they are received. A parent captures the consequences of a teacher's well-meaning overconcern and overprotectiveness:

At first she babied him, was scared of him, and afraid to touch him. He was fragile to her. He sensed this and used this to his advantage.

Several youngsters also report teacher overprotectiveness:

I felt I got a little teacher overprotection.

I usually ended up as a coach in gym. I couldn't do a lot of things that the other kids did. I got an automatic "A" in the course.

When they find the school staff too eager to help them, some youngsters deliberately seek to avoid unnecessary dependency.

I would tell my teachers not to baby me and that I was just like everyone else.

I tried to keep my problems from them so I wouldn't develop a crutch to lean on.

It is wise for ill youngsters to fear overprotection. If worried parents and teachers buffer them too much and overprotect them, youngsters may receive a message of their extreme vulnerability and may become hesitant and cautious about behaving normally (Spinetta et al., 1976). Parents provide examples of the benefits of the school staff treating the child as normally as possible.

They just made her comfortable. They treated her like the rest of the kids with a few exceptions. That was real important to her.

They treated her normally, with no favors, which is what she and I wanted.

At times, parents and professionals may go too far in the opposite direction. By denying that problems exist, parents and school staff may fail adequately to protect ill children. Many children need preparation and protection to face ignorance, cruelty, or inflexibility on the part of peers, neighbors, or even the school staff.

Several examples of the insensitive actions of school administrators and a rigid adherence to rules of the school bureaucracy left parents outraged and upset.

A year and a half ago I went over to school and asked about his credits and being able to graduate. They looked at the records and the counselor said he was fine and he'd be able to graduate with his class. Then he did well in school and all was forgotten until the first semester of the 12th grade. I received a letter stating he had no 9th grade English credit, and he'd have to go to night school to graduate. He enrolled in night school and attended. The more he thought about it, the more he said, "The hell with it, they lied to me, said I could graduate, and now they say I can't unless I do extra work." At that point, he dropped out of school. We went to the school for help and they denied it. It disgusts me. He worked his hind end off to maintain his grades and then they screw up down there.

The hospital sent the school a letter regarding his absences and that he was in the hospital. Teachers called to offer assistance, but the principal gave them a lot of hassles regarding taking his final exams. He missed the last week of school and the principal wanted him to take the tests right away. The principal didn't want the teachers to take them to the hospital and administer them either. Also, he was very sick and not up to taking them. The teachers tried to help him, but the principal was the problem.

Principal should have been better informed about help available to sick kids — like a homebound teacher. We didn't find out about it for a while.

The school bureaucracy, like the hospital bureaucracy, sometimes fails to anticipate and respond to individual youngsters' needs.

There is a delicate tension or balance among the behaviors parents identify in Table 11.3. If caring and giving special help are positive, too much of it may be overprotective. If treating the child as normal is positive, too much of that (in the face of the child's specialness) may be insensitive. Van Eys summarizes this dilemma (1977a):

If the cancer were ignored by well-meaning people, the child's reality would be distorted and he would not be accepted as the person he is. On the other hand, when the cancer is made the overwhelming concern, the "normal" in the child that wants to be recognized is ignored. Either produces despair. (p. 168)

Siblings

We report (Chapter 6) that siblings often appear to be the most left-out family members and to receive the least attention at home. Some parents note the problems this creates at school and are concerned about the school staff's sensitivity to siblings.

The school let me down when they didn't understand my sick kid's older brother. I mean, a nice boy like that, who's never done anything wrong before, suddenly acting out. You'd think they would have anticipated some changes and been on the lookout, or at least been more sensitive when it happened.

The little one feels he isn't getting enough attention at home, and he's right. I need some extra help from the school on this one.

In addition to home and family strains, siblings also react to the peer issues that the ill child encounters at school. When siblings are taunted with the refrain "Your brother's going to die," or when they see their brother or sister being teased, they may respond with vigorous action.

Her brother is often getting into fights because he can't stand the other kids teasing her . . . about her hair and everything.

Moreover, when parents of peers restrain their children from playing with children with cancer (or do not encourage them to play with ill children), peers may also withdraw from siblings.

These reports suggest that school-related problems exist not only in the ill child's behavior or attitudes but also in the reactions of the child's teachers, peers, parents of peers, own parents, and siblings. If all attempts to moderate the stress of school reentry are directed toward the sick child, or even to the sick child's family, without attention to peers and educators, significant sources of stress will remain unresolved and interventions will be incomplete and ineffective.

HELP PROVIDED BY THE SCHOOL STAFF

Three fourths of the educators report that they provide emotional comfort and support to the family, and a substantial number report listening to parents' problems and holding them or crying together. In addition to providing help to parents, over one third of the teachers report reaching out to the ill child by visiting or taking assignments to the hospital, and by providing emotional and social support, as well as academic assistance, in the classroom. Sometimes this help is delivered on a one-on-one basis, teacher to student; at other times teachers organize others to provide support.

I went over to her house when she was isolated. I took her some papers and talked to her. She was getting quite lonesome for her friends and her mother said it was a very hard two weeks for her.

The school sent flowers right away. We spent a lot of time talking with the kids about whether they would be going to the funeral and whether they had ever been to one before. I felt very good that on the day of the funeral many of the children in my class went and some of them also went to visit at the funeral home. A lot of the teachers from the school, as well as the principal and the secretary, went. The school also collected money for a memorial fund and got people involved in helping to make food for the funeral and the brunch to follow. The teachers brought dishes and the cooks prepared things as well. There was a lot of involvement that way.

These actions are confirmed by parents' and staffs' reports in Tables 11.3 and 11.4. In addition, parents note the things the school staff does in school that make the transition to school easier:

She's just a super person. She gives him his medication and vitamins every day. If he's had a bad day (after chemo) she sends his homework home. She's very understanding.

I told his teacher that he had cancer and that if anyone sneezed on him he'd be sick. If a mother sent her child to school with a cold the teacher called me to take him home.

They've done things that have made him more comfortable. Like they have a rule that you can't wear hats in school but when he lost his hair he could wear his hat. When he was tired, they had a rug in the back of the room, which they called the reading area, and as long as he was caught up and had his work done, he could go take a nap if he was exceptionally tired. At first he would do that quite often but he doesn't do that too much anymore. He's got more energy.

Table 11.4
Staff Members' Reports of Help They Provided
to Families of Children with Cancer

Type of Help Provided	Percent Reporting Providing this Help (N=29, 100%)
Emotional comfort or support	76.2%
Listening to parents' problems	47.6
Holding parent or child	42.9
Taking assignments to hospital	38.1
Providing extra academic assistance to child	38.1
Crying together with parents	33.3
Solving problems of child discipline	33.3
Playing with ill child	33.3
Looking up information	28.6
Visiting child in hospital	14.3
Asking doctor for information	14.3
Raising money	4.8

One quite extraordinary instance of how helpful and thoughtful the school staff can be is contained in the following parent's report:

> *After several relapses we brought my son home from the hospital. We all knew he was dying, but he wanted to spend his last weeks at home and we all agreed. He could not go back to school, however, and we were unsure how he could say goodbye to his old friends and teachers. But on Halloween we had a grand time. The school always has a costume day on Halloween, and all the kids get dressed up. It was a nice day, and my son's teacher had all the children in his class walk the three blocks from the school right past our house — all in costume. They all waved to my son as they went past, and he felt part of the class and part of the festivities even though he wasn't in school anymore. In fact, he got dressed up in a costume of his own and waved back to all the kids from just inside our front door. He had great fun with his skeleton's costume.*

This family, this teacher, and other members of the community remember this event long after the death of the young man. The memory of the march through the neighborhood is a symbol of how much the school cared for that ill child and how warmly the family and the school collaborated in expressing that caring.

Adolescents generally view the school staff's attempts to help quite favorably. Their positive evaluations of the staff's behavior center around the flexibility that teachers have for schoolwork deadlines while they are in treatment, and the direct help teachers give them while they are in the hospital. One student missed two and one-half months of school during her 10th grade but was able to complete the most essential course work. Students also appreciate teachers who take the initiative to help the class understand cancer and its treatment. Other forms of help strongly appreciated by students include:

> *Taping class lectures and making them available to students who are at home or in the hospital;*

> *Allowing students to focus on main concepts or skills and omitting supplementary requirements when time is limited;*

> *De-emphasizing the importance of grades;*

> *Using discretionary power to waive formal examinations if the student is hospitalized or undergoing chemotherapy;*

> *Sending cards to the hospitalized student;*

Providing the student with an extra set of books to leave at home if the student is on crutches;

Demonstrating the use of prostheses to the class;

Communicating directly and honestly with the student.

These actions by teachers also make it much easier for the students' peers to accept and to be direct with students with cancer upon their return to school.

Some parents suggest dealing with the complex school organization by nurturing a relationship with one staff member who will take the role of advocating and facilitating school life for the child.

Have one person at the school responsible for knowing the status of your child—school nurse, classroom teacher or school psychologist. Keep in touch so there is a free flow of information, especially if the child is absent frequently.

A close connection with one strong and compassionate advocate is especially important if parents cannot count on such behavior from the entire staff.

Who Receives Help from the School Staff?

Over 50% of the parents describe the school people as being very or quite helpful to them and their child; but just less than half describe the staff as not helpful or only a little helpful. Parents of ill children over 11 years of age report slightly more helpful responses from educators than do elementary school parents. Perhaps these children and their parents have more experience with the school and know how to assert themselves to get appropriate help.

More highly educated parents report receiving helpful responses from school people significantly more often than do parents with less educational background (chi square=9.9, $df=2$, $p. <.01$). Several different factors related to educators, the child, and the parent may account for this finding: School people may respond more positively to parents of the same or higher status as themselves; children of more highly educated parents may do better in school and be seen as better bets for educators to invest their time and energy on; parents with more educational experience may be more assertive about asking for help for their children or appreciate the help they receive more than other parents.

Helpfulness of school people may matter! Parents who report that school people are "very" or "quite" helpful are slightly more likely to feel that their children are caught up with their classmates. The number of children who are described by their parents as not caught up with their classmates is too small for numerical analysis (6 of 59=10%), but the trend is clear nevertheless. Using a larger sample, Feldman (1980) reports that students with cancer from families with higher educational backgrounds are more likely than students from other families to improve their academic performance upon their reentry to school. If higher educational background is related to parents' perception of helpfulness from the school, and if more helpfulness is related to the child's stable or even improved performance on reentry, then this finding makes good sense.

STAFF STRESSES AND COPING PATTERNS

Most research on school reentry of children with cancer overlooks the personal emotional issues that confront teachers and administrators of seriously ill children. Since childhood cancer is a shared experience, educators, like the child's parents, the family's friends, and the child's playmates, are affected by the child's impaired health status and by the struggle of living with a serious and chronic illness. Some educators report strong personal reactions, such as concern about death and dying and feelings of pity for the child and parents. These reactions often are marked by a combination of sadness, fear, and anger – many of the same feelings that parents experience upon learning about the diagnosis.

> *I was surprised because he seemed like such an average, normal student and he didn't have any real personal problems. No one ever said anything to me about it. It seems to be happening more and more and it comes closer to you. You can't assume that it is on the other side of the fence – you have to deal with the situation. With any disabled student, it makes you aware that this is a reality of life and there for the grace of God, go I.*

> *I really felt bad – like it wasn't fair . . .the usual reaction that someone so young is not going to grow up. He was a very responsible little boy. I guess the greatest thing was that my emotions would come in – feeling sorry for him and pity. I guess I was having a hard time dealing with my emotions.*

A significant proportion of the school staff is forced by this experience to grapple with the meaning of life and death, and to place many issues in a new personal perspective. For example, a majority of school staff members report a marked increase in patience (60%), faith in God (57%), sympathy for the sick (54%), and understanding of death (54%) as a result of having a child with cancer in their classroom. Like parents and friends of the family, educators working with children with cancer re-examine attitudes and values that go unchallenged in the normal course of life.

The challenges associated with school reentry often require a more intense involvement between family and school staff and a redefinition of the entire family-school relationship. Many school personnel report wondering how helpful they should try to be to the sick child and how much they should extend themselves to the family. Many report fearing that parents or colleagues would resent meddling or overinvolvement. If some teachers and school administrators are uncertain about how the ill child's parents will react, they may refrain from taking the initiative.

Even the best prepared and experienced teachers walk a thin line in deciding how to act, and in acting, in ways that are truly helpful to returning students and their families. Teachers new to and inexperienced in these situations often respond in anxious and fearful ways, either ducking and ignoring issues or paying too much attention to imagined difficulties and problems. Those professionals who define their roles narrowly often feel they are unable to be as helpful as they might have been or wish to be. When parents or youngsters do not confide in the staff, or do not indicate directly that they are receptive to and appreciative of help, school staff members face an especially difficult situation. With the notable exceptions of providing emotional support, holding a parent or child, and crying together with parents, most of the common helpful behaviors in Table 11.4 are in keeping with educators' typical professional roles. However, the reentry of the ill child is handled most smoothly when school personnel go beyond the normal boundaries of their professional roles. When school staff members are unable to resolve the dilemma regarding their professional roles and personal feelings, less successful transitions are reported. Some teachers express this dilemma:

> *I felt helpless at times. . . . I didn't feel that there was anything I could do. I didn't feel very involved and I wanted to be more involved. He never confided or shared his feelings with me, but now and then I wonder if I had let him get away with something that others didn't.*

> *I really feel that I should have visited her in the hospital, which I did not do. My experience of 34 years in a school system is that regardless of how sick a child is they really enjoy contact with their*

teachers or principal and cards from the kids. Why I didn't go, I really don't know, but it wasn't the easiest year for me.

If teachers are isolated from the family and unable to create or respond to conversations about the child's condition and needs, their discomfort and these problems are exacerbated.

School staff members who report their stresses related to a child with cancer in class (see Table 11.5) often feel they lack specific details about the child's health status (60%) and knowledge about the disease itself (43%). The staff's lack of information increases the stress of the child's school reentry because staff members do not know what to expect and have few guidelines for their own behavior. This lack of knowledge contributes to two other problems that teachers often mention as serious: uncertainty about how demanding to be (50%) and uncertainty about how to discipline the child (50%).

When parents actively communicate with the school, and when the school uses the information, many important benefits result. As two teachers note:

The parents came in to talk to me several times and I brought up the topic with them also. The closeness between the parents and the school and the whole atmosphere made her a good normal person. I maintained steady contact with the parents and they told

Table 11.5
Percent of School Staff Reporting Personal Stresses
or Problems (N=29)

Personal Stresses or Problems	Serious Problem	Slight Problem	No Problem
Lack of specific details about child's health status (N=25)	60%	12%	28%
Uncertainty about how to discipline the sick child (N=18)	50	6	44
Uncertainty about how demanding to be of the sick child (N=18)	50	11	39
Lack of general knowledge about cancer (N=21)	43	24	33
Personal concern about death/dying (N=24)	16	46	38
Tendency to pity (N=21)	10	38	52
Absence of support from other teachers/principal (N=23)	0	39	61

me whenever her medicines were changed and if she had had a bad or good day or night. What the parents did was wonderful—they told me everything that was happening and there was close communication between the home and the school.

The previous teachers had told me that the mother had been in very close contact with them and sure enough, within the first two days of school she called and wanted to know if she could come in and sit down and talk with me about it. And she did within three days. She said that if at all possible he would be in school because he really liked it and he didn't particularly like going in for treatments. She gave me a booklet for the teacher of a child with cancer and she invited me to attend a lecture on the topic with her. That happened to be a night that I was attending a class so I couldn't go. She gave me a lot of information about his exact case and said that if I had any questions she would be happy to help me with anything she could. Shortly after that she saw me again and wanted me to talk to my class because he said that he had frequently been teased about his hair loss. We discussed the way that he wanted me to tell the class. When the mother first talked to me and gave me all kinds of details, I wondered to myself how she could be so matter of fact and thought it was probably because she had done this so many times with so many people. I was somewhat amazed by her openness. I questioned her about how he felt about all of this and I wanted to know if he would ever talk about it or share it with me or with the other students or if he would write about it. She told me some of the things that he told the family at that time but not much. I thought she was an incredibly strong person. After he became terminally ill and I started visiting their home I saw the kind of strength in that home. When I visited there, they gave me the strength that I needed because I didn't know how I would get through that visit when I laid eyes on him. I was ready to just leave the room because it really bothered me and I didn't know what to say or what to do but his family made it easy for me. They were so uplifting. And after that I visited him on a number of occasions and I got to know them so much better. Since then they have become very close friends of mine.

As educators attempt to deal with these personal stresses, some feel they receive considerable help. Most report receiving support from the child's family (90%) or from the child (71%). Thus, informed and effective parental behavior may affect the ability of the school staff to cope with their own stresses, as well as with child and classroom problems.

A little more than half of the educators report getting support from the school principal (54%) and from their peers (57%).

*The greatest help you get is from other teachers or the principal.
The social workers just can't feel the impact of it like another
teacher who's there every day. The social workers deal in isolated
situations and they feel it differently.*

When peer support is available it is extremely important in helping
teachers gain perspective and balance. One teacher, in whose class a
student with cancer died during the school year, comments on the
importance of the help and consolation that were provided by her professional peers.

*The support of the other teachers meant a great deal to me. I came
back to school very late on the day of the funeral to return some
pans, and people were surprised to see me. His previous teacher
came over to me and said something to me and I started crying
all over again. The principal also came over. Two of the middle-aged
teachers said that it must have been a very hard day for me, and
that never in their years of teaching had they experienced the death
of a student, and that people can teach for years and years and
never have that experience. People came up to me and were very
understanding.*

However, peer and administrative support is not universal. In some
cases, teachers find very little support from the principal or other
teachers.

*The principal would have gone to pieces and been so upset that
he would not have been able to give me any special help. I would
not have gone to either of the two teachers she had previously because I did not agree with some of the things they did.*

Although a few teachers also report receiving assistance and support
from school social workers and school nurses, these staff members are
not available in most schools. In addition, very few educators report
receiving help from the medical staff. At the time this study was conducted the local medical center had no systematic outreach program to
the schools that their patients attended, and all direct or indirect contact
with the medical staff was on an individual family basis.[8] Educators are
not always comfortable relying upon the family for accurate and complete medical information. Some teachers aren't sure that parents have
the answers to questions about the child's medical condition or future,
and others do not wish to intrude or ask awkward or threatening questions of parents. A number of major medical centers that treat large

numbers of children with cancer sponsor special conferences or in-service training programs for educators. Sometimes these events are initiated or co-sponsored by local parent self-help groups, school systems themselves, or the American Cancer Society. Tables 11.6, 11.7, 11.8, and 11.9 provide examples of these programs.

Table 11.6

THE CHILD WITH CANCER IN THE CLASSROOM
sponsored by Candlelighters and American Cancer Society
Oregon Medical Association, Portland, Oregon
Friday, October 8, 1982

OBJECTIVES:
*to further the understanding of pediatric cancer and its treatments.
*to understand the feelings and fears shared by both teacher and student.
*to answer your questions and concerns about the children you deal with.
*to increase the school effectiveness in dealing with death or life-threatening
 disease.

Presentations:

CHILDHOOD CANCERS: TREATMENT AND PHYSICAL
SIDE-EFFECTS
—Robert Neerhout, M.D.
Chief of Pediatric Hemotology & Oncology
Oregon Health Sciences University

PSYCHOLOGICAL IMPACT OF CANCER AND TREATMENT
—William Sack, M.D. and 3 Parents
Child Psychiatrist
Oregon Health Sciences University

AMERICAN CANCER SOCIETY COMMUNITY RESOURCES
—Margaret McCreedy, R.N., B.S.
Educational Services Coordinator, VNA

DR. SACK TALKS TO CHILDREN WITH CANCER
—William Sack, M.D.
Child Psychiatrist
Oregon Health Sciences University

WHAT ABOUT SIBLINGS?
—Mary McBride, R.N., M.S.
*Assistant Professor—*School of Nursing
Oregon Health Sciences University

HELPING YOUR CLASS DEAL WITH DEATH
—Beverly Chappel, R.N.
Volunteer Counselor & Speaker
Public Schools

Table 11.7

THE CHILD WITH LIFE-THREATENING DISEASE
sponsored by Milwaukee Public Schools Workshop

Spring 1981

Instructors: Mary Lauer, R.N., Gordon S. Leonard, Ph.D.

SESSION I   February 18, 1981
Topics:
1. Introductions
2. Overview of workshop: the purpose, objectives, and topics
3. Workshop requirements
4. The Medical Aspects of Childhood Cancer

SESSION II   February 25, 1981
Topics:
1. The Nursing and Practical Aspects of Childhood Cancer
2. Impact of the Treatment Process on Neuropsychological Functioning

SESSION III   March 4, 1981
Topics:
1. Psychological patterns of adjustment in families of children with cancer
2. Enhancing the functioning and coping abilities within families of children
   with cancer.

SESSION IV   March 11, 1981
Topics:
1. Communicating with parents of children with life-threatening diseases
2. Open discussion with some parents of children with cancer regarding
   specific parent-teacher-student concerns
3. Class reaction to parent discussion

SESSION V   March 18, 1981
Topics:
1. Exploring your own feelings
2. Defining the teacher's role
3. Presentation of workshop projects

SESSION VI   March 25, 1981
Topics:
1. Continuation of workshop project presentations
2. Discussion of community resources
3. Collection of written projects
4. Evaluation of workshop

Table 11.8

SCHOOL: OBSTACLE OR OPPORTUNITY?
sponsored by
American Cancer Society
Hamilton County Unit
and
Division of Hematology-Oncology
Children's Hospital Medical Center

Raymond Walters College, Cincinnati, Ohio
October 26, 1982

Presentations:
Childhood Cancer: The Changing Story
Beatrice Lampkin, M.D. Prof. of Pediatrics
Chemotherapy And The Classroom
Pamela Flummerfelt Rappaport, R.N. MSN, CPNP
Understanding Radiation Therapy
Carolyn Hollan, Dir. Radiation Therapy Tech.
Today's Crisis, Tomorrow's Challenge
But What About Death?
Frank Schmidt
Work Session:
The Concerns Identified
Panel Discussion:
Speaking From Experience
Seminar:
Special Needs, Special Solutions

ACTION STEPS

These multiple perspectives of parents, school personnel, and students demonstrate a remarkable consistency in their perception of the reentry problems that exist and the ways in which all parties would prefer to deal with them. All argue for normalization of the child's environment and experience and for direct and well-coordinated communication among parents, educators, and medical staff. However, each group has its own set of problems to deal with, and therefore views the situation from a slightly different perspective.

All parties agree that school can normalize life for the child with cancer, and that the child should be treated as a normal student in school, provided with opportunities for experiences as identical as possible with those of other children. Normalization also requires avoidance of stigma and negative social reactions that unduly single out ill children and deny them access to important resources. Thus, it involves chal-

Table 11.9

BACK TO SCHOOL MEETING
FOR PARENTS, SCHOOL TEACHERS, STAFF
sponsored by
Candlelighters of Rhode Island, Inc.
(Parents Allied To Help—PATH)

Rhode Island Hospital
Thursday, October 14, 1982

Parents are urged to attend and bring along someone from their child's school—
a classroom teacher, school nurse, principal, guidance counselor, psychologist,
etc.

We hope to share information about the importance of school for the child with
cancer. We will be discussing ways to optimize the school experience, how siblings fare, and various medical issues which might be of concern to school personnel.

Our primary purpose is to open up a dialogue and to improve school/hospital
communication.

---

lenging stereotypes and behaviors that suggest that children with cancer are fragile, incapacitated, or doomed to academic failure. In some
cases, of course, lowered or relaxed requirements and special care are
necessary and appropriate. Normalization does not mean denial of the
seriousness of these children's conditions, nor denial of physical or psychological differences that may affect the administration of classroom
rules and regulations. Most importantly, it does not mean treating all
children with cancer like all other children, as in one parent's report that
the *hospitalized* child was required to take his final examination at the
same time and place as all other students in the class.

Comments from the interviews led to the following recommendations for school staffs, parents, and medical staffs.

Recommendations to the School Staff

Advanced preparation can make a substantial difference in the ease
and effectiveness of school reentry for children with cancer. Such preparation can provide school staff members with information on the illness,
course of treatment, and potential effects on the child's school behavior.
Some of this information can be provided by parents, but many teachers
would prefer verifying it from medical sources. Although written information can be helpful, meetings with nurses, social workers, and doctors
on the hospital staff are much more so. Acknowledgment of their own

personal stresses and emotional reactions to childhood cancer can help educators share their feelings and gain the support and help they need. It is important for teachers and principals to build an organizational climate that reduces stress and helps solve school problems faced by the child with cancer and the staff dealing with the child.

The staff also must play an active role in preparing classmates for the reentry of the child with cancer. After checking with the child and family, classmates can be told about the ill child, that he or she may have lost hair, may appear obese, or may have lost a limb. Sharing information and open discussion may forestall some gawking stares, teasing, and student fears or anxieties about speaking to the ill child. Classmates and their parents can be forewarned that cancer is not contagious, and that radiation treatment does not pose a danger to others. It is important that other families keep the school informed regarding infectious illness that classmates bring to school, since exposure to chicken pox, shingles, and flu can be a serious threat to the life of a child whose immune system is suppressed by cancer treatment. Classmates can be involved in discussions of cancer and in science projects that increase their understanding of the illness. Isolation and exclusion of the sick child from school events can be avoided, or compensations can be made in the form of hospital or home visits organized by the class. Especially when the ill child is separated from the class, an active stance by the school staff can ensure that this psychological lifeline is maintained.

Recommendations to Parents

Parents play an active role in the school reentry of their children: They may make the crucial difference between good and poor adjustment and achievement. In those cases in which children's ability to learn is seriously compromised by the disease or the side effects of their treatment, parents and children need direct help from the school staff. Information for parents of these children on what and how to get this help is presented in the Candlelighters Foundation Quarterly Newsletter (Doerr & Doerr, 1984).

The local school district is responsible for making certain that appropriate educational services are available to all school-age children whose families or legal guardians reside in the district. If you feel that your child is having some difficulty at school, you should actively seek help for your child.

Not all health impaired children need the services of such agencies but agencies should be made aware of the child's condition so

*that if in the future help is needed (for example, speech and lan-
guage therapy, physical/occupational therapy, tutoring, and psychological counseling), it can be obtained.*

*Try to have the school treat the child as an equal not a "special
child." Our children have a great need to be accepted by their
friends and to be treated like the rest of the class.*

*Make yourself aware of the services of the school and don't feel
like you are asking for excessive help. The services are there to help
your child get the education to which he or she is entitled by law.*

*A child doesn't need to attend a full day of school if they tire
easily. A more flexible day can be arranged so that they can be a
part of school for a specific time and still get the necessary rest
for their health. (p. 3)*

Because they spend so much time with the ill child and know the child
well, parents have insights that may be useful to teachers in helping
them decide how to help the child grow academically. Parents can provide advance warning about external events that might cause a child
to be upset or in an unusual mood; they can acquaint the staff with the
child's medication and hospitalization schedule, and when the child may
be worried about medical test results. Regular contact between parents
and teachers is essential. Parents must appreciate the educators' need
for information about childhood cancer and its treatment, and the
teachers' struggles with their own emotional reactions to cancer and the
threat to the child's life. Parents can help educators find a balance
between being overprotective or seeming to show a lack of concern for
the child.

Parents can solicit or encourage the involvement of medical personnel
in helping to plan or manage the child's return to school. As the natural
link between the hospital and the school, parents are in the best position
to create or maintain an open system of communication and contact
between personnel in both institutions.

Recommendations to the Medical Staff

The medical staff typically encourages children's return to school as
quickly as possible and helps parents keep track of health problems that
may keep a child out of school. Professionals can also help parents and
teachers by sharing information regarding the child's health status with
the school in a way that is understandable and useful to a nonmedical
audience. The medical staff also can assist educators in dealing with
their fears, stereotypes, and concerns about the reactions of other students, other parents, and colleagues. Discussions of specific techniques

of behavior management and classroom organization are also necessary and appropriate.

Currently there are several models of medical outreach to schools. At Children's Hospital of Philadelphia this function is carried out by the social work staff; at Children's Hospital in Cincinnati a health educator performs this role; at Children's Hospital at Stanford the discharge nurse on the pediatric hematology-oncology unit serves as the liaison between the hospital and school and provides consultation to family and school on reentry issues; in other hospitals parent groups run programs to educate school personnel and classmates (see Tables 11.6 and 11.9); some hospitals have no outreach programs at all. Outreach by the medical staff is a critical ingredient in helping the school staff anticipate and plan adequately for the child's return to school.

Concern for the normal growth of a child with cancer is shared among many people. A major obstacle to realizing this goal is the tendency of each party to view his/her contribution in isolation. Significant strides can be made toward successful school reentry if greater attention is paid to coordinating the efforts of family, school, and hospital. Open and regular contact between the medical care organization, the school, and the family can create a partnership that will make the child's reentry in school more comfortable and productive.

CHAPTER NOTES

1. In addition to data from the sample of parents and youngsters described previously, we conducted interviews with 29 teachers, administrators, and school health professionals who had experience with the children in this sample in school. Elementary, junior high, and high school educators were interviewed; different ones had contact with children with cancer at various stages of their illness – at diagnosis, during remission or just prior to the child's death. All educators were nominated by the parents in this study, and all who were contacted agreed to an interview.

2. See, for example, Lansky, Lowman, Vats, and Gyulay (1975), Futterman and Hoffman (1970).

3. Several researchers argue that others' reactions constitute the most serious reentry problems for children with cancer (Cyphert, 1973; Greene, 1975; Katz, 1980). Although there is little systematic empirical research on the actual reactions of peers and educators, the issues are discussed in some detail in several publications (especially regarding peers, see Katz et al., 1977; Moore & Triplett, 1980; Zwartjes, 1978; especially regarding educators, see Cyphert, 1973; Deasy-Spinetta & Spinetta, 1980; Feldman, 1980; Kaplan, Smith, and Grobstein, 1974).

4. Deasy-Spinetta and Spinetta (1980) report the responses of teachers of 42 school-age cancer patients who completed questionnaires comparing the functioning of a typical student to a student with cancer. Teachers did not rate students with cancer as different from students without cancer on academic motivation and behavior, but they were seen as lower in attendance, concentration, energy, risk taking, and emotional expressiveness.

5. Missing "much" schooling is defined here as more than a few days a month on a continual basis, excluding the diagnosis and early treatment period.

6. The data in Tables 11.1 and 11.2 (and 11.3 and 11.4) are not strictly comparable, since the questions were posed to parents and to teachers in different formats. Parents were asked to respond to an open-ended question describing what, if any, problems their child encountered in schooling. Teachers were provided with a closed-ended list of problems and asked to rate the seriousness of each.

7. This situation is not unlike that faced by close friends as they decide whether to take a risk by seizing the initiative, whether to reach out and help without being asked (Chapter 9). Signs from parents and youngsters about how close and accessible they want to be often are subtle and difficult to read. Closely related issues in ill adolescents' relationships with their peers also are discussed in Chapter 8.

8. Since then the medical center has developed more systematic communication with the schools youngsters with cancer attend, and has also convened outreach events and conferences for local educators.

CHAPTER 12

Families' Responses to the Challenge of Childhood Cancer

In this chapter we integrate families' reports of stress, coping, and social support. The analysis of research results is combined with the wisdom that parents have accumulated as a result of their experience with cancer. We also discuss action that parents, medical staffs, family members, and friends can take to deal with the illness's psychosocial impact. The result is an overview of the ways that families experience and respond to the challenge of childhood cancer.

THE LINKAGES OF STRESS, COPING, AND SOCIAL SUPPORT

Throughout this book we address the stresses faced by families of children with cancer, the many ways in which parents, youngsters, and other family members cope with the illness and its psychosocial impact; and the varieties of social support family members reach out for and utilize. Table 12.1 provides an overview of the ways in which different kinds of stress, coping strategies, and sources of social support may be linked.

Intellectual stresses stem from large amounts of new and technical information, confusion, and lack of clear criteria on which to make sound judgments. These stresses are especially severe in the early weeks and months of a child's illness and tend to abate somewhat as parents find

Table 12.1

Stresses, Coping Strategies, and Social Support for Parents of Children with Cancer

Categories of Stress (Chapters 2, 3, 4)	Individual and Family Coping Strategies (Chapters 5, 6, 7, 8)	Sources of Social Support (Chapters 9, 10, 11)
Intellectual		
Confusion	Seek information about the illness, treatment, prognoses	Medical staff
Ignorance of medical terms	Seek information about the hospital	Social workers
Ignorance about where things are in the hospital	Get help in understanding jargon	Scientists and researchers
Ignorance about who the physicians are	Share confusion with others and learn together	Parent group education programs
Lack of clarity about how to explain the illness to others	Have open communication with the ill child	
Instrumental		
Disorder and chaos at home	Seek information about finances and insurance coverage	Social workers
Financial pressures	Get help at home and at work change work schedule	Family members
Lack of time and transportation to the hospital	Divide labor and solve household problems cooperatively	Friends
Need to monitor treatments	Get information about treatments and symptoms	Neighbors/co-workers
	Care for the ill child	Community agencies
	Find new financial resources	Parent group programs
Interpersonal		
Needs of other family members	Get help from spouse, close friend, and family	Family members
Friends' needs and reactions		Close friends

Challenges	Coping strategies	Resources
Relations with the medical staff	Be optimistic with others, especially medical staff	Medical and social work staff
Behaving in public as the parent of an ill child	Get help from medical staff	Other parents of ill children
	Deny relationship problems	Religious congregation
	Make time to be close with spouse and siblings	
	Find people who care who will listen, who will "be there"	
	Coordinate coping strategies with other family members	
Emotional		
Shock	Deny personal problems . . . deny feelings	Close friends
Lack of sleep and nutrition	Get physical and psychological "checkup"	Spouse
Feelings of defeat, anger, fear, powerlessness	Accept the reality of the illness	Social worker/psychologist
Physical or psychosomatic reactions	Maintain hope, optimism, and emotional balance	Other parents of ill children
	Express feelings of fear, anger, joy	Clergy, fellow congregants
	Participate in care of the child	
	Live one day at a time	
	Get close to the ill child	
	Rely on spouse . . . or distance from spouse	
	Eat right, sleep nights, meditate, and exercise	
Existential		
Confusion about "why this happened to me"	Trust in God . . . or reexamine faith	Clergypeople
Uncertainty about the future	Seek information about illness cause	Fellow congregants
Uncertainty about God and fate and a "just world"	Pray together with family members	Philosophers
	Share the struggle with others	

effective ways to gather information. Some parents actively read about the illness and its treatments, both from highly technical medical books and articles and from publications oriented to laypersons. Medical staff, especially junior physicians, nurses, and medical social workers are important sources of this kind of support.

Instrumental stresses come from practical challenges and pressures, including the need to monitor medical treatments, balance household and child-care tasks, and maintain financial security. Coping with these practical stresses also requires dealing with the intricacies of hospital billing and insurance repayment processes, appealing to public or private charities, rearranging traditional roles and chores in the family, and finding low-cost temporary housing, perhaps at a Ronald McDonald House or its equivalent. Families also must become competent medical-care providers for their child, providing treatment, reporting new symptoms, and arranging checkups. The support of others outside the immediate family, in the form of extra labor for household maintenance, child care, and transportation, is often invaluable, as is assistance from staff members and representatives of school or community agencies.

Interpersonal stresses generally stem from the reactions of other persons in the family's social environment. Responding to these others' ongoing needs, as well as to the way the crisis of cancer affects them personally, is a constant pressure. In addition to pressures from previously established relationships, parents must deal with the medical staff, strangers who have life and death power over the ill child. Some parents cope with interpersonal stress by maintaining a positive and optimistic stance on the child's current and future status. In the press of a crisis, denial may be quite effective; however, there also is a potential "pile-up" effect, whereby multiple interpersonal demands accumulate and have to be dealt with later. Just as every close relationship is potentially stressful, every interpersonal stressor is a potential source of help and support. The most important helpers appear to be spouses, close friends, and medical staff members, although other family members, other parents of ill children, neighbors, and members of social or religious organizations may also be important. It is especially important for husbands and wives to make time together to be nurturant, caring, and supportive of one another, and for parents to make time to care for their other children. Some supporters are helpful because they just listen or "are there"; others penetrate deeply into parents' hearts and minds, providing deep affection and affirmation.

Emotional stresses begin with the sense of shock, anxiety, and numbing terror that accompany the initial diagnosis. Over time these feelings fade somewhat, but parents indicate that anxiety, anger, and a sense of powerlessness often stay with them. Emotional stresses may create other stresses, as constant tiredness and irritability lead to new or escalated interpersonal problems with friends, family members, or medical staffs. Some parents cope with these emotional stresses of childhood cancer by not feeling, or by denying strong feelings. Others do their best to be optimistic and hopeful about their child's progress and future. Maintaining emotional balance and avoiding the roller-coaster ride of great hope and great depression is achieved by parents who take "one day at a time." By living in the present, focusing on immediate tasks, they avoid extreme fears and fantasies. The experience of "feeling like I am going crazy" is quite common for many parents; friends, other parents, or expert professionals sometimes provide a fresh perspective, or even a formal physical or psychological checkup. Other parents of children with cancer may be in a good position to be sensitive and compassionate helpers, since they themselves share much of the painful and stressful reality that parents experience. Some parents also find it useful to seek help from staff members such as social workers and psychologists.

Existential stresses include threats to parents' basic belief systems and to their established ways of dealing with the world. Coping with such uncertainty and confusion often triggers a reexamination of prior religious beliefs, usually (but not always) resulting in a greater reliance on faith and prayer. Even if religion itself is not a coping aid, an exploration of core questions of identity and social community is typical. The crisis leads some parents to reevaluate the direction and meaning of their lives, and to rethink their work and career goals and priorities, especially those that limit the time and energy available for children and family members. Parents also seek factual information about the nature of the illness and its probable consequences to help resolve some of these uncertainties. Social support sources particularly relevant to coping with these existential stresses include members of the clergy.

THEMES IN THE REPORTS OF PARENTS AND CHILDREN

Throughout parents' discussions of their struggles with stress, coping, and social support, several major themes emerge. These themes constitute the collective wisdom of these families and embody their goals and survival techniques: They describe how people "meet the challenge."

Seeking Normalcy

The data on stress indicate that the diagnosis and treatment of childhood cancer threaten everyone's ability to continue with life as it existed prior to the illness. As parents seek to normalize their family life while dealing with the illness, they proceed down one of two paths: maintaining the family in a pre-illness situation (accepting that prior state as normal), or adjusting their lives to the new context of illness (redefining normalcy to include the illness situation). Few parents are ever able to go back to life as it was before the illness, but most do try to balance these two paths by finding new ways to do old things: sharing intimate feelings with their spouses, nurturing and supporting their other children, rearing the ill child in consistent ways, and encouraging the child to return to an active social and school life.

Youngsters want to be treated like the same people they were before the illness and not solely like a patient or a "person with cancer." However, they also know they now are different in important ways. Thus, for many parents and children seeking a normal life does not necessarily mean a life like everyone else. Rather, it means a life that is not totally focused on the illness, a life that deals with issues (intimacy, child rearing, schooling) that other families also deal with, and a life that supports positive relationships within the family and between the family and the external environment.

The issue of normalcy, of returning to the past versus growing toward the future, also arises when parents are asked, "How are you doing?" Most parents respond that they are coping quite well; indeed, many parents report that their personal wisdom and skills, as well as their family relations, have been strengthened and deepened as a result of their experience with childhood cancer. Many youngsters with cancer, moreover, feel more mature and wiser than their physically healthy peers, and this judgment is echoed by their parents. Thus, many people manage not merely to survive the challenge of childhood cancer but also to grow from it; they alter the threat or challenge to a growth opportunity. All life is a growth process, of course, and to cease growth leads inevitably to death – death of the spirit if not the body. Being normal never means being the same as others, nor does it mean being the same as before.

Most parental reports, and most recent research, indicate that these parents and children do live relatively normal, although somewhat different, lives. Most importantly, parents and children dealing with childhood cancer do not necessarily become psychologically abnormal, nor are families necessarily split or destroyed. Most recent research, and certainly the evidence from this study, reveal that although the stresses of childhood cancer are painful and create problems for all involved, neither children surviving this illness nor their parents or families are emotionally crippled or candidates for psychological disaster.

Taking One Day at a Time

Many parents discuss the importance of not planning too far ahead when dealing with the unknown and unknowable situation of childhood cancer. They argue that they have to take one day at a time and stay anchored in the present. Great hopes for the future and/or great pessimism both get in the way of the many daily tasks required to take care of the child, maintain the family, and go on with employment. Moreover, many parents suggest, there are many joys to be gained from present interactions with their ill child, regardless of the long-term future.

The 50% five-year survival rate for children with cancer also means that 50% of those youngsters diagnosed with cancer will not survive five years after diagnosis. And some of the survivors beyond the fifth year will relapse and die as well. Even those youngsters who are long-term survivors, who have been off all treatment for five years and may be considered cured, have a significant potential for late effects of treatment, and for contracting a second cancer. Psychological and practical problems also may arise later in life, as an adult who had cancer as a child seeks employment, applies for insurance, marries, wishes to have children, experiences marital stress, contracts an illness reminiscent of the cancer, and so on.

The continuing impact of the childhood cancer experience is also discussed by parents of children who have died from cancer. Their child's death is not the end of their struggle. Many issues must still be dealt with, such as managing and maintaining memories, rebuilding a family that now has one less member, and living in the present rather than the past. As parents think about the future without their loved child, they often cannot imagine "going on." As they live this future in the present, most do go on.

Taking one day at a time does not mean ignoring the future, but it does mean focusing upon the feelings and issues at hand, enjoying one's child and one's life at the moment, and creating opportunities for pleasure and growth in the present. Many families of children with cancer take vacations together as soon as their child is healthy enough to travel, instead of waiting until their years of treatment are over; they insist on good behavior from their ill child right now, rather than assuming that after the illness is over they will reinstitute good child-rearing practices; and they try to make each day a good day, rather than assuming that good days will only be possible after their child has been cured.

Finding Different Ways to Cope

Some parents deny or avoid discussions of the illness, whereas others attend to every detail and take every opportunity for conversation. Some reach out to friends and neighbors for help, others manage very privately. Some complain and cry out in pain or anger, others passively or stoically endure. Every person experiencing or observing families of children with cancer has his/her own preferences regarding what coping strategies work best, or which do not work at all. There is as yet little sound evidence on this issue, except that different people utilize quite different coping strategies, making it very difficult and perhaps even dangerous to judge different individuals' coping success on the basis of generalized standards and criteria. The majority of parents feel that they cope quite well. However, parents' judgments of the effectiveness of their coping are qualified and comparative. Parents do not charac-terize their situations as rosy — they are not; rather they contrast their situation with how bad things could be. Whatever strategies they use, most parents feel that they are able to keep their heads above water and go on with the tasks of life. Although no particular coping strategy is able to sufficiently neutralize the overwhelming reality of the illness to make a big difference, almost any coping strategy can help a little.

Three patterns of coping stand out as especially effective for many parents: the use of active and assertive styles; the creation of open family communication; and the presence of a coherent belief system. Although many parents report the positive value of adopting an active coping style in dealing with the varied stresses of childhood cancer, not all parents are active in the same ways. Some become active information seekers; some work actively to care for their child at home, in school, and in the hospital; others actively seek emotional or material help from professionals, friends and neighbors, and members of their extended family; some actively organize (or reorganize) family chores, work rela-tionships, and solutions to financial problems; some actively tend to their own health, utilizing meditation, exercise, prayer, and counseling to promote their physical and emotional well-being. Not all parents are active doing all these things at once; most pursue some of these tasks actively and passively let others go by. The typical notion of active versus passive coping styles needs to be reconsidered in light of the many different tasks facing parents of children with cancer.

Many parents emphasize open communication as a cornerstone of effective personal and family coping with childhood cancer. Parents often report their preference for accurate information and two-way communication with the medical staff, and for good communication with one's spouse, the ill child, the immediate family, friends, and the school staff. Youngsters often report a desire for open and honest communication about their illnesses. Not all parents and children pursue open communication with all these people with equal fervor, however. Whereas open communication is greatly valued, its use varies considerably.

As the existential challenge of childhood cancer threatens one's understanding of the natural order of life and death, of innocence and suffering, it becomes important to have a set of understandings that helps make sense of this chaos. Many parents rely upon or develop a strong and consistent belief system, a way of thinking that explains and gives meaning to the world, their place in it, and the illness. For many parents this belief system is rooted in religious faith and a relationship with God that provides a theological interpretation or response to the illness. Being part of a religious congregation or spiritual community helps support such interpretations. Other parents find similar comfort and aid in a more secular tradition, in thinking through anew their notions of a good life and what a good person does when confronted with unreasonable suffering.

Relying on Others

Parents report the great effect of childhood cancer on others than the individual child and his/her parents. Siblings, grandparents, and other relatives are also concerned and upset, and their lives are often traumatized and altered by the demands of the illness and their concern for the ill child; neighbors and friends may mirror parents' reactions in their own stress and anxiety; teachers, medical staff members, and others who come into regular contact with the ill child often find themselves in great pain and great concern. Figure 12.1 depicts the widespread impact of childhood cancer.

The reactions of this broader network play a significant role in shaping the ill child's quality of life, since many of these people and groups are sources of potential personal and family support for the child. This reality establishes a reciprocal or mutual system of helping, with parents both providing help to others and relying on them for assistance.

No parent manages to deal with this chronic and serious illness alone. Everyone reaches out for help, although the sources of help vary, as do the kinds of help sought. Most parents report that their spouse is a

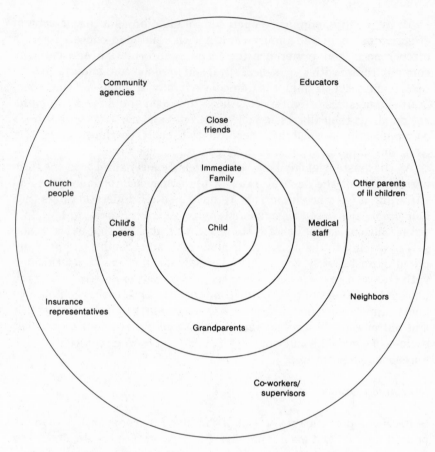

Figure 12.1. The widespread impact of childhood cancer

great source of help and support, although it sometimes is difficult for
parents to take time and energy from new child care and household
tasks to fully care for one another. Some find their own parents a great
comfort, whereas others find their parents' reactions quite distressing
and difficult to deal with. Other parents primarily reach out to their
friends, who provide them with both tangible and intangible support,
including helping with child care and household chores, and providing
listening ears and affirmation. In relying on friends and family, however,
parents often struggle with concern about others' energy and feelings,
their own level of openness and vulnerability, and whether others really
can be effective helpers. Professional services, in the person of social
workers and psychologists, represent an important source of help for

some parents, although a relatively small number overall use these services. Some parents also reach out for help from other parents of children with cancer, either on an individual basis or in mutual support groups. Parents who have the same experiences, some of whom have dealt with issues that others are only beginning to encounter, often provide a very special resource. Getting help, and having an opportunity to give help to others, is an especially important aspect of peer support and self-help.

Another important source of help that parents rely upon is the medical staff treating their child. Dealings with the medical staff are complex, and parents often indicate the mix of positive and negative feelings with which they perceive and approach physicians and nurses. Although most parents are grateful and appreciative of the medical and psychosocial aid their child receives, many also are quite uncomfortable with the staff's overall approach and are reluctant to ask for special help. Some parents indicate that they fear the staff's power over their child, and potential retaliation should the staff's authority be threatened. Such dependency is escalated when it is embedded in the larger impersonal bureaucracy of a major hospital. Bureaucratic procedures, which may interfere with their child's particular needs, often fail to make good sense to parents. Parents are most pleased when they can combine their reliance on the staff's help with their own ability to offer valuable help to the staff in the treatment of their child. This is a specific example of the general phenomenon that many observers report: Effective help requires a sharing of resources and the establishment of reciprocal helping relationships.

Becoming a Partner in Health Care

Many parents seek to become partners with the professional staff in the provision of medical and psychosocial care. Whereas professionals are acknowledged to be experts in medical problems and treatments, parents feel they are experts in the physical and psychological makeup of their own child. Both forms of expertise are critical for the child's long-term welfare.

In order to create an effective partnership, both parents and professionals need to feel potent and useful as they each try to do their best for the child and for one another. A partnership relationship provides parents assurance that their insights about the needs of their child will influence the treatment plan, and enables them to feel competent in their efforts to cope with the illness. Parental assistance may relieve busy nurses for more essential medical duties, and parent cooperation may make it easier to secure cooperation from a frightened and reluctant child. Thus, new partnerships entail not simply a revision of existing roles, but a new vision of how professionals and the people they care for relate to one another. Such visions of a more egalitarian physician-patient relationship, a more symmetrical conception of expertise and power, already characterize some staff-parent relations.

Successful implementation of a partnership role requires parental education regarding the nature of childhood cancer, its treatments and side effects, and the psychosocial and medical problems. Armed with this information, parents can work closely with the treatment team to formulate and select alternatives, make decisions, and help monitor and implement treatment. Parents can play an especially crucial role in learning and then teaching the child how to use self-administered pain control techniques such as relaxation and visual imagery.

Some medical care organizations make it easier for parents to become well informed and active participants – partners – in the medical and psychosocial care of their child; some do not. At the Seattle Children's Orthopedic Hospital, a staff team has developed an information program designed for parents of children with cancer.[1] Much more extensive than the annual or biannual lecture by a local oncologist, these materials provide parents with a great deal of information about medical and psychosocial issues. In discussion groups led by experienced parents and/or trained professionals, parents gain the information required for them to take educated and active roles. This information package, and others like it, are beginning to be made available to parents whose children are being treated at medical centers around the nation.[2] Unfortunately, we have a long way to go before such information packages and materials, or effective combinations of parental and professional resources, will be available to support all children with cancer.

A partnership also can operate at a group or organizational level, as when professionals ask experienced parents of children with cancer to meet with parents of newly diagnosed children. Young people with cancer also may meet with newly diagnosed youngsters with cancer or with their parents. It often is tremendously comforting for a parent of a newly diagnosed child to meet someone "who has been there." This is a normal feature of self-help sessions, and illustrates the potent role that self-help groups play in assisting individual parents and the medical staff. When the hospital itself supports or encourages such individual or group activities, it takes one step further toward establishing an effective partnership with parents.

Parents with special expertise have joined some medical staffs, in volunteer or semiprofessional capacities, to improve the quality of the health care delivery system from within.[3] As advocates of parents' interests, and as links to parents at large, their presence on the staff clearly reflects a new form of partnership. They both keep the staff informed of parental concerns and special needs and inform parents about the issues faced by the health care staff.

Even when parents and staff agree about the need for new programs to benefit children and their families, local financial resources may not be sufficient to take appropriate action. In some instances, parent groups take an active role by helping to raise funds to support hospital programs or to finance new programs. The development of Ronald McDonald Houses is one splendid example of parent-professional-community partnership, but it is not the only example of self-help activities that benefit the hospital, the child, and the family. Sometimes parents and parent groups are not only fund-raisers but also partners in the process of deciding how to spend funds to improve hospital services and facilities.

Despite the positive potential of parent-professional partnerships, a number of objections exist. Table 12.2 presents parents' and medical staffs' views of some of the positive and negative aspects of such an approach to health care for children and families. On the negative side, parent-professional partnerships may be viewed as intrusions into staff roles and responsibilities, as unnecessary and dangerous options for untrained persons, and as the expressions of a small and vocal minority of parents, perhaps parents responding inappropriately to the stress of their child's illness. Thus, much of the medical staff's reluctance to embrace active parent involvement may be related to their expectations that the primary consequences of partnerships are negative. Parents also may be hesitant, as they fear their own lack of skills, time and energy overcommitment, and resistance from the staff.

On the positive side, some staff members and parents see partnerships as a fruitful way to join hands in multiplying the resources available to ill children. They may also see it as a way to deal with current problems of misinformation, grievance, and low energy or burnout. Thus, their interest in active parent involvement is related to expectations of positive consequences of partnership, and perhaps to new and different visions of the medical care system.

The creation of parent-professional partnerships on the health care team will require exploiting these payoffs and overcoming these barriers. They may include new forms of parental involvement in the provision of care that do not yet commonly exist in health care delivery settings. They require parent and staff acceptance of different forms of expertise, and the establishment of a more egalitarian view of pa-

Table 12.2
Views of the Positive or Negative Aspects of
Parent-Professional Partnerships

Positive or supportive views of partnerships	Negative or cautious views of partnerships
Aid to medical system	Challenge to medical system
Learn about often unaddressed issues	Some things parents cannot and do not need to understand
	Unrealistic demands create a fuss
Information leads to helpful action, and improves choices	Misinformation and simplistic views or fads might be spread
	Comparisons create anxiety and thwart research protocols
Parents are a unique source of information	Parents are an important source of information but lack objectivity
Clarify parent fears and misinformation	Intrudes on staff or patient privacy
Positive outlet for staff and parents' energy	Lack of parent skill in dealing with medical and emotional problems
Channel for dealing with grievances	Sap energy from more important things
Increase funds and support for the medical system	Arguments about who gets the credit and who controls funds
	Heighten parent–staff conflict
Can cooperate to create a better system	Direction of medical system is a staff prerogative
Useful for most parents	Great potential for mobilizing anger and "acting out"
Represent a constituency often without access	Active parents are special interest group not necessarily representative

tients' rights and status (Bakker & Karel, 1983).[4] Clear boundaries, as well as meaningful responsibilities, and an agreed-upon division of labor are essential if conflicts are to be avoided. In the end, the value of these collaborative roles will be their own reward, insofar as they harness the resources of parents and professionals to help with the crucial problem of maintaining a high quality of life for the child, family, and staff.

Are These Themes Credible and Typical for All Parents?

The stresses, coping strategies, and social support reported by parents in this study reflect typical issues experienced by all parents of children with cancer. However, each family's experience is somewhat different, and various personal and social factors influence people to respond quite differently to the threats and challenges of this illness. In addition, there are some important limits to the sample and inquiry methods on which this research is based, and these limits mandate caution in generalizing about families' experiences, about these themes, and about the suggestions that follow.

First, this sample of parents is overwhelmingly white/Anglo, and does not reflect the experience of black, Hispanic, Asian, and native American peoples. These latter groups often have fewer educational and economic resources, and thus more limited access to high-quality medical and psychosocial services. In addition, their socioeconomic and cultural status may generate different stresses, different coping strategies, and different social support patterns than those common in a white population. In particular, they may affect the roles parents play in relationships with the health care staff and community, and the way in which various institutions (medical and educational) interact with them.

Second, the relatively small size of this sample makes it difficult to compare and contrast effectively the experiences of parents of children who have different types of cancer. This problem is exacerbated by our lack of direct conversation with parents about the difference that different diagnoses make. Although many of the dynamics of stress, coping, and social support appear to be quite similar regardless of the specific diagnosis, this is not true in all circumstances. For instance, since children with brain tumors have a relatively low rate of long-term survival and children with Wilms' tumors have a relatively high rate, more extensive comparisons of the experiences of a larger number of these parents might be very instructive. An in-depth comparative analysis also could help us understand potential differences between the experiences of parents of adolescents with bone cancer and those with Hodgkin's disease.

Third, all the parents in this sample sought treatment for their child at a single major medical center. Parents' experiences at other medical centers, or at smaller community hospitals, might be substantially different. This is especially possible with regard to parents' relationships with the members of the medical staff and the medical bureaucracy itself. Although we think that the depth of our analysis of parents' experiences with the medical system identifies and explains issues that occur regardless of particular parents and particular medical settings, we cannot yet be certain.

Obviously there are many more things to learn about the psychosocial aspects of childhood cancer, and about how parents and children (and friends, extended family members, educators, and so on) respond to the stresses associated with this illness. Although the themes generated by this research appear to be typical of a wide variety of parents and families, there are still many unanswered questions.

PRACTICAL SUGGESTIONS FOR PARENTS

One way of summarizing the research findings is to address questions parents raise as they consider how to meet the challenge of childhood cancer. In the following, we articulate parents' typical questions, and answers provided by our research, indicating chapters in which each issue is discussed. These suggestions or action guides are just that, guides; they are not inflexible rules or guaranteed paths to success.

1. *How can the medical staff help me? How can I best manage my relationship with the staff?* (Chapters 4 and 5) It is natural for the medical staff to focus its primary attention on the ill child's physical condition. Staffs that have become more sophisticated, and that have added pediatric social workers (and other ancillary staff such as psychologists and child life workers), have developed programs aimed at meeting both the child's and parents' psychological needs as well. There is some evidence that staffs relate best with parents who have relatively passive and optimistic coping strategies; at least parents adopting those strategies report better relations with the staff. But this does not mean that parents who wish to know more about the illness and its treatments, or wish to play an active role in medical care, should not assert themselves by asking questions or making suggestions.

Parents' questions may extend from requests for written information about the illness and treatments to questions about nutrition, feeding, and child-rearing practices. Parents who have questions would do well to write them down and bring them to an information session with the staff. In this way important issues will not be forgotten. Active parental participation in care may extend from monitoring drug dosages and watching for returning symptoms to attendance in treatment rooms and holding the child while blood is withdrawn or bone marrow aspirations are performed. Parents have much to offer to the staff and to the treatment process; as experts on their own child, they may help the staff modify or apply standard regimens to fit their child's unique styles or needs.

As parents express their own or their child's needs and desires to the medical staff it is useful for them to remember that the staff, too, is busy and under emotional stress. Not only does the staff see many young patients under trying circumstances but they also care about their young patients and so suffer many of the emotional stresses common to parents. The staff can best be approached in a gentle but firm manner. Physicians and nurses do not like being attacked or harassed any more than anyone else. On the other hand, care for the staff's feelings should not lead parents to stifle their own questions or desires to play an active role in the treatment process.

Parents' feelings of intimidation and fears of retaliation if they should offend the staff are common. Most staff members would not consciously retaliate against a child for a parent's offense, and most are not deliberately intimidating, but parental worry about this issue often deters effective staff-parent communication and problem solving.

Parents are the guardians and protectors of their children, and this role does not cease when a child is diagnosed with cancer or when a physician takes on the battle for the child's life. In the best situations, parents and staff members are able to combine their different roles and expertise in a lasting partnership to provide effective physical and psychosocial care. They often care for each other as well as for the ill child.

2. *What should I keep in mind regarding my child's adjustment? What does my ill child need from me?* (Chapter 7) Parenting continues even when a child is ill. The stress of a serious illness creates considerable confusion for the child, and this is a time for clear and firm parenting, perhaps even more than when the child was healthy. The basic guidelines by which a positive parent-child relationship existed prior to an illness need not change in the face of cancer. In fact, some observers argue that a dramatic change, such as a relaxation of all expectations, may have negative impact, as it may be a signal to the child that something quite terrible is wrong. A nonhospitalized and nondisabled child – a child with cancer in remission – can be expected to perform a reasonable number of typical household and family chores. Moreover, the ill child can be encouraged to reengage and maintain normal social relations with friends and classmates.

One hallmark of a healthy parent-child relationship is clear and open communication between parent and child. Since many things may be happening to the child that he or she may not understand, open communication is especially critical during the early days of the experience with cancer. At this time the child is especially dependent upon parents to share information about the illness and its meaning. Most observers now agree that children of school age should know the nature of their illness, treatment, and prognosis, although many parents and staff members are still reluctant to share such information with young children.

The stress that the child is under is exacerbated when loved ones are not available for the maintenance of a loving and caring relationship. Thus, it is important for parents to be constant and attentive visitors for the ill child, as much as that is possible. Parents also can create loving support by encouraging the child's siblings and friends to visit and/or to send cards and letters. Some parents of children who are terminally ill have elected to have their child die at home, just so the child may be surrounded by a loving family environment in the last days of his/her life.

Finally, we emphasize that a child with cancer is not necessarily dying, is not likely to be useless, and is not likely to be an emotional cripple. With proper medical care and some luck, with firm parenting, with good communication, and with love, many children will recover and live long, happy and useful lives. Even those who do not recover are still children and need to be treated as such.

3. *What does my child think about all that is happening to him or her? How can I best talk with my ill child?* (Chapters 7 and 8) Youngsters with cancer often want to talk with their parents about their illness. In some families these conversations can be very open and direct. However, sometimes parents find these conversations to be difficult, and youngsters may sense their parents' discomfort or unwillingness to talk about painful topics. Thus, partly in an effort to protect or shield their parents, older children often do not talk about their concerns openly. Adolescents with cancer may be especially reluctant to talk openly because of their normal concerns about privacy and independence.

Younger children often rely upon denial as a dominant coping strategy. Perhaps not understanding the full implications of the illness, or perhaps understanding it full well, these youngsters may not want to talk. Then, parents who do wish to talk may find it difficult to take their cue from these children, and to permit them their own space and their use of denial. Youngsters who are not able or who do not wish to talk with their parents may find it useful to discuss their concerns with social workers or psychologists, with nurses, with other ill children, or with their friends. Child life workers can provide play situations in which children may easily express many of their concerns. Parents can be helpful in encouraging their children to make use of these resources.

4. *How can I deal with my other children's reactions? What are the needs of siblings of ill children?* (Chapter 6) Increasing attention is now being paid to siblings' reactions and needs and to encouraging parents

to recognize and deal with these other youngsters' jealousies, fears, and feelings of being left out.

Siblings need to be loved and they need this love in the midst of a family illness just as they needed it prior to an illness. In a family atmosphere of love and open communication, siblings can both meet their needs and play a useful role in helping the ill child, parents, and other family members. If they are informed about the illness, siblings often can be involved in visiting and helping to care for their ill sister or brother, in picking up — temporarily — a larger share of family chores, and in carrying messages to and from extended family members, neighbors, and classmates. If the ill child dies, the siblings may become a source of support, and a model of courage for parents.

5. *How can I best facilitate my child's progress in school? How can I help schoolpeople work well with my ill child?* (Chapter 11) Since school is the normal extrafamilial environment for children between the ages of 6 and 18, it is important for the ill child to return to school as soon as he or she is able. It indicates to everyone — child, classmates, school, family — that the ill child is going on with the normal business of life. Parents can help their children deal with their fears about their appearance, peer teasing, or rejection, and falling behind in work with family conversations, linkage to educators for up-to-date assignments, and maintenance of peer contact. In order to avoid loneliness and isolation for a hospitalized child, classmates can be urged to write notes or visit. Parents can urge the medical staff and educators to meet together to plan for the child's reentry to school. In cases in which a reentering child is visibly changed or disabled, it is worthwhile to prepare the child's classmates as well as the child. Effective preparation can prevent the worst forms of peer teasing and rejection and can help develop a sense of mutual responsibility and caring among an entire class of youngsters.

In addition to supporting the child, parents often must support educators as well. Teachers and administrators who are unfamiliar with cancer or other chronic and serious illnesses in children may not know how to deal with the ill child. They may overreact by overprotecting the child, or they may underreact by refusing to deal with the child's real limitations and needs. Meetings with educators and the medical staff, with or without the child present, may help to create an information flow and a pattern of joint planning that helps the child adapt to the school situation. Be assertive!

6. *How can I best deal with this terrible crisis? What do I need?* (Chapter 5) No one knows anyone else's answer to these questions.

Almost all parents report that at times they were overwhelmed or thought they wouldn't "make it in one piece." However, to the extent that parents understand their needs and their traditional ways of coping with stress, they may be able to respond more effectively. Most parents cope with the situation quite well, although some plans are delayed or even shelved permanently. Even when a child dies, most parents and families survive the pain and suffering; life continues and most parents' lives return to normal. However, normal does not mean the same as before the illness.

Some people exercise and work off their internal tension. Others seek friends or family members with whom to talk. Many people try to focus on the present, "take one day at a time," and deny or refuse to deal with longer-term issues and implications – for themselves, their child, or their family. Others rely on a religious belief system, faith in God, and a community of fellow congregants to provide spiritual and existential relief and support. Still others try to adopt a "happy face" and create an optimistic environment for themselves and others. Some seek professional counseling as a way of learning new ways of coping with stress.

7. *What can I do to preserve the best in my relationship with my spouse during this difficult period? What do I need from my spouse?* (Chapter 6) People need the same things from their spouses that have always been at the core of good marital relations: time together, affirmation and mutual regard, a sense of pulling together, commitment to the long haul, and intimate sharing. Given the strain that childhood cancer puts on all people and relationships, these issues become even more important. Above all, husbands and wives indicate that it is critical to make time for themselves, time when they can share information with one another, buttress and support one another, love one another, and plan joint action. In these intimate times, husbands and wives also can share the feelings – anger and fear, joy and hope, pain and promise – that they cannot share easily with others. A couple must also be accepting of each other's different responses and differing timing – one may be grieving while another is using optimism to sustain her/himself. The time needed for this sharing is so critical it may have to be taken at the expense of extra time with the ill child, with the rest of the family, or with work responsibilities.

Husbands often indicate that they are especially threatened or pained when their wives spend a great deal of time with the ill child at the hospital, leaving them out of this information network and requiring them to pick up a great deal of slack at home. Wives, on the other hand, indicate that they are most pained when their husbands do not ask about or spend time at the hospital, appearing not to care about the ill child, and dumping too much medical responsibility on them. The child is, after all, the product of both their bodies and both their hearts, and both parents must be involved in medical care and in home maintenance. Husbands can make sure that they express care and visit their wives and ill children. Wives can make sure they include their husbands in their expressions of caring, and take time off from the children's bedside to be with their husbands and other family members at home. It is not easy to leave the bed of an ill child. But that child is still only one member of a larger marital and family system, others of whom also have important needs for sharing and a life together.

Single parents carry the same burden, often without the financial and social resources of an adult partner. For them, the help of extended family, friends, and community resources is particularly important. The ability to reach out and negotiate help from one's social network may be the most crucial determinant of long-term adjustment in the single adult household.

8. *Can my religious beliefs help me at this time? How can I get comfort from religion?* (Chapter 5) Many parents indicate that their religious beliefs and associations are very helpful. Some report an increase in their religious faith and commitment. Not all parents find comfort in religion; some feel that their religious commitments were tested in this experience and failed. Others who had not found religion important to them previously did not rely upon it during the illness.

Some parents report that their religion helps them make sense out of their child's experience with cancer, that it provides "reasons" for the illness and so eases their existential stress. Others report that a direct personal relationship with a loving God supports them emotionally; they feel less alone and adrift as a result of constant prayer and communication with God. Still other parents report that the most meaningful aspect of their religion is fellow church members who lend a helping hand, listen, pray with them, and provide a sense of being part of a community of faith. Religious beliefs and concerns take on special importance at the time of a child's death, when questions about life after death or relations with God and the hereafter become even more poignant. These positive functions of religion stay with some parents long after the illness, even after the death of their child, providing new meaning and direction to their lives.

9. *Can my friends make a difference? How can I best reach out to my friends for help and support?* (Chapter 9) Parents report receiving many

different kinds of help from their close friends. Emotional sharing and affirmation, practical aid with family and household chores and transportation, and assistance in the care of the ill child are important resources that friends are able to provide. However, not all friends are able to or wish to "be there" for parents of children with cancer, and the withdrawal of some close friends is often a source of disappointment, pain, and added stress.

One of the critical steps in gathering help and support from friends comes early in the experience with childhood cancer – at the time of diagnosis. Parents who quickly share information about the diagnosis often are able to involve friends in dealing with the emotional trauma of the illness. To the extent that parents are able to be clear about their needs, and about who could meet which needs, their friends are more likely to be well informed and able to provide help.

Four actions that parents can take with friends are (1) telling friends about the diagnosis, perhaps with the aid of medical staff members who can answer a wide variety of questions; (2) discussing openly the level of pain and shock everyone is experiencing; (3) providing clear cues regarding the kinds of help that is needed, and from whom; and (4) providing clear feedback regarding the effectiveness or utility of help that has been provided.

10. *What help can I get from other parents of children with cancer? How can I help others?* (Chapter 10) Many parents who have been active in self-help or mutual support groups indicate that they both give and get from these groups. In fact, "giving is getting" is a common refrain. Among the benefits parents receive in such formal or informal settings are affirmation that their feelings of guilt, fear, anger, and powerlessness are normal; information from others who understand problems in the medical situation, marital relationships, and child rearing; a listening ear and a helping hand from others who truly know what living with childhood cancer feels like; emotional comfort and comradeship during the hard times of surgery, relapse, or death; an opportunity to help others by making a contribution to the medical care system; a sense that they are coping well if they still have the energy and skill to be helpful to others.

11. *How can I help coordinate care for my child and family?* (Chapters 11 and 12) Many medical and psychosocial staff members, educators, and community agency staffs will try their best to provide effective care for the child with cancer and the child's family. However, these groups seldom are experienced in working together, and their care often is less

effective because of a lack of coordination. Parents usually are responsible for connecting all these professionals, and for providing the information, direction, and focus to their efforts. Parents can call a meeting at which members of the hospital staff and the school staff share information and plans for the medical and school treatment of the child. Likewise, medical services and community services to families must be coordinated by parents or it is not likely to happen. The day when medical and psychosocial care are delivered in a sophisticated and coordinated manner as a matter of course is not yet here. It is still up to parents to make their own and their child's needs known, to advocate for their own and the child's welfare, and to guarantee the effective delivery of a full range of care. Parents who are unsure how to take these steps should consult sensitive medical staff members, other parents of ill children who know this "game," the American Cancer Society, or the Candlelighters Childhood Cancer Foundation.

All these suggestions, and the responses to all these questions, represent families' efforts to meet the challenge of childhood cancer.

CHAPTER NOTES

1. Pendergrass et al. (1982); Rudolph et al. (1981).

2. Staff members at Children's Hospital, Los Angeles, have built on the resources and materials used in Seattle to develop a 6-week, 12-hour educational program for families of children with cancer ("We Can Cope"). An evaluation of this program showed education to be successful in reducing parents' self-reported anxiety, depression, anger, and lack of vigor (Ruccione, 1985).

3. Pitel et al. (1985) describe and evaluate one example of this strategy, the parent-advocate role, in a major medical setting.

4. In the language of Borman (1979), partnerships require a new definition of the professional as a collaborator instead of a controller of care, a virtual paradigm shift in the conceptualization of human sources.

Appendix:
Methods of Inquiry

To provide maximum readability throughout this volume, many technical details regarding research methods have been eliminated from the text and placed in this Appendix. For the same reason, extended references to other scholarly works and technical commentaries on scientific issues are placed in notes at the conclusion of each chapter.

Readers wishing to know more about the methods utilized in the study on which this book is primarily based can, in the following pages, find details on: the approach; the sample; interviews and data-gathering procedures; data-analysis techniques; and interview and questionnaire forms. This material extends information presented in abbreviated form at the conclusion of Chapter 1.

PRIOR WORK AND THE APPROACH USED IN THIS STUDY

Our review of prior research on psychosocial aspects of childhood cancer indicates it has been limited by several ideological or methodological premises:

1. A focus on problems of death and dying;
2. The utilization of a medical model that assumed passive and compliant (but occasionally reactive) family interactions with benevolent and powerful health care professionals;
3. A concern about pathology in individual (child or parent) and family adjustment/coping, and for identifying better ways health professionals could prevent these problems or help these problem individuals;

4. The use of highly structured questionnaires that failed to inquire into or respond to informants' unique or divergent concerns and experiences;

5. The use of clinical and projective instruments that emphasized individual reactions and that promoted comparisons with pathologic populations;

6. A retrospective approach to families' experiences;

7. The use of small samples, generally located at a single medical institution.

Our own effort avoids some, but not all, of these problems. For instance, we do not focus primarily on death and dying, nor do we utilize a traditional medical model of research. We do not assume that patient/family pathology is a given. We try to avoid the twin dangers of overstructured instruments or excessively clinical and anecdotal data collection devices by drawing from both traditions. However, this study still is limited by its retrospective rather than longitudinal approach, its focus on a sample drawn from a single treatment facility, the lack of a racially diverse sample, and the use of a sample that is still rather small by conventional social scientific standards.

As Spinetta notes in his lucid discussion of research techniques in the area of pediatric oncology, the area needs now to "combine the best qualities of both intra-individual and normative research strategies" (1984, p. 2223). He reviews the problems inherent in standardized tests comparing patients with cancer to "so-called normal controls," and suggests that, "A valuable supplementary method of study would be to use the cancer population as its own control . . . " (p. 2223). In pursuing just such a strategy we combine individual and aggregate analysis procedures, analyzing data with both quantitative and qualitative techniques. Moreover, we utilize elements of both a deductive and an inductive approach. We wanted parents of children with cancer (and in some cases, children with cancer themselves, their siblings, their school staffs, and their parents' friends) to "speak for themselves." That required allowing them to define the problems and issues involved in the experience of childhood cancer. Thus, formal hypotheses and well-defined instruments could not be generated prior to investigation of the phenomena of parents' and youngsters' experiences. At the same time, we did not wish to conduct a large number of completely unique interviews and conversations. Our compromise was to begin with a semistructured interview, and to ask questions in a way that permitted and encouraged informants to answer these questions and to pose issues in ways that they felt were most realistic. Thus, informants wander from our format at times, and provide us with material we could not anticipate ahead of time. The same desire to be sensitive to individual variations means that not all parents answered all questions, creating the missing N problem in several tables.

As noted in Chapter 1, we began this process by first embedding ourselves in the phenomena of childhood cancer, spending time informally interacting with parents, children, and medical staff members. We also reflected on our own experience, as it compares and contrasts with others' reports. As Featherstone says regarding her own powerful and important work on family life with a disabled child, "I begin to judge an idea by asking whether it makes sense in the context of my own life and in that of my husband and children. . . . My own experience has helped to form the grid through which I listen to other people's stories" (1981, p. 9). Most people operate in this manner in their daily lives, and make sense of others' experiences partly through this process of mutual identification and comparison. In the effort to be as objective as possible, however, many scientists overreact to this common-sense approach and seek to limit or totally deny this avenue of personal insight and learning. Without being captive to or blinded by our own experience as parents of ill children, but using the lessons and insights gained therein, we self-consciously utilize personal knowledge as part of the current study.

When we were ready to proceed with the more formal aspects of this research we enlisted the assistance of several articulate parents of children with cancer in the generation of a list of important issues, and used this list to create a draft version of the interview form. These same parents were a test population on which interviewers practiced both the interview form and their own style. Experience with these pilot interviews led to redesign of the interview and questionnaire.

THE STUDY SAMPLE

The sample of informants from families of children with cancer is presented in Table A.1. As indicated in Chapter 1, the pool of potential informants was stratified on the basis of the age and life-status characteristics of children with cancer. Within each age and life-status grouping in the total pool, a sample was selected on the basis of assignment by means of a table of random numbers. Whenever a family that was part of the sample declined to participate (15 families declined out of the 70 families contacted), or could not be located, we made substitutions from the pool to match the original sample as closely as possible.

Other demographic characteristics of the sample are presented in Table A.2. This table also indicates the percentages of parents of chil-

Table A.1
The Sample for This Study

Child Status	Total Families	Both Parents	One Parent	Children with Cancer	Siblings	Total Persons
Living, under 6 yrs.	9	7×2=14	2	0	1	17
Living, 6–11 yrs.	17*	13×2=26	4	15	7	52
Living, 11–21 yrs.	17	12×2=24	5	11	7	47
Deceased	12**	9×2=18	2	0	8	28
Total	55	41×2=82	13	26	23	144

*In one family the mother's interview was so incomplete that it has been omitted from all quantitative analyses, resulting in an effective N of 94 parents in 54 families for these purposes.
**In one family the mother refused to be interviewed at the last moment and an older sibling of the ill child, who had adopted a maternal role, substituted.

Table A.2
Medical and Sociodemographic Characteristics of the Sample

	N of Parents (N=95)	% of Parents
Medical Characteristics		
Child's Health Status		
Initial remission	62	65
In remission but had relapsed	13	14
Deceased	20	21
Child's Diagnosis		
Leukemia	32	34
Lymphomas	18	19
Neuroblastoma	12	13
Wilms' tumor	8	8
Osteosarcoma	9	9
Brain or central nervous system	6	6
Other	10	11
Sociodemographic Characteristics		
Parent Gender		
Male	42	44
Female	53	56
Marital Status		
Married	82	86
Single	13	14
Parental Education		
High School graduate or less	30	32
Some college	26	27
College graduate	29	30
No report	10	11
Parental Income		
Less than $15,000	17	18
$15,000–$25,000	36	38
Over $25,000	35	37
No report	7	7

dren with different diagnoses of childhood cancer. If, instead of listing percentages of parents of children, we list percentages of children themselves, the sample contains the following distribution: leukemias—35%, brain tumors—7%, neuroblastomas—11%, lymphomas—18%, Wilms' tumors—7%, osteosarcomas—9%, others—13%. When these sample characteristics are compared with national incidence data (see Table 1.1), it is clear that the sample roughly approximates national figures, except that it includes proportionately more youngsters with lymphomas (18% vs. 11%) and fewer with brain and spinal cord cancers (7% vs. 20%). The sample also is skewed in the direction of relatively fewer parents of children who are deceased or who have relapsed.

These features of the sample (fewer parents of deceased children, fewer parents of children who have relapsed, and fewer parents of children with brain tumors – a relatively unfavorable prognosis) may imply that the general experiences of parents in this sample are not as stressful as would be the case in a more representative sample of parents of children with cancer. As a result, our findings may portray an unduly optimistic picture. This concern has two important implications. First, when we make aggregate statements (e.g., 81% of parents report they are coping well or extremely well) we must acknowledge that they are not based upon a truly representative and comprehensive sample (e.g., representative of all parents of children with cancer). There are very few places in this volume in which such aggregate statements are made, and they usually are accompanied by efforts to examine whether different circumstances (such as having a living or deceased child with cancer) influence the findings.

Second, we should conduct detailed comparisons, insofar as possible, between parents with children with different diagnoses, prognoses, and outcomes. Although we have tried to create such analyses, the small sample and limited depth of discussion with parents about illness distinctions make such efforts quite difficult and the results tentative. Most researchers constantly wish for larger and more representative samples, with greater depth of inquiry, and we are no exception. However, comparisons within and between representative samples of families is not the only way to generate understanding of the psychosocial dynamics of childhood cancer, and this in-depth exploration of a small sample obviously provides important insights and lessons.

The procedures utilized to identify the special samples of friends of parents and of school personnel are specified in Chapters 9 and 11.

INTERVIEW PROCEDURES

Once the sample was selected, all parents in the sample were sent a letter describing the study and requesting their participation. About two weeks after this letter was sent, families were contacted by telephone and asked to agree to the interview. Written consent forms were signed by all informants prior to the interviews.

Interviews were conducted by specially trained university students, students who had prior experience working as volunteers with seriously ill children and their families at the hospital. A mix of graduate and undergraduate students, they read about the issues that these families faced, role-played the interview process, and practiced a pilot series of interviews. A continuing seminar was held during the interview stage of the study, and interviewers constantly were debriefed, both with regard to their own reactions and to any problems they experienced relating with parents and children in the study. Although interviewers were pressed to follow the semistructured format of the instrument, they also were instructed to be responsive to informants' desires to tell about their experiences in the ways that they themselves wished.

It is clear that the interviews were successful. In addition to providing rich and detailed data, they also often were a fruitful experience for informants and for interviewers. In the mail-back questionnaire parents were asked about their reactions to the study and to the interview.

a. In response to the questions about informants' feelings after the interview:
   almost all said they were glad they had done it;
   most said that they were glad to have the chance to talk about the issues again.
b. In response to questions about their reactions to the interview:
   66% said the interviewer made them feel very comfortable and relaxed;
   34% said they felt fairly comfortable;
   none said they were not very comfortable at all.
c. When asked how complete a picture of their feelings and experience we received:
   60% said it was excellent coverage of most issues;
   33% said it was fairly good coverage, with some parts missing;
   7% said it was sketchy coverage of only a small part of the issue.
d. When asked whether family members talked about their interviews with one another afterwards:
   73% said yes;
   everyone who responded to the question of whether talking with family members was good or bad said it was good.

Several parents report that their participation in the interview was cathartic, indicating that at times it was painful, but also that it was a helpful avenue of release or reconceptualization.

I think it is great that you people are gathering this information because everyone who has experienced such an illness has something to share with others. It sure should be helpful to others.

I am glad I participated in the interview because it helped to get in touch with and express many feelings that I had buried.

I remembered the love shared by many and all the positive coping that was done.

We talked about it afterwards, and we never really did talk about it very much before.

Our oldest child revealed hidden hurts and feelings with us after the interview.

Interviewers' comments indicate that they, too, felt the interviews were an effective device; they reported that:

a. 76% of informants had a good and clear understanding of most questions;
   23% of informants had a moderate understanding;
   1% of informants had little understanding of the questions.

b. 56% of informants appeared to be relaxed throughout the interview;
   39% of informants got more relaxed as time went on;
   1% of informants got less relaxed as time went on;
   4% of informants appeared uneasy throughout the interview.

c. 82% of informants appeared to be friendly and eager to talk;
   18% of informants were cooperative but not particularly eager;
   none were indifferent or suspicious.

Both interviewers and informants report occasional episodes of tearfulness or crying during interviews. Clearly, the interviews were deeply emotional experiences for some informants. Our understanding of interviewers' and informants' reports is that this experience was emotionally coherent and positive in almost all cases.

All interviews were tape recorded, and interviewers listened to these tapes in reconstructing their conversations in written form on the interview schedule/instrument.

DATA ANALYSIS

The reconstructed interview material was subject to both qualitative and quantitative analysis. In the qualitative approach we first read through the entire interview, noting major themes in parents' (or youngsters' or siblings') responses that cut across the separate interview questions. These major themes, once identified, were used as search categories or "magnets" around which we organized the interview material and looked for variation on each theme. For instance, if parents' concerns about the medical staff is a major theme, the seven specific issues comprising this concern are the variations around it (Chapter 4). Likewise, if parents' concerns about their friends is a major theme, the five issues presented in Chapter 9 are the variations around it. From the collection of responses to any given variation or subtheme, such as parents' concerns about staff empathy with the child (Chapter 4), or parents' fears about friends' emotional burden (Chapter 9), we selected some representative quotes for use in the volume. This is, in essence, a coding process, but a process that generates categories from the data rather than placing data into categories developed ahead of time (Charmaz, 1983; Miles & Huberman, 1984). It also codes on the bases of whole ideas or patterns present in the data rather than on small bits of a response.

Data were prepared for quantitative analysis using a coding process as well, but within a more reductionist framework. In examining informants' answers to a particular question (e.g., who was hard to tell about the illness?), all responses to this question were laid out on a chart, and the major categories were identified. Then individual responses were placed into these categories, assigned numerical codes, and entered into the computer for analysis. In the case of structured questions, such as those in the questionnaire, precoded categories were available on the basis of the question/answer format.

The prestructured questionnaire items often did miss the mark, and were much less helpful in understanding and interpreting parents' experiences than was the rich detail in the open-ended interview questions. Their positive value, on the other hand, lies in verifying some of the findings developed through analysis of the interview questions and in identifying issues that needed to be pursued and verified through the interview material.

The size of the sample and the intended audience directed the statistical procedures we could or did perform in the quantitative analysis. For purposes of readability by a wide audience, we have generally limited the statistical techniques reported in this volume to Chi squares, correlations (rank-order and product-moment), and Means' tests. On appropriate occasions, and in other analyses reported in technical papers, we have utilized regression, ANOVA and MANOVA techniques.

The fact that all the data were collected at one time means that the analyses are correlational or associational. Although we can discover important relationships among variables, we often cannot tell what "causes" what. For instance, in Chapters 4 and 5 we discuss the relationship between negative experiences or problems with the medical care system, parents' higher level of education, and use of an active coping style. Although these three variables occur together, it is difficult to say what causes or leads to what. Since parental level of education occurs temporally prior to the experience with childhood cancer, we are certain that negative experiences with the medical system do not cause education; nor is it likely that an active style of coping with a child's illness causes higher education. On the other hand, it is reasonable to conclude that education may lead one to more critical views of the health care system and therefore to report more negative medical experiences. Or, higher education may lead to a more active coping style. Or it may lead to both at once. In addition, perhaps an active coping style leads to more tense and negative relations with the medical staff, especially if the staff prefers more passive and compliant styles. Or, perhaps more negative staff relations leads to a more active coping style. Although we can say that these variables are related closely to one another, and occur together for parents, we cannot ascertain with any certainty which causes which, or whether both are caused by yet another important factor. Such conclusions will have to wait for another study, hopefully one that is longitudinal in character, or that asks parents directly about these causal connections.

INSTRUMENTS

In the following pages we present the three major instruments used in the study: (1) the semistructured interview form utilized with parents of living children; (2) the semistructured interview form utilized with parents of deceased children; and (3) the structured questionnaire form utilized with both sets of parents. Other instruments, such as those used with children with cancer, siblings of these children, educators working with ill children, and friends of parents, are roughly similar.

**SEMISTRUCTURED INTERVIEW FORM FOR
PARENTS OF LIVING CHILDREN**

Informant:

Interviewer:

Date:

Time:

Place:

Thank you for agreeing to talk to us.

1. How many children do you have, and how old are they?
   _____

   Do they all live at home?
2. Can you tell me what happened when _____
   was diagnosed?
   > When was that?
   > Symptoms?
   > Prognosis given?

   2a. Did you have any choices or decisions to make at
   that time?
3. What did it feel like at this time? What was the impact
   on you of the diagnosis?
   > Anger?
   > Confusion?
   > Sleep?
   > No sleep?
   > Hope?

   3a. How did you deal with these feelings?
4. Is there anything that might have made this period of
   diagnosis easier for you?
   > Doctors?
   > Friends?
   > Family?
5. What did you tell your child about her/his illness?

   5a. Was there anything he/she was not told? Why or
   Why not?

   5b. What was _____'s reaction?
6. How did you tell other family members?

   6a. Spouse (or the child's other parent if separated)

   6b. Other child

6c. Grandparents
   Were any problems created?
6d. Who was the hardest to tell?
7. Was it difficult to share the diagnosis with friends?
   7a. How did they react?
      Were they helpful? How?
      What was not helpful?

      Give me a concrete example
8. Is there anything else that stands out in your mind about the time of diagnosis?
   8a. How long did it take to get over the shock, and to begin to really deal with what you had to do?

Let's talk now about some of the general issues and problems that may have started at diagnosis, and may continue today.

9. What have been the toughest problems or the toughest times during your child's illness?
      How did you deal with them?
   9a. When else?

HAND OUT THE STRESS CHART AND GO OVER THE INSTRUCTIONS. HELP THEM FILL IT OUT!

10. What are some good or positive things that have come out of this period of illness, for you or your family?
      How is that positive?
   10a. Anything else?
      Discover strengths?
11. In general, how do you feel you're handling your child's illness?
   11a. What things are you doing best? What are your strengths?
   11b. What areas are you managing less well?
   11c. Have some of these changed over time? Have you gotten stronger in some and less good in others?
      If yes, how?
   11d. Are there any kinds of help and support that might make it easier?
      Friends?
      Family?
      Others?

Now I'd like to understand more about _____'s treatment.

12. Has he/she been hospitalized much?
    12a. For what? For how long?
         Treatment (chemotherapy, surgery)?
         Pneumonia or other infections?
    12b. Did you live/sleep in the hospital during the time _____
         was hospitalized?

         If yes, who took care of the family?

         Work out OK?
13. Have you ever had any problems with any of the doctors or services in the hospital?
         Emergency Room?
    13a. How about the nursing staff?
14. Some parents remember times when they "stepped in" to prevent a "mistake" from being made, or to suggest a better way of treating or dealing with their child. Do you remember anything like that happening to you, or to your child?
         If yes, what happened?
15. Has your child had a relapse or recurrent of the disease?
    15a. If yes, in what ways was the relapse like the original diagnosis time?
         In what ways was it different?
         Do you think a lot about the possibility of another one?
    15b. If no, do you think a lot about the possibility of a relapse?
    15c. Does your child seem to fear a (another) relapse?
         Do you and she/he talk about this?
16. I know it's difficult to ever guess what will be, but when you think about _____'s future, what sort of pictures come to your mind?
    16a. What kinds of things do you think will happen?
         School?
         Work?
         Family?
17. Everyone in this position has to sometimes think that their child may not survive this terrible illness. When those thoughts are in your mind, is there anything that makes you feel better, or more optimistic?
    17a. Is there any person who can help you in these times?
18. Have your religious beliefs or practices changed over the time of the illness? (If mentioned previously, ask for summary.)
    If yes, how?
         Have they helped you through the hard times?

19. Do you ever wonder why this happened to your child?
    19a. How do you explain it to yourself?

Now I'd like to ask you some questions about everyday life in your family.

20. Aside from the times when _____ has been hospitalized, how has the illness affected family routines?
    20a. Who is generally responsible for _____'s medical care? Does this interfere with other family jobs?
    20b. Has the illness affected the amount or quality or time and attention you give to the other children?
    20c. How has the illness affected the way you spend your vacations?
    20d. Has it affected other routines and chores? Does _____ do the same chores he/she did before the illness?
21. In some families where a child has a chronic illness, the family grows closer together, and in other families people grow further apart. Are there some ways in which this family has changed?
    21a. Are there some ways in which this family has grown closer?
    21b. Are there some ways in which this family has grown further apart?
22. How about _____'s brother(s) and sister(s)? How do they feel about _____?
    22a. Are they closer now than before the illness began? Or are they further apart?
    22b. Do they understand the seriousness of the illness?
    22c. Do they show any special feelings about the treatment and attention he/she gets?
        Jealousy? Guilt? Love? Caring? Left out?
        Have these feelings changed over time?
    22d. What have been the most difficult parts of the experience for them?
    22e. Do you think they've learned anything from this entire situation?
23. How has your child responded to his/her illness?
    23a. What behaviors are you most pleased or satisfied with?
    23b. What behaviors bother you most?
    23c. Is he/she developing similarly to others of his/her age?
        If different, how so?
        If similarly, how did you manage that?
24. Has the illness affected the way you do your daily job or work?

24a. Have you had to change any of your goals or plans for the future as a result of the illness?

  If yes, in what ways?

24b. Have you had to reduce your working hours outside of the home, or your working responsibilities, as a result of the illness?

  If yes, in what ways?

24c. Have you gotten support from your co-workers and/or supervisors?

  What have they done that helped?

  Did they make it tougher in any ways?

Now let's talk a bit about school. FOR NURSERY AGES AND UP.

25. After the initial diagnosis (or after a serious relapse or recurrence), did you inform the school of your child's illness?

  If yes, whom did you tell?

25a. How did that work out?

25b. Were you child's classmates told?

  If yes, by whom?

  How has that worked out?

25c. Have there been any unusual reactions from classmates or their parents?

25d. Are you satisfied with the ways the teacher(s) responded?

  If yes, what did they do that was good?

  If no, what happened?

  Is there anything you would have liked them to do differently?

26. How is _____'s classwork going? Is he/she caught up?

26a. Is his/her schoolwork going any differently now than before the illness?

  If yes, how and how come?

27. Has your child experienced any special problems at school since the time he/she was diagnosed?

27a. If yes, can you give me some examples?

27b. Has _____ missed much school?

  If yes, how much?

  Why has she/he missed school?

   Illness?

   Low counts?

   Treatment?

   Fear of contagion?

27c. Do you feel any of these problems are directly related to
_____'s illness?

27d. How have you handled any of these problems? Have you gotten any help from school officials?

27e. Would you have wanted (or want now) any help from a doctor, nurse, social worker, or a hospital liaison person? How might they have helped?

28. If it had been freely and easily available, would you have wanted to talk with a social worker or psychologist about any of the issues you mentioned throughout our conversation?

28a. Did you ever speak with a counselor, social worker, etc.?
If yes, was it helpful? In what ways?

28b. Would you want to speak with someone like this now?
Why or why not? About what issues?

I understand that some of the parents and inpatients get to know each other pretty well, and that they help each other through some tough times.

29. Suppose you were asked for advice, what are the most important things you'd say to a parent whose child had just been diagnosed with a disease like your child's?

29a. What should they do or not do?

29b. What would you tell them about hope/optimism/faith?

29c. What would you tell them about pain/sorrow/struggle?

29d. What would you warn them about?
About the disease?
About the treatment?
About people?

30. Do you think your child would like to talk to other children with the same or similar illness?
Why or why not?

30a. Do you personally think it would be good for him/her?
Why or why not?

31. Do you know of the activities of the parents' group, _____?

31a. Do you receive their newsletter?
If yes, what do you think of it?

31b. Have you gone to any of their meetings?
Why or why not?
If yes, what was your reaction?
Did your spouse go too?

31c. What else could they be doing to help people like you and your child?

31d. Would you ever like to talk to other parents of children with cancer?

Why or why not?

Do you ever get much of a chance?

32. Is there anything else you think I should know before we end this conversation? Do you think I have a fairly accurate picture, even in this brief time, of what it's been like for you and your family, as you've dealt with your child's illness? If there anything you'd like to add?

THANK YOU VERY MUCH FOR YOUR TIME!

HAND OUT QUESTIONNAIRE WITH RETURN ENVELOPE.

Here is a chart, a timeline, that can be used to describe the time that has elapsed from before you learned the diagnosis until now.

1. Mark on this line the critical events or stages in your experience with your child's cancer. Indicate the approximate date of each.

Before
the
diagnosis_____now

2. Which of these events or stages were most stressful? Draw an arrow for each event, indicating with a high line the highest stress times or events, and with a low line the lesser stress times or events.

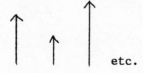

etc.

Post-Interview Questions for the Interviewer

1. How much privacy was there in the interview situation?
   No one else around _____ Young child around _____
   Other adults or children within earshot _____
         Sometimes _____   Often _____
   Child with cancer around _____
   Parent around _____
2. How much disturbance was there during the interview?
   Telephone calls _____
   Visitors _____
   Children demanding attention _____
   Adult moving in _____
3. What was the informant's ability to understand the questions?
   Little understanding of most questions _____
   Moderate understanding of most questions _____
   Good and clear understanding of most questions _____
4. During the interview, did the informant:
   seem nervous or agitated _____
   have a sad or tearful expression _____
   talk about serious issues with no emotion _____
   act inappropriately cheerful _____
   show a sense of humor _____
   smoke heavily _____
   seem tired and without energy _____
   appear interested in questions _____
5. Did the informant try to make *you* feel comfortable?
6. How "at ease" was the informant?
   Relaxed throughout _____
   More relaxed as time went on _____
   Less relaxed as time went on _____
   Uneasy throughout _____
7. What was the informant's posture toward the interview?
   Friendly and eager to talk _____
   Cooperative but not particularly eager _____
   Indifferent _____
   Resentful and suspicious _____

SEMISTRUCTURED INTERVIEW FORM FOR
PARENTS OF DECEASED CHILDREN

The interview format for parents of deceased children follows closely the format of the interview for parents of living children. We present here only the ways in which it differs from the prior format: (1) questions 5, 6, 7, 8, 12, 14, 15, 20, 23, 25, 27, 30 were not asked of parents of deceased children; (2) some other questions were asked in slightly different wording; and (3) questions listed in the following pages were added specifically to explore the experiences of parents of deceased children.

1. What kind of child/person was _____? What was he/she like?
   1a. What things did she/he enjoy doing?
2. In general, how do you feel you handled your child's illness and death?
   2a. What did you do best? Or what are you doing best? What are your strengths?
   2b. In what areas or what ways did or do you manage less well?
   2c. Have these ways changed over time?
       If yes, how?
3. Did _____ ever ask if he/she was going to die?
       If yes, what was your answer?
   3a. Did you feel you were completely honest at that time?
       Why or why not? Was that important?
4. When did _____ die?
   4a. Where did she/he die?
   4b. How did you prepare yourself and your family for death?

ASK ONLY IF THERE ARE OTHER LIVING CHILDREN

5. I can imagine that dealing with a child's death must be very hard for the parents, but also for sisters and brothers.
   How did _____'s sisters and brothers react to his/her illness and death?
   5a. Was their schoolwork affected?
       How are they doing in school now?
   5b. What has been the most difficult part of the experience for them?
   5c. Have you been able to do anything to help them with their feelings?
       Do you want to?
   5d. Was there anything that might help you deal with them and their feelings?

6. Do you know of the activities of the parents'/families' group,
   _____?

   6a. Have you seen their newsletter?

      What do you think of it?

   6b. Do you know of the Bereaved Parents Group that is part of it?

      If yes, have you ever gone to any of their meetings?

      What was your reaction?

   6c. What else could a group like that be doing to help families like yours?

   6d. Do you think your children would like to talk with other brother and sisters of children who have died?

      Why or why not?

QUESTIONNAIRE FORM FOR PARENTS
OF CHILDREN WITH CANCER

Name: _____. We need your
name in order to coordinate this form with the earlier interview. As soon
as we do that we will tear off this front sheet, and no one will know any-
body's name, or who said what.

On the pages that follow are a series of short questions. Most of them
can be answered by placing a check on the appropriate line. We would
appreciate your taking the time to fill out these items. It is quicker this
way than continuing with a long interview. It also gives you a chance
to reflect on the interview and to add any new thoughts or things we
missed.

If you do not wish to answer some questions, feel free to skip them; if
you want to write in longer answers, please do so . . . use the reverse
or margins or whatever. When you are finished, place this form in the
attached self-addressed envelope and mail it to us.

THANKS VERY MUCH!

1. Here is a list of some of the ways in which some parents report that
their experience with childhood cancer may have changed their lives.
Some of these changes may have happened for you or have not happened for you. Please indicate with a check in the appropriate column
whether you now do have much more, more, less, much less, or about
the same of each of these feelings or concerns as you used to.

	Much More	More	About The Same	Less	Much Less
a. sympathy for the sick	___	___	___	___	___
b. ability to cope with tragedy	___	___	___	___	___
c. desire to help others	___	___	___	___	___
d. desire to spend time with others	___	___	___	___	___
e. patience with minor problems	___	___	___	___	___
f. time with myself	___	___	___	___	___

	Much More	More	About The Same	Less	Much Less
g. desire to make a lot of money	___	___	___	___	___
h. understanding of death	___	___	___	___	___
i. anger toward fate	___	___	___	___	___
j. anger toward the medical system	___	___	___	___	___
k. concern about polluting the environment	___	___	___	___	___
l. concern about nuclear energy	___	___	___	___	___
m. faith in God	___	___	___	___	___
n. desire to spend time with close friends	___	___	___	___	___
o. desire to make new friends	___	___	___	___	___
p. concern about my health	___	___	___	___	___
q. feeling good about my spouse	___	___	___	___	___
r. feeling good about doctors	___	___	___	___	___
s. feeling I can control my life	___	___	___	___	___
t. willingness to ask friends for help	___	___	___	___	___
u. going out to the movies or out to eat	___	___	___	___	___
v. taking vacations with family	___	___	___	___	___
w. being impatient with minor problems	___	___	___	___	___
x. going to useless meetings	___	___	___	___	___
y. spending extra time at work	___	___	___	___	___

	Much More	More	About The Same	Less	Much Less
z. willingness to get psychological help	_____	_____	_____	_____	_____
aa. respect for the medical system	_____	_____	_____	_____	_____

2. In "times of difficulty," many of us seek out support and help from others. In the chart below, we have listed several potential sources of help. Please place a check on the line that represents how helpful each of these sources has been for you, in general. If you have had no contact with these, check that line.

	Very Helpful	Quite Helpful	Somewhat Helpful	A Little Helpful	Not Helpful	No Contact
a. Spouse	_____	_____	_____	_____	_____	_____
b. Social worker	_____	_____	_____	_____	_____	_____
c. Close friends	_____	_____	_____	_____	_____	_____
d. My parents	_____	_____	_____	_____	_____	_____
e. My other children	_____	_____	_____	_____	_____	_____
f. Psychiatrists, Psychologists	_____	_____	_____	_____	_____	_____
g. Other relatives	_____	_____	_____	_____	_____	_____
h. Other friends	_____	_____	_____	_____	_____	_____
i. Physicians	_____	_____	_____	_____	_____	_____
j. Other parents with ill children	_____	_____	_____	_____	_____	_____
k. Neighbors	_____	_____	_____	_____	_____	_____
l. Church leader	_____	_____	_____	_____	_____	_____
m. Nurses	_____	_____	_____	_____	_____	_____
n. School-people	_____	_____	_____	_____	_____	_____
o. Other (Who)	_____	_____	_____	_____	_____	_____
(Who)	_____	_____	_____	_____	_____	_____

3. When we deal with childhood cancer, there are many kinds of stress we each experience. Some of these stresses are worse than others. Please rate the following list of potential stresses in terms of whether they were very strong stresses for you, moderate stresses, or not strong stresses for you at all.

	Very Strong	Moderate	Not Strong
a. the fact my child had cancer	_____	_____	_____
b. my child's reaction to the drug	_____	_____	_____
c. fear my child would learn how serious the disease is	_____	_____	_____
d. my fear of my child's death	_____	_____	_____
e. tense relations with medical staff	_____	_____	_____
f. financial problems	_____	_____	_____
g. concern that if something happened to me it would be hard on the rest of the family	_____	_____	_____
h. fear my child might have a relapse	_____	_____	_____
i. marital problems	_____	_____	_____
j. sibling problems	_____	_____	_____
k. fear that one of my other children might get very sick	_____	_____	_____
l. relations with my parents (child's grandparents)	_____	_____	_____
m. relations with friends and neighbors	_____	_____	_____
n. fear of nervous breakdown	_____	_____	_____
o. worry about the effect on my other children	_____	_____	_____
p. fear of "spoiling" the child with cancer	_____	_____	_____

4. We have a few questions about the financial impact of childhood cancer on your family.
   a. Approximately what percent of your child's medical bills have been covered by insurance? _____%
   b. To date, about how much has your child's illness cost you, out of your pocket? $_____
   c. How would you describe the financial impact of your child's illness?

____ none ____ slight ____ somewhat serious
____ serious ____ a disaster

d. Have you had to make adjustments in your standard of living?
____ Yes ____ No
If yes. for instance:

5. Does/did your child know her/his diagnosis? ____ Yes ____ No
   a. If yes, who informed him/her?
   ____ you ____ your spouse ____ you and spouse
   ____ family doctor or pediatrician ____ hospital doctor
   ____ other (specify)
   b. If yes, how soon after you learned the diagnosis was the child told?
   ____ immediately, same time and place ____ later that day
   ____ within a week ____ a few months later
   ____ has never been told

6. Now we have a few brief questions about you and your background.
   a. What is your religious preference? _____
   b. When were you born (year)? _____
   c. Are your parents living?
   Mother: ____ living ____ deceased
   Father: ____ living ____ deceased
   d. If your mother/father are living, where do they live now?
   (town and state) _____
   e. What is your current marital status?
   ____ single ____ married ____ separated
   ____ divorced ____ widowed
   f. How long have you been? (whatever answer to 6e) _____
   g. What is the highest level of schooling you have completed?
   ____ 8th grade ____ some high school
   ____ graduated from high school ____ some college
   ____ graduated college ____ post-college study
   h. What is your job or occupation? _____
   i. What is your approximate family income (last year)?
   ____ less than $5,000 a year
   ____ between $5,000–$15,000 a year
   ____ between $15,000–$25,000 a year
   ____ between $25,000–$40,000 a year
   ____ more than $40,000 a year

7. And finally, we have a few questions to ask about the interview itself.

   a. To what extent did the interviewer help you feel comfortable and relaxed during the conversation?

     ____ not very comfortable at all

     ____ fairly comfortable

     ____ very much, really made it relaxed

   b. Were most of the questions easy to understand, clear or not?

     ____ hard to know what you were after

     ____ some easy to know what to say, others hard to figure

     ____ easy to see what you wanted to know

   c. How did you feel about the conversation?

     ____ sorry I had done it   ____ glad I had done it

     ____ like it was a waste of time

     ____ gave me some new ideas   ____ pleased to help out

     ____ sorry I had to go over these issues and feelings again

     ____ glad to have the chance to talk about these things again

   d. Did members of your family talk about their interviews with each other afterwards?

     ____ Yes   ____ No

     ____ If yes, has that been ____ good or ____ bad

   Please explain your answer a little:

   e. How complete a picture of your experience and feelings did we get?

     ____ Pretty sketchy, only covered a small part

     ____ Fairly good coverage, some parts skipped

     ____ Excellent, covered most issues

   f. What things did we miss that we should be sure to ask about if there were a next time?

   g. Are there any things you've thought about since the conversation that you want to add to what you said before? For instance?

THANK YOU VERY MUCH. THANKS FOR THE INTERVIEW AND FOR FILLING OUT THIS FORM. WE APPRECIATE YOUR TIME AND PATIENCE AND ENERGY. PLEASE PLACE THIS FORM IN THE ENCLOSED SELF-ADDRESSED ENVELOPE AND MAIL IT OFF TO ME.

Bibliography

Abramson, L., Seligman, M., & Teasdale, J. Learned helplessness in humans: Critiques and formulation. *Journal of Abnormal Psychology*, 1978, 87:49–74.

Adams, D. *Childhood Malignancy: The Psychosocial Care of the Child and His Family*. Springfield: Charles C Thomas, 1979.

Adams, D., & Deveau, E. *Coping with Childhood Cancer*. Reston, Va.: Reston, 1984.

Adams, M. Helping the parents of children with malignancy. *Journal of Pediatrics*, 1978, 93 (5):734–738.

Anderson, B., & Auslander, W. Research on diabetes management and the family: A critique. *Diabetes Care*, 1980, 3(6):696–702.

Antonovsky, A. Conceptual or methodological problems in the study of resistance resources and stressful life events. In B. Dohrenwend & B. Dohrenwend (Eds.), *Stressful Life Events: Their Nature and Effects*. New York: Wiley, 1974.

Antonovsky, A. *Health, Stress, and Coping*. San Francisco: Jossey-Bass, 1980.

Back, K., & Taylor, R. Self-help groups: Tools or symbol. *Journal of Applied Behavioral Science*, 1976, 12 (3):295–309.

Baker, L. *You and Leukemia*. Philadephia: Saunders, 1978.

Bakker, B., & Karel, M. Self-help: Wolf or Lamb? In D. Pancoast, P. Parker, & C. Froland (Eds.), *Rediscovering Self-Help: Its Role in Social Care*. Beverly Hills, Calif.: Sage, 1983.

Banhoff, E. Widow groups as an alternative to informal social support. In M. Lieberman & C. Borman (Eds.), *Self-help Groups for Coping with Crises*. San Francisco: Jossey-Bass, 1979.

Barbarin, O., & Chesler, M. *Children with Cancer: School Experiences and Views of Parents, Educators, Adolescents, and Physicians*. Maywood, Ill.: Eterna Press, 1983.

Bateson, G. *Steps to an Ecology of Mind*. New York: Ballantine Books, 1972.

Becker, M., & Maiman, L. Strategies for enhancing patient compliance. *Journal of Community Health*, 1980, 6:113–135.

Belle-Isle, J., & Conradt, B. Report of a discussion group for parents of children with leukemia. *Maternal-Child Nursing Journal*, 1979, 8 (1):49–58.

Binger, C., Albin, A., Feuerstein, R., Kushner, J., Zoger, S., & Mikelsen, C. Childhood leukemia: Emotional impact on patient and family. *New England Journal of Medicine*, 1969, 280:414–418.

Binger, C. M. Jimmy: A clinical case of child with a fatal illness. In E. Anthony & C. Koupernick (Eds.), *The Child in His Family: The Impact of Disease and Death*, Vol. 2. New York: Wiley, 1973.

Bloom, J., Ross, R., & Burnell, G. The effect of social support on patient adjustment after breast surgery. *Patient Counselling and Health Education*, 1978, 1 (2):50–59.

Bluebond-Langner, M. I know, do you?: Awareness and communication in terminally ill children. In B. Schoenberg, A. Carr, D. Peretz, & A. Kutscher (Eds.), *Anticipatory Grief*. New York: Columbia University Press, 1974.

Bluebond-Langner, M. *The Private Worlds of Dying Children*. Princeton, N.J.: Princeton University Press, 1978.

Blum, R., & Chang, P. A group for adolescents facing chronic and terminal illness. *Journal of Current Adolescent Medicine*, 1981, 3:7–12.

Borman, L. Characteristics of growth and development. In M. Lieberman & L. Borman (Eds.), *Self-Help Groups for Coping with Crisis*. San Francisco: Jossey-Bass, 1979.

Borman, L. Self-help skills: Leadership in self-help/mutual aid groups. *Citizen Participation*, 1982, 3(3):26, 30–31.

Boyle, I., Sant'Agnese, P., Sack, S., Millican, F., & Kulczycki, L. Emotional adjustments of adolescents and young adults with cystic fibrosis. *Journal of Pediatrics*, 1976, 88 (2):318–326.

Brickman, P., Kidder, L., Coates, D., Rabinowitz, V., Cohn, E., & Karuza, J. The dilemmas of helping: Making aid fair and effective. In J. Fisher, A. Nadler & B. DePaulo (Eds.), *New Directions in Helping*, Volume I. New York: Academic Press, 1983.

Brickman, P., Rabinovitz, V., Karuza, J., Coates, D., Cohn, E., & Kidder, L. Models of helping and coping. *American Psychologist*, 1982, 37:368–384.

Burke, R., & Weir, T. Husband-wife helping relationships: The mental hygiene function of marriage. *Psychological Reports*, 1976, 40 (3):911–925.

Burke, R., & Weir, T. Patterns in husbands and wives coping behaviors. *Psychological Reports*, 1979, 44 (3):951–956.

Burton, L. *The Family Life of Sick Children*. Boston: Routledge & Kegan Paul, 1975.

Buttino, L. *For the Love of Teddi*. Rochester, N.Y.: Mohawk, 1983.

Cairns, N., Clark, G., Smith, S., & Lansky, S. Adaptation of siblings to childhood malignancy. *Journal of Pediatrics*, 1979, 95 (3):484–487.

Campbell, J. The child in the sick role. *Journal of Health and Social Behavior*, 1978, 19:35–51.

Camps for children with cancer and their siblings. *Candlelighters Foundation Quarterly Newsletter*, 1983, 7 (2):1, 4.

Cancer Facts and Figures. New York: American Cancer Society, 1984.

Caplan, G. *Support Systems and Community Mental Health*. New York: Behavioral Publications, 1974.

Caplan, R. Patient, provider, and organization: Hypothesized determinants of adherence. In S. Cohen (Ed.), *New Directions in Patient Compliance*. Lexington, Mass.: Heath, 1979.

Cassileth, B., & Hamilton, J. The family with cancer. In B. Cassileth (Ed.), *The Cancer Patient: Social and Medical Aspects of Care*. Philadelphia: Lea and Febiger, 1979.

Charmaz, K. The grounded theory method: An explication and interpretation. In R. Emerson (Ed.), *Contemporary Field Research*. Boston: Little, Brown, 1983.

Chesler, M., & Anderson, B. Chronically ill adolescents as health care consumers. Ann Arbor, Mich.: CRSO Working Paper, #329, 1985.

Chesler, M., & Barbarin, O. Relating to the medical staff: How parents of children with cancer see the issues. *Health and Social Work*, 1984, 9 (1):49–65.

Chesler, M., & Yoak, M. Self-help groups for families of children with cancer: Patterns of stress and social support. In H. Roback (Ed.), *Helping Patients and Their Families Cope with Medical Problems* (pp. 481–526). San Francisco: Jossey-Bass, 1984.

Clapp, M. Psychosocial reactions of children with cancer. *Pediatric Clinics of North America*, 1976, 23(1):225–232.

Clark, M. Reactions to aid in communal and exchange relationships. In J. Fisher, A. Nadler, & B. DePaulo (Eds.), *New Directions in Helping*, Volume 1. New York: Academic Press, 1983.

Coates, D., Renzaglia, G., & Embree, M. When helping backfires: Help and helplessness. In J. Fisher, A. Nadler, & B. DePaulo (Eds), *New Directions in Helping*, Volume I. New York: Academic Press, 1983.

Collins, A., & Pancoast, D. Natural Helping Networks. Washington D. C.: *National Association of Social Workers*, 1976.

Comaroff, J., & Maguire, P. Ambiguity and the search for meaning: Childhood leukemia in the modern clinical context. *Social Science and Medicine*, 1981, 15B:115-123.

Cook, J. Influence of gender on the problems of parents of fatally ill children. *Journal of Psychosocial Oncology*, 1984, 2 (1):71-91.

Coping with Cancer. Bethesda, Md.: U.S. Department of Health and Human Services (National Cancer Institute 80-2080), 1980.

Cornils, M. My own story. *The Candlelighters Foundation Quarterly Newsletter*. 1981, 5 (4):5.

Craig, S. Eight hours of agony: Investment of a lifetime. *Candlelighters Foundation Youth Newsletter*, 1983, 5(2):1-2.

Crain, A., Sussman, M., & Weil, W. Effects of a diabetic child on marital integration and related measures of family functioning. *Journal of Health and Human Behavior*, 1966, 1:122-127.

Cyphert, F. Back to school for the child with cancer. *Journal of School Health*, 1973, 43:215-217.

D'Angio, G. Late sequellae after cure of childhood cancer. *Hospital Practice*, 1980:109-121.

Datan, N., & Ginsberg, L. (Eds). *Life-span Developmental Psychology*. New York: Academic Press, 1975.

Davis, J., Eckert, P., Golden, D., & McMillan, S. Families with newly diagnosed handicapped infants. In P. Azarnoff and C. Hardgrove (Eds.), *The Family in Child Health Care*. New York: Wiley, 1981.

Deasy-Spinetta, P. The adolescent with cancer: A view from the inside. In J. Spinetta & P. Deasy-Spinetta (Eds.), *Living with Childhood Cancer*. St. Louis: C. V. Mosby, 1981.

Deasy-Spinetta, P., & Spinetta, J. The child with cancer in school: Teachers' appraisal. *American Journal of Pediatric Hematology/Oncology*, 1980, 2:89-94.

Decade of Discovery. Rockville, Md.: National Cancer Institute (USDHHS 81-2323), 1981.

Desmond, H. Two families: An intensive observation study. In J. Kellerman (Ed.), *Psychological Aspects of Childhood Cancer*. Springfield, Ill.: Charles C Thomas, 1980.

de Traubenberg, N. Psychological aspects of congenital heart disease in the child. In J. Anthony & C. Koupernick (Eds.), *The Child in His Family: The Impact of Disease and Death*, Vol. 2. New York: Wiley, 1973.

DiMatteo, M. A social psychological analysis of physician-patient rapport: Toward a science of the art of medicine. *Journal of Social Issues*, 1979, 35 (1):12-33.

DiMatteo, M., & Hays, R. The significance of patient's perception of physician conduct: A study of patient satisfaction in a family practice center. *Journal of Community Health*, 1980, 6:18-34.

DiMatteo, M., & Hays, R. Social support and serious illness. In B. Gottlieb (Ed.), *Social Networks and Social Support*. Beverly Hills, Calif.: Sage, 1981.

Doerr, J., & Doerr, R. Back to school. *Candlelighters Foundation Quarterly Newsletter*, 1984, 8 (3):3.

Dohrenwend, B., & Dohrenwend, B. Overview of prospects for research on stressful life events. In B. Dohrenwend & B. Dohrenwend (Eds.), *Stressful Life Events: Their Nature and Effects*. New York: Wiley, 1974.

Dohrenwend, Barbara. Social class and stressful events. In E. Hare & J. Wing (Eds.), *Psychiatric Epidemiology*. New York: Oxford University Press, 1970.

Dohrenwend, Bruce. Problems in defining and sampling the relevant population of stressful life events. In B. Dohrenwend & B. Dohrenwend (Eds.), *Stressful Life Events: Their Nature and Effects*. New York: Wiley, 1974.

Dory, F., & Riessman, F. Training professionals in organizing self-help groups. *Citizen Participation*, 1982, 3 (3):27-28.

Duffner, P., Cohen, M., & Flannery, J. Referral patterns of childhood brain tumors in the state of Connecticut. *Cancer*, 1982, 50:1636.

Dunkel-Schetter, C. Social support and cancer: Findings based on patient interviews and their implications. *Journal of Social Issues*, 1984, 40 (4):77–98.

Durman, E. The role of self-help in service provision. *Journal of Applied Behavioral Science*, 1976, 12:433–443.

Edelstyn, G. The physician and the family. In L. Burton (Ed.), *Care of the Child Facing Death*. Boston: Routledge and Kegan Paul, 1974.

Edwards, G. Who goes to alcoholics anonymous? *Lancet*, 1966, 2:382.

Eickhoff, T., & Eickhoff, A. Parent's corner. *Cope Torch*, 1985, 9 (4):4.

Eiser, C. Intellectual abilities among survivors of childhood leukemia as a function of CNS radiation. *Archives of Diseases of Childhood*, 1978, 53:391–395.

Ellenberg, L., Kellerman, J., Dask, J., Higgins, G., & Zeltzer, L. Use of hypnosis for multiple symptoms in an adolescent girl with leukemia. *Journal of Adolescent Health Care*, 1980, 1:132–137.

Evans, A., If a child must die. *New England Journal of Medicine*, 1968, 278:138–142.

Farrell, F., & Hutter, J. Living until death: Adolescents with cancer. *Health and Social Work*, 1980, 5:35–38.

Featherstone, H. *A Difference in the Family*. New York: Penguin, 1981.

Feldman, F. *Work and Cancer Health Histories* (Abridged). Oakland, Calif.: American Cancer Society, 1980.

Fisher, J., Nadler, A., & Whitcher-Alagna, S. Four theoretical approaches for conceptualizing reactions to aid. In J. Fisher, A. Nadler, & B. DePaulo (Eds.), *New Directions in Helping*, Volume 1. New York: Academic Press, 1983.

Franz, T. *When Your Child Has a Life-Threatening Illness*. Washington, D.C.: Association for the Care of Children's Health, 1983.

Freudenberger, H. Staff burn-out. *Journal of Social Issues*, 1974, 30:159–165.

Friedman, S., Chodoff, P., Mason, J., & Hamburg, D. Behavioral observations on parents anticipating the death of a child. *Pediatrics*, 1963, 34 (4):610–625.

Friedson, E. *Profession of Medicine*. New York: Dodd, Mead, 1970.

Froland, C., Pancoast, D., Chapman, N., & Kimboko, P. *Helping Networks and Human Services*. Beverly Hills, Calif.: Sage, 1981.

Futterman, E., & Hoffman, I. Transient school phobia in a leukemic child. *Journal of the American Academy of Child Psychology*, 1970, 9:477–493.

Futterman, E., & Hoffman, I. Crisis and adaptation in the families of fatally ill children. In J. Anthony & C. Koupernick (Eds.), *The Child in His Family: The Impact of Death and Disease*, Vol. 2. New York: Wiley, 1973.

Gartner, A., & Riessman, F. *Self-help in the Human Services*. San Francisco: Jossey-Bass, 1977.

Geist, R. Onset of chronic illness in children and adolescents. *American Journal of Orthopsychiatry*, 1979, 49 (1):4–23.

Gilder, R., Buschman, P., Sitarz, A., & Wolff, J. Group therapy for parents of children with leukemia. *American Journal of Psychotherapy*, 1976, 30:276–287.

Glaser, B., & Strauss, A. *Awareness of Dying*. Chicago: Aldine, 1965.

Glaser, B., & Strauss, A. *The Discovery of Grounded Theory*. Chicago: Aldine, 1967.

Goffman, E. *Stigma: Notes on the Management of Spoiled Identity*. London: Penguin, 1968.

Gogan, J., Koocher, G., Foster, D., & O'Malley, J. Impact of childhood cancer on siblings. *Health and Social Work*, 1977, 2:41–57.

Gottlieb, B. The development and application of a classification scheme of informal helping behaviors. *Canadian Journal of Behavioral Science*, 1978, 10:105–115.

Gottlieb, B. (Ed.). *Social Networks and Social Support*. Beverly Hills, Calif.: Sage, 1981.

Gouldner, A. The norm of reciprocity: A preliminary statement. *American Journal of Sociology*, 1960, 25:161–178.

Gourash, N. Help-seeking: A review of the literature. *American Journal of Psychology*, 1978, 6 (5):413–423.

Greeley, J., & Mechanic, D. Social selection in seeking help for psychological problems. *Journal of Health and Social Behavior*, 1976, 17 (3):249–262.

Greene, P. The child with leukemia in the classroom. *American Journal of Nursing*, 1975, 75:86–87.

Griffel, M. Wilms' tumor in New York State, epidemiology and survival. *Cancer*, 1977, 40:3140.

Griffin, B. Having a child with cancer: A mother's story. *Candlelighters Foundation Quarterly Newsletter*, 1982, 6(3):1, 4–5.

Halpern, R. Physician-parent communication in the diagnosis of child handicap: A brief review. *Children's Health Care*, 1984, 12 (4):170–173.

Hamburg, B., & Inoff, G. Coping with Predictable crises of diabetes. *Diabetes Care*, 1983, 6(4):409–416.

Hamburg, D., & Adams, J. A perspective on coping behavior: Seeking and utilizing information in major transitions. *Archives of General Psychiatry*, 1967, 17:277–284.

Hamovitch, M. *The Parent and the Fatally Ill Child*. Durante, Calif.: City of Hope Medical Center, 1964.

Harris, R. Improving patient satisfaction through action research. *Journal of Applied Behavioral Science*, 1978, 14 (3):382–399.

Hatfield, E., & Sprecher, S. Equity theory and recipient reactions to aid, In J. Fisher, A. Nadler, & B. DePaulo (Eds.), *New Direction in Helping*, Volume 1. New York: Academic Press, 1983.

Haug, M., & Lavin, B. Methods of payment for medical care and public attitudes toward physician authority. *Journal of Health and Social Behavior*, 1978, 19:279–281.

Haug, M., & Sussman, M. Professional autonomy and the revolt of the client. *Social Problems*, 1969, 17: 153–160.

Havighurst, R. *Developmental Tasks and Education*. New York: Longman's Green, 1951.

Heffron, W. Group therapy sessions as part of treatment of children with cancer. In C. Pockedly (Ed.), *Clinical Management of Cancer in Children*. Acton, Mass.: Science Group, 1975.

Hewett, S., & Newson, J. *The Family and the Handicapped Child*. Chicago: Aldine, 1970.

Hilgard, J., & LeBaron, S. Relief of anxiety and pain in children and adolescents with cancer: Quantitative measures and clinical observations. *International Journal of Clinical and Experimental Hypnosis*, 1982, 30:417–442.

Hirsch, B. Natural support systems and coping with major life changes. *American Journal of Community Psychology*, 1980, 8:159–172.

Holmes, H., & Holmes, F. After ten years, what are the handicaps and life styles of children treated for cancer? *Clinical Pediatrics*, 1975, 14:819–823.

Homans, G. *Social Behavior: Its Elementary Forms*. New York: Harcourt Brace, 1961.

House, J. *Work, Stress and Social Support*. Reading, Mass.: Addison-Wesley, 1981.

Howarth, R. The psychiatric care of children with life-threatening illnesses. In L. Burton (Ed.), *Care of the Child Facing Death*. London: Routledge and Kegan Paul, 1974.

Howell, D. A child dies. *Journal of Pediatric Surgery*, 1966, 1:2–7.

Hughes, W. Early side effects in treatment of childhood cancer. *Pediatric Clinics of North America*, 1976, 23 (1):225–232.

Hymovich, D. Parents of sick children: Their needs and tasks. *Pediatric Nursing*, 1976, 2:9–13.

Jackson, D. Family rules: The marital quid pro quo. *Archives of General Psychiatry*, 1965, 12:589–594.

Jacobs, J. *The Search for Help: A Study of the Retarded Child in the Community*. Washington, D.C.: University Press of America, 1982.

Jaffe, N. Late sequalae of cancer therapy. In W. Sutow, D. Fernbach, & T. Vietti (Eds.), *Clinical Pediatric Oncology*. St. Louis: Mosby, 1984.

Jahoda, M. Toward a social psychology of mental health. In A. Rose (Ed.), *Mental Health and Mental Disorder*. New York: Norton, 1955.

Jay, S., & Elliot, C. Psychological intervention for pain in pediatric cancer patients. In

G. Humphrey, L. Dehner, G. Grindey, & R. Acton (Eds.), *Pediatric Oncology*. Boston: Martinus Nijhoff, 1983.

Kagan-Goodheart, L. Re-entry: Living with childhood cancer. *American Journal of Orthopsychiatry*, 1977, 47:652–658.

Kalnins, I. Cross-illness comparison of separation and divorce among parents having a child with a life-threatening illness. *Child Health Care*, 1983, 12 (2):72–77.

Kaplan, D., Smith, A., & Grobstein, R. School management of the seriously ill child. *Journal of School Health*, 1974, 44:250–254.

Kaplan, D., Smith, A., Grobstein, R., & Fishman, S. Family mediation of stress. *Social Work*, 1973, 18 (4):60–69.

Karon, M., & Vernick, J. An approach to the emotional support of fatally ill children. *Clinical Pediatrics*, 1968, 7:274–280.

Kartha, M., & Ertel, I. Short-term group therapy for mothers of leukemic children. *Clinical Pediatrics*, 1976, 15:803–806.

Katz, A. Self-help and mutual aid: An emerging social movement? *Annual Review of Sociology*, 1981, 7:129–155.

Katz, A., & Bender, E. Self-help groups in Western society: History and prospects. *Journal of Applied Behavioral Sciences*, 1976, 12 (3):265–282.

Katz, E. Illness impact and social reintegration. In J. Kellerman (Ed.). *Psychosocial Aspects of Childhood Cancer*. Springfield, Ill.: Charles C Thomas, 1980.

Katz, E., & Jay, J. Psychological aspects of cancer in children, adolescents, and their families. *Clinical Psychology Review*, 1984, 4:525–542.

Katz, E., Kellerman, J., Rigler, D., Williams, K., & Siegel, S. School intervention with pediatric cancer patients. *Journal of Pediatric Psychology*, 1977, 2:72–77.

Katz, E., Varni, J., & Jay, S. Assessment and management of pediatric pain. In M. Herson, R. Eisler, & P. Miller (Eds.), *Progress in Behavior Modification and Therapy*. New York: Academic Press, 1984.

Kellerman, J. Comprehensive psychological care of the child with cancer: Description of a program. In J. Kellerman (Ed.), *Psychological Aspects of Childhood Cancer*. Springfield, Ill.: Charles C Thomas, 1980.

Kellerman, J., & Katz, E. The adolescent with cancer: Theoretical, clinical, and research issues. *Journal of Pediatric Psychology*, 1977, 2:127–131.

Kellerman, J., Zeltzer, L., Ellenberg, L., Dash, J., & Rigler, D. Psychological effects of illness on adolescence, Part I: Anxiety, self, and perception of control. *Journal of Pediatrics*, 1980, 97(1):126–131.

Killilea, M. Mutual help organizations: Interpretations in the literature. In G. Caplan & M. Killilea (Eds.), *Support Systems and Mutual Help*. New York: Grune and Stratton, 1976.

King, S., & Meyers, R. Developing self-help groups: Integrating group work and community organization strategies. *Social Development Issues*, 1981, 5(2):33–46.

Kjosness, M., & Rudolph, L. *What Happened to You Happened to Me: A Book for Young People with Cancer*. Seattle: Children's Orthopedic Hospital and Medical Center, 1980.

Klagsbrun, S. Cancer, emotions and nurses. *American Journal of Psychiatry*, 1970, 126: 1273–1344.

Klagstad, N. Anger. *Candlelighters Foundation Quarterly Newsletter*, 1982, 6 (3):3.

Kleiman, H., Mantell, J., & Alexander, E. Collaboration and its discontents: The perils of partnerships. *Journal of Applied Behavioral Sciences*, 1976, 12 (3):403–409.

Knapp, V., & Hansen, H. Helping the parents of children with leukemia. *Social Work*, 1973, 18 (4):70–75.

Koch, C., Hermann, J., & Donaldson, M. Supportive care of the child with cancer and his family. *Seminars in Oncology*, 1974, 1:1.

Koocher, G. Coping with survivorship in childhood cancer: Family problems. In A. Christ & K. Flomenhaft (Eds.), *Childhood Cancer: Impact on the Family*. New York: Plenum, 1984a.

Koocher, G. The crisis of survival. In A. Christ & K. Flomenhaft (Eds.), *Childhood Cancer: Impact on the Family*. New York: Plenum, 1984b.

Koocher, G., & O'Malley, J. *The Damocles Syndrome: Psychological Consequences of Surviving Childhood Cancer.* New York: McGraw-Hill, 1981.

Koocher, G., & Sallan, S., Pediatric oncology. In P. Magrab (Ed.), *Psychological Management of Pediatric Problems.* Baltimore: University Park Press, 1978.

Kübler-Ross, E. *On Death and Dying.* New York: Macmillan, 1969.

Kulka, R., Veroff, J., & Douvan, E. Social class and the use of professional help for personal problems: 1957 and 1976. *Journal of Health and Social Behavior,* 1979, 20 (1):2-17.

Kupst, M., & Schulman, J. Family coping with leukemia in a child: Initial reactions. In J. Schulman & M. Kupst (Eds.), *The Child with Cancer.* Springfield, Ill.: Charles C Thomas, 1980.

Kupst, M., Schulman, J., Honig, G., Maurer, H., Morgan, E., & Fochtman, D. Family coping with childhood leukemia: One year after diagnosis. *Journal of Pediatric Psychology,* 1982, 7 (2):157-174.

Kushner, H. *When Bad Things Happen to Good People.* New York: Avon, 1981.

Lang, P., & Mitrowski, C. Supportive and concrete services for teenage oncology patients. *Health and Social Work,* 1981, 6:42-45.

Lansky, S., Cairns, N., Clark, G., Lowman, J., Miller, L., & Trueworthy, R. Childhood cancer: Non-medical costs of the illness. *Cancer,* 1979, 43:403-408.

Lansky, S., Cairns, N., Hassamien, R., Wehr, J., & Lowman, J. Childhood cancer: Parental discord and divorce. *Pediatrics,* 1978, 62:184-188.

Lansky, S., Lowman, J., Vats, T., & Gyulay, J. School phobia in children with malignant neoplasms. *American Journal of Disabled Children,* 1975, 129:42-47.

Lascari, A., & Stehbens, J. The reactions of families to childhood leukemia. *Clinical Pediatrics,* 1973, 12 (4):210-214.

Lawrence, S. Results: Candlelighters discipline questionnaire. *Candlelighters National Newsletter,* 1978, 2(2):2.

Lazarus, R. *Psychological Stress and the Coping Process.* New York: McGraw-Hill, 1966.

Lazarus, R. The costs and benefits of denial. In J. Spinetta & P. Deasy-Spinetta (Eds.), *Living with Childhood Cancer.* St. Louis: C. V. Mosby, 1981a.

Lazarus, R. The stress and coping paradigm. In C. Eisdorfer, D. Cohen, A. Kleinman, & T. Maxin (Eds.), *Models for Clinical Psychopathology.* New York: Spectrum, 1981b.

Lazarus, R., & Launier, R. Stress-related transactions between person and environment. In L. Pearlin & M. Lewis (Eds.), *Perspectives in Interactional Psychology.* New York: Plenum, 1978.

Leiken, S., & Hassakis, P. Psychological study of parents of children with cystic fibrosis. In J. Anthony & C. Koupernick (Eds.), *The Child in His Family: Impact of Disease and Death.* Vol. 2. New York: Wiley, 1973.

Lenrow, P., & Burch, R. Mutual aid or professional services: Opposing or complementary? In B. Gottlieb (Ed.), *Social Networks and Social Support.* Beverly Hills, Calif.: Sage, 1981.

Levine, A. Support systems for the patient with cancer: Future prospects. *Cancer,* 1975, 36:813-820.

Levine, A. (Ed.). *Cancer in the Young.* New York: Masson, 1982.

Levy, L. Self-help groups: Types and psychological processes. *Journal of Applied Behavioral Science,* 1976, 12:310-322.

Levy, L. Self-help groups viewed by mental health professionals: A survey and comments. *American Journal of Community Psychology,* 1978, 5:305-313.

Lewis, S. Cancer in adolescents. In H. Roback (Ed.), *Helping Patients and Their Families Cope with Medical Problems.* San Francisco: Jossey-Bass, 1984.

Li, F., Cassady, J., & Jaffe, N. Risk of second tumors in survivors of childhood cancer. *Cancer,* 1975, 35:1230-1235.

Li, F., & Stone, R. Survivors of cancer in childhood. *Annals of Internal Medicine,* 1976, 84:551-553.

Lieberman, M. Help-seeking and self-help groups. In M. Lieberman & L. Borman (Eds.), *Self-help Groups for Coping with Crisis.* San Francisco: Jossey-Bass, 1979.

Lieberman, M., & Borman, L., Epilogue: Self-help and social research. *Journal of Applied Behavioral Science*, 1976, 12(3):17–30.

Lieberman, M., & Borman, L. (Eds.). *Self-Help Groups for Coping with Crisis*. San Francisco: Jossey-Bass, 1979.

Lysen, N. Siblings. *Candlelighters Foundation Quarterly Newsletter*, 1982, 6(4):7.

Maccoby, E. *Social Development: Psychological Growth and the Parent-Child Relationship*. New York: Harcourt Brace Jovanovich, 1980.

Manchester, P. The adolescent with cancer: Concerns for care. *TCN Oncology* 1981:31–36.

Marcus, L. Patterns of coping in families of psychotic children. *American Journal of Orthopsychiatry*, 1977, 47: 338–399.

Marten, G. Psychologic effects of cancer in the adolescent: Clinical management and challenge for research. in J. Schulman & M. Kupst (Eds.), *The Child with Cancer*. Springfield, Ill.: Charles C Thomas, 1980.

Martinson, I. The child with leukemia: Parents help each other. *American Journal of Nursing*, 1976, 76 (7):1120–1122.

Maslach, C. Burn-out. *Human Behavior*, 1976, 5 (9):16–22.

Massie, R., & Massie, S. *Journey*. New York: Warner Books, 1976.

Masters, J., Cerreto, M., & Mendlowitz, D. The role of the family in coping with childhood illness. In T. Burish & C. Brodley (Eds.), *Coping with Chronic Disease*. New York: Academic Press, 1983.

Mattsson, A. Long-term physical illness in childhood: A challenge to psychosocial adaptation. In C. Garfield (Ed.), *Stress and Survival: The Emotional Realities of Life-Threatening Illness*. St. Louis: C. V. Mosby, 1979.

Mattsson, A., & Gross, S. Adaptational and defensive behavior in young hemophiliacs and their parents. *American Journal of Psychiatry*, 1966, 122:1349.

McCollum, A. *Coping with Prolonged Health Impairment in Your Child*. Boston: Little, Brown, 1975.

McCollum, A., & Schwartz, A. Social work and the mourning patient. *Social Work*, 1972, 17 (1):25–36.

McCubbin, H., & Patterson, J. Family adaptation to crisis. In H. McCubbin, A. Cauble, & J. Patterson (Eds.), *Family Stress, Coping, and Social Support*. Springfield, Ill.: Charles C Thomas, 1982.

McFate, P. Ethical issues in the treatment of cancer patients. In B. Cassileth (Ed.), *The Cancer Patient: Social and Medical Aspects of Care*. Philadelphia: Lea and Febiger, 1979.

Mead, G. *Mind, Self, and Society*, Chicago: University of Chicago Press, 1934.

Meadow, R. Parental response to the medical ambiguities of congenital deafness. *Journal of Health and Social Behavior*, 1968, 9 (4):299–309.

Meadows, A., Hopson, R., Lustbader, E., & Evans, A. Survival in childhood acute lymphocytic leukemia (ALL): The influence of protocol and place of treatment. *Proceedings of the American Society of Clinical Oncology* (Abstract C-554), 1979, 20:425.

Mechanic, D. The influence of mothers on their children's health attitudes and behaviors. *Pediatrics*, 1964, 33:444–453.

Mechanic, D. *Medical Sociology*. (2d Ed.). New York: Free Press, 1978.

Miles, M., & Huberman, M. *Qualitative Data Analysis: A Sourcebook of New Methods*. Beverly Hills, Calif.: Sage, 1984.

Miller, D., & Haupt, E. Clinical cancer research: Patient, parent, and physician interactions. In A. Christ & K. Flomenhaft (Eds.), *Childhood Cancer*. New York: Plenum, 1984.

Miller, L., & Miller, D. The pediatrician's role in caring for the child with cancer. *Pediatric Clinics of North America*, 1984, 31(1):119–132.

Miller, R., & McKay, F. Decline in US childhood cancer mortality:1950 through 1980. *Journal of the American Medical Association*, 1984, 251:1567–1570.

Minuchin, S. *Families and Family Therapy*. Cambridge, Mass.: Harvard University Press, 1974.

Moldow, D., & Martinson, I. *Home care: A Manual for Parents*. Minneapolis: University of Minnesota Press, 1979.

Moore, I., & Triplett, J. Students with cancer: A school nursing perspective. *Cancer Nursing*, 1980, August: 265–271.

Morrissey, J. Death anxiety in children with a fatal illness. In H. Parad (Ed.), *Crisis Intervention: Selected Readings*. New York: Family Service Association of America, 1965.

Morrow, G., Hoagland, A., & Morse, I. Sources of support perceived by parents of children with cancer: Implications for counseling. *Patient Counseling and Health Education*, 1982, 4(1):36–40.

Mulhern, R., Crisco, J., & Camitta, B. Patterns of communication among pediatric patients with leukemia, parents and physicians: Prognostic disagreements and misunderstandings. *Journal of Pediatrics*. 1981, 99 (3):480–483.

Myers, J., Lindenthat, J., & Pepper, M. Social class, life events, and psychiatric symptoms. In B. Dohrenwend & B. Dohrenwend (Eds.), *Stressful Life Events: Their Nature and Effects*. New York: Wiley, 1974.

Nelcamp, B. Into the light, Part II: A mother's feelings. *Cincinnati Horizons*, 1980, 9 (5):12–13.

Nelcamp, G. Into the light, Part II: A father's feelings. *Cincinnati Horizons*, 1980, 9 (5):10–12.

Nelcamp, V. Into the light. *Cincinnati Horizons*, 1980, 9 (4):13–17, 49–50.

Newman, H. Helping siblings in the family with childhood cancer. *Candlelighters Foundation Quarterly Newsletter*, 1981, 5 (2):5.

Obetz, S., Swenson, W., McCarthy, C. Gilchrist, G., & Burgert, E. Children who survive malignant disease: Emotional adaptation of the children and their families. In J. Schulman and M. Kupst (Eds.), *The Child with Cancer*. Springfield, Ill.: Charles C Thomas, 1980.

Oliff, A., & Levine, A. Late effects of anti-neoplastic therapy. In A. Levine (Ed.), *Cancer in the Young*. New York: Masson, 1982.

O'Malley, J., Koocher, G., Foster, D., & Slavin, L. Psychiatric sequallae of surviving childhood cancer. *American Journal of Orthopsychiatry*, 1979, 49 (4):608–616.

Oncology Handbook for Parents. Cincinnati: COPE-Cincinnati Oncology Parents Endeavor, 1978.

Oncology Handbook for Parents. Milwaukee: LODAT-Living One Day at a Time, 1977.

Oncology Handbook for Parents. Candlelighters of South Florida, 1976.

Orbach, C., Sutherland, A., & Bozeman, M. The adaptation of mothers to the threatened loss of their children through leukemia; Part II. *Cancer*, 1955, 8 (1):20–33.

Orr, D., Hoffmans, M., & Bennetts, G. Adolescents with cancer report their psychosocial needs. *Journal of Psychosocial Oncology*, 1984, 2(2):47–59.

Panke, C. Adolescent videotape program. *Candlelighters Childhood Cancer Foundation Newsletter*, 1985, 9 (2/3):6.

Pearlin, L. Sex roles and depression, In N. Datan & L. Ginsberg (Eds.), *Lifespan Developmental Psychology*. New York: Academic Press, 1975.

Pearlin, L., & Lieberman, M. Social sources of emotional distress. *Research in Community and Mental Health*, 1979, 1:217–248.

Pearlin, L., & Schooler, C. The structure of coping. *Journal of Health and Social Behavior*, 1978, 19:2–21.

Pendergrass, T., Rudolph, T., Clark, J., Wallace, M., & Kjosness, M. *Coping with Childhood Cancer: Information for Parents of Children with Cancer – Leader's Manual*. Seattle: Children's Orthopedic Hospital, 1982.

Pendleton, E. *Too Old to Cry . . . Too Young to Die*. Nashville, Tenn.: Thomas Nelson, 1980.

Pilisuk, M., & Froland, C. Kinship, social networks, social support, and health. *Social Science and Medicine*, 1978, 12B:273–280.

Pitel, A., Pitel, P., Richards, H., Benson, J., Prince, J., & Forman, E. Parent consultants in pediatric oncology. *Children's Health Care*, 1985, 14 (1): 46–51.

Plank, E. Death on a children's ward. *Medical Times*, 1964, 92:638–644.

Pless, B. Clinical assessment: Physical and psychological functioning. *Pediatric Clinics of North America*, 1984, 31(1):33–45.

Pless, I., & Pinkerton, P. *Chronic Childhood Disorder: Promoting Patterns of Adjustment.* Chicago: Kimpton, 1975.

Potter, D. Specific problems related to the age of the child. In *Nursing Problems of Children with Cancer.* New York: American Cancer Society, 1974.

Powell, T. The use of self-help groups as supportive reference communities. *American Journal of Orthopsychiatry,* 1975, 45 (5):756–764.

Reigel, K. Adult life-crisis: A dialectic interpretation of development. In N. Datan & L. Ginsberg (Eds.). *Lifespan Developmental Psychology.* New York: Academic Press, 1975.

Reinharz, S. The paradox of professional involvement in alternative settings. *Journal of Alternative Human Services,* 1981, 7:21–24.

Reiss, D. *The Family's Construction of Reality.* Cambridge, Mass.: Harvard University Press, 1978.

Richmond, J., & Waisman, H. Psychologic aspects of management of children with malignant diseases. *American Journal of Diseases of Children,* 1955, 89:42–47.

Ries, L., Pollack, E., & Young, J. Cancer patient survival: Surveillance, epidemiology and end results program, 1973–1979. *Journal of the National Cancer Institute,* 1983, 70:693–707.

Riessman, R. The "helper-therapy" principle. *Social Work,* 1965, 10, 2:27–32.

Roach, N. The last day of April. *American Cancer Society,* 1974.

Robison, L., Nesbit, M., Sather, H., Meadows, A., Ortega, J., & Hammond, D. Factors associated with IQ scores in long-term survivors of childhood acute lymphoplastic leukemia. *American Journal of Pediatric Hematology/Oncology,* 1984, 6:115–121.

Rook, K., & Dooley, P. Applying social support research: Theoretical problems and future directions. *Journal of Social Issues,* 1985, 41(1):5–28.

Ross, J. Social work intervention with families of children with cancer. *Social Work in Health Care,* 1978, 3 (3):257–282.

Ross, J. Coping with childhood cancer: Group intervention as an aid to parents in crisis. *Social Work in Health Care,* 1979, 4(4):381–391.

Ross, J. Childhood cancer: The parents, the patients, the professional. *Issues in Comprehensive Pediatric Nursing,* 1980, 4(1):7–16.

Rothenberg, M. Reactions of those who treat children with cancer. *Pediatrics,* 1967, 40 (3):507–519.

Ruccione, K. *We Can Cope: A Program for Parents of Children with Cancer* (Progress Report). Los Angeles: Children's Hospital of Los Angeles, 1985.

Rudolph, L., Pendergrass, T. Clarke, J., Kjosness, M., & Hartman, J. Development of an education program for parents of children with cancer. *Social Work in Health Care,* 1981, 6 (4):43–54.

Rutherford, W. The institutional organization: Self-serving or patient-serving? In J. Van Eys (Ed.), *The Truly Cured Child.* Baltimore: University Park Press, 1977.

Sabbeth, B. Understanding the impact of chronic childhood illness on families. *Pediatric Clinics of North America,* 1984, 31 (1):47–58.

Schiff, H. *The Bereaved Parent.* New York: Penguin, 1978.

Schontz, F. Reaction to crisis. *The Volta Review,* 1965, May:364–370.

Schulman, J., & Kupst, M. (Eds.). *The Child with Cancer.* Springfield, Ill.: Charles C Thomas, 1980.

Schwartz, S. Normative influences on altruism. In L. Berkowitz (Ed.), *Advances in Experimental Social Psychology,* Vol. 10. New York: Academic Press, 1977.

Schweers, E., Farnes, P., & Foreman, E. *Parents' Handbook on Leukemia,* Providence, R.I.: American Cancer Society, 1977.

Seltzer, B. Thoughts. *Candlelighters Foundation Teen Newsletter,* 1983, 5 (1):3.

Share, L. Family communication in the crisis of a child's fatal illness: A literature review and analysis. *Omega,* 1972, 3 (3):187–201.

Showalter, J. The child's reaction to his own terminal illness. In B. Schoenberg, A. Carr, D. Peretz, & A. Kutscher (Eds.), *Loss and Grief: Psychological Management in Medical Practice.* New York: Columbia University Press, 1970.

Sigler, A. The leukemic child and his family: An emotional challenge. In M. Debuskey (Ed.), *The Chronically Ill Child and His Family*. Springfield, Ill.: Charles C Thomas, 1970.

Silberfarb, P. Research in adaptation to illness and psychosocial intervention. In Procedures of the Working Conference on the Psychological Social and Behavioral Medicine Aspects of Cancer. *Cancer*, 1982, 50 (9):1921–1925 (Supplement).

Silverman, P. Mutual help. In R. Hirschowitz & B. Levy (Eds.), *The Changing Mental Health Scene*. New York: Spectrum, 1976.

Simone, J., Aur, R., Hustu, H., Verzosa, M., & Pinkel, D. Three to ten years after cessation of therapy in children with leukemia. *Cancer*, 1978, 42:839–844.

Singer, J. Some issues in the study of coping. In Proceedings of the Working Conference on Methodology in Behavioral and Psychosocial Cancer Research – 1983. *Cancer*, 1984, 53:2303–2313 (Supplement).

Slavin, L., O'Malley, J., Koocher, G., & Foster, D. Communication of the cancer diagnosis to pediatric patients: Impact on long-term adjustment. *American Journal of Psychiatry*, 1982, 139 (2):179–183.

Smith, D., & Pillemer, K., Self-help groups as social movement organizations: Social structure and social change. In L. Kriesberg (Ed.), *Research in Social Movements: Conflict and Change*, 1983, 5:203–233.

Sontag, S. Illness as metaphor. *Cancer News*, 1979, 33 (1):6–12.

Sourkes, B. Siblings of the pediatric cancer patient. In J. Kellerman (Ed.), *Psychological Aspects of Childhood Cancer*. Springfield, Ill.: Charles C Thomas, 1980.

Sourkes, B. *The Deepening Shade: Psychological Aspects of Life-Threatening Illness*. Pittsburgh: University of Pittsburgh Press, 1982.

Spinetta, J. The dying child's awareness of death: A review. *Psychological Bulletin*, 1974, 81:256–260.

Spinetta, J. Communication patterns in families dealing with life-threatening illness. In O. Sahler (Ed.), *The Child and Death*. St. Louis: C. V. Mosby, 1978.

Spinetta, J. Disease-related communication: How to tell. In J. Kellerman (Ed.), *Psychological Aspects of Childhood Cancer*. Springfield, Ill.: Charles C Thomas, 1980.

Spinetta, J. The sibling of the child with cancer. In J. Spinetta & P. Deasy-Spinetta (Eds.), *Living with Childhood Cancer*. St. Louis: C. V. Mosby, 1981.

Spinetta, J. Development of psychometric assessment methods by life cycle stages. *Cancer*, 1984, 53(10), 2222–2225.

Spinetta, J., & Deasy-Spinetta, P. (Eds.). *Living with Childhood Cancer*, St. Louis: C. V. Mosby, 1981.

Spinetta, J., Deasy-Spinetta, P., McLaren, H., Kung, F., Schwartz, D., & Hartman, G. The adolescent's psychosocial response to cancer. In C. Tebbi (Ed.), *Major Topics in Pediatric and Adolescent Oncology*. Boston: Hall, 1982.

Spinetta, J., Rigler, D., & Karon, M. Anxiety in the dying child. *Pediatrics*, 1973, 52:841–845.

Spinetta, J., Rigler, D., & Karon, M. Personal space as a measure of the dying child's sense of isolation. *Journal of Consulting and Clinical Psychology*, 1974, 42:751–756.

Spinetta, J., Spinetta, P., Kung, F. & Schwartz, D. *Emotional Aspects of Childhood Cancer and Leukemia: A Handbook for Parents*. San Diego: Leukemia Society of America, 1976.

Spinetta, J., Swarner, J., & Sheposh, J. Effective parental coping following the death of a child from cancer. *Journal of Pediatric Psychology*, 1981, 6 (3):251–263.

Stein, R., & Jessop, D. General Issues in the Care of Children with Chronic Physical Conditions. *Pediatric Clinics of North America*, 1984, 331 (1):189–198.

Steinman, R., & Traunstein, D. The self-help challenge to the human services. *Journal of Applied Behavioral Science*, 1976, 12:347–362.

Stolberg, A., & Cunningham, J. Support groups for parents of leukemic children. In J. Schulman & M. Kupst (Eds.), *The Child with Cancer*. Springfield, Ill.: Charles C Thomas, 1980.

Stone, G. Patient compliance and the role of the expert. *Journal of Social Issues*, 1979, 35 (1):156–184.

Straus, S. My story. *Candlelighters Foundation Teen Newsletter*, 1983, 5(1):2-3.

Strong, P. *The Ceremonial Order of the Clinic*. London: Routledge & Kegan Paul, 1979.

Stuetzer, C. Support systems for professionals. In J. Schulman & M. Kupst (Eds.), *The Child with Cancer*. Springfield, Ill.: Charles C Thomas, 1980.

Sussman, E., Hollenbeck, A., Nannis, E., & Strope, B. A developmental perspective on psychological aspects of childhood cancer. In J. Schulman & M. Kupst (Eds.), *The Child with Cancer*. Springfield, Ill.: Charles C Thomas, 1980.

Sutow, W. General aspects of childhood cancer. In W. Sutow, D. Fernbach, & T. Vietti (Eds.), *Clinical Pediatric Oncology*. St. Louis: C. V. Mosby, 1984.

Sutow, W., Fernbach, D., & Vietti, T. (Eds.). *Clinical Pediatric Oncology*. St. Louis: C. V. Mosby, 1984.

Szasz, T., & Hollander, M. A contribution to the philosophy of medicine: Basic models of doctor-patient relationships. *Archives of Internal Medicine*, 1956, 97: 585-592.

Tavormina, J., Kastner, L., Slater, P., & Watt, S. Chronically ill children: A psychologically and emotionally deviant population? *Journal of Abnormal Child Psychology*, 1976, 4 (2):99-110.

Taylor, S. Hospital patient behavior: Reactance, helplessness, or control? *Journal of Social Issues*, 1979, 35 (1):156-184.

Taylor, S. Adjustment to threatening events: A theory of cognitive adaptation. *American Psychologist*, 1983, 38 (11):1161-1173.

Taylor, S. Response. In Proceedings of the Working Conference on Methodology in Behavioral and Psychosocial Cancer Research – 1983. *Cancer*, 1984, 53:2313-2315 (Supplement).

Tebbi, C. (Ed.). *Major Topics in Pediatric and Adolescent Oncology*. Boston: G. K. Hall, 1982.

Teta, M., Delpo, M., Kasl, S., Meigs, J., Myers, J., & Mulvihill, J. Psychosocial consequences of pediatric cancer survival. Presented to meeting of the Society for Epidemiologic Research. Houston, 1984.

The Chronically Ill Child and Family in the Community. Washington, D.C.: Association for the Care of Children's Health, 1982.

Thomas, L. Patient groups for children who have cancer. In J. Schulman and W. Kupst (Eds.), *The Child with Cancer*. Springfield, Ill.: Charles C Thomas, 1980.

Toch, R. Management of the child with a fatal disease. *Clinical Pediatrics*, 1964, 3, 418-427.

Tracy, C., & Gussow, Z. Self-help health groups: A grass roots response to a need for services. *Journal of Applied Behavioral Science*, 1976, 12 (3):381-397.

Tucker, J. *Ellie: A Child's Fight Against Leukemia*. New York: Holt, 1982.

Tylke, L. Family therapy with pediatric cancer patients: A social work perspective. In J. Schulman & M. Kupst (Eds.), *The Child with Cancer*. Springfield, Ill.: Charles C Thomas, 1980.

Vachon, M., Lyall, W., & Freeman, S. Measurement and management of stress in health professionals working with advanced cancer patients. *Death Education*, 1978, 1:365-375.

Van Eys, J. The outlook for the child with cancer. *Journal of School Health*, 1977a, 47:165-169.

Van Eys, J. What do we mean by "The truly cured child?" In J. Van Eys (Ed.), *The Truly Cured Child*. Baltimore: University Park Press, 1977b.

Vaughn, C. Camp – a great experience. *Candlelighters Childhood Cancer Foundation Youth Newsletter*, 1985, 7(1):6.

Vaux, A. Variations in social support associated with gender, ethnicity, and age. *Journal of Social Issues*, 1985, 41(1): 89-110.

Vaux, K. Life-threatening disease in children: The challenge to personal and institutional values. In J. Van Eys (Ed.), *The Truly Cured Child*. Baltimore: University Park Press, 1977.

Vernick, J. Meaningful communication with the fatally ill child. In J. Anthony & C. Koupernick (Ed.), *The Child and His Family: The Impact of Disease and Death*, Vol. 2. New York: Wiley, 1973.

Vernick, J., & Karon, M. Who's afraid of death on a leukemia ward? *American Journal of Diseases of Children*, 1965, 109:393-397.

Videka-Sherman, L. Effects of participation in a self-help group for bereaved parents: Compassionate friends. *Prevention in Human Services*, 1982, 1(3):69–78.

Voysey, M. Impression management by parents with disabled children. *Journal of Health and Social Behavior*, 1972, 13 (1):80–89.

Waechter, E. Children's awareness of fatal illness. *American Journal of Nursing*, 1971, 71: 1168–1172.

Wheat, P., & Lieber, L. *Hope for the Children*. Minneapolis: Winston, 1979.

White, R. Strategies of adaptation. In R. Moos (Ed.), *Human Adaptation*. Lexington, Mass.: D. C. Health, 1976.

Wilbur, J. Rehabilitation of children with cancer. *Cancer*, 1975, 36:809–812.

Wilson, B. Pediatric cancer hospital lobby and waiting rooms. *Candlelighters Foundation Quarterly Newsletter*, 1982, 6(4):6.

Worchel, F., & Copeland, D. Psychological intervention with adolescents. *Cancer Bulletin*, 1984, 36 (6):279–284.

Wortman, C. Social support and the cancer patient: Conceptual and methodological issues. In Proceedings of the Working Conference on Methodology in Behavioral and Psychosocial Cancer Research – 1983. *Cancer*, 1984, 53(10), 2339–2360 (Supplement).

Wortman, C., & Dintzer, L. Is an attributional analysis of the learned helplessness phenomenon viable? A critique of the Abraham-Seligman-Teasdale reformulation. *Journal of Abnormal Psychology*, 1978, 87(1):75–90.

Wortman, C., & Dunkel-Schetter, C. Interpersonal relationships with cancer: A theoretical analysis. *Journal of Social Issues*, 1979, 35 (1):120–125.

Yoak, M., & Chesler, M., Alternative professional roles in health care delivery: Leadership patterns in self-help groups. *Journal of Applied Behavioral Science*, 1985, 21(4):427–444.

Young Board Member Plans for Youth Groups. *Candlelighters Foundation Teen Newsletter*, 1983, 5(1):1.

Yudkin, S. Children and death. *Lancet*, 1967, 1:37–41.

Zeltzer, L. Chronic illness in the adolescent. In J. Shenker (Ed.), *Topics in Adolescent Medicine*. New York: Grune and Stratton, 1978.

Zeltzer, L., Kellerman, J., Ellenburg, L., Dash, J., & Rigler, D. Psychosocial effects of illness in adolescence, Part II: Impact of illness on crucial issues and coping styles. *Journal of Pediatrics*, 1980, 97:132–138.

Zwartjes, W. Education of the child with cancer. Presented at the American Cancer Society National Conference on the Care of the Child with Cancer. Boston, 1978.

Name Index

Subject Index